AMBASSADORS IN WHITE

Books by

CHARLES MORROW WILSON

Ambassadors in White
Central America: Challenge and Opportunity
Cornbread and Creek Water: Landscape of Rural Poverty
Backwoods America
Roots of America
Rabble Rouser
Ginger Blue
Aroostook
Country Living
Acres of Sky
Meriwether Lewis

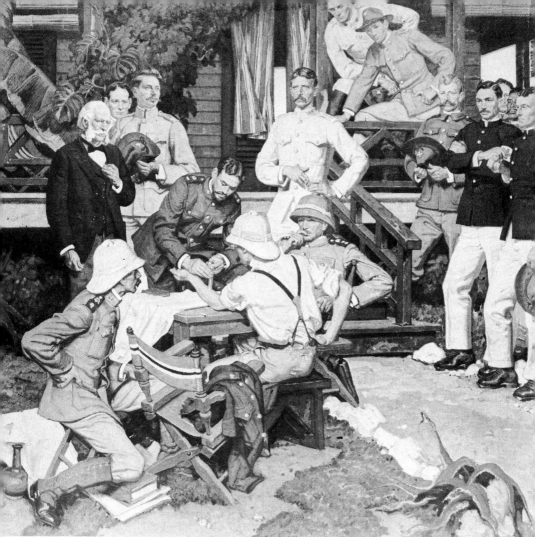

CONQUERORS OF YELLOW FEVER

Painting by Dean Cornwell, N.A.

At table: (left) Major Jefferson R. Kean, Chief Surgeon of the Department of Western Cuba: (Seated with arm extended for mosquito bite inoculation) Dr. James Carroll: (administering infected mosquito in test tube) Dr. Jesse W. Lazear: (Seated onlooker) Major General Leonard Wood, Governor-General of Cuba.

Standing: (Extreme left) Dr. Carlos Finlay; Lieutenant Albert E. Truby; Dr. Aristides Agramonte; Dr. Walter Reed.

Looking on from Porch: Dr. Roger P. Ames and Dr. Robert P. Cooke: (Standing) Private Warren G. Jernegan, Army Hospital Corps; Private John J. Moran, and Private John R. Kissinger, also of the Army Hospital Corps.

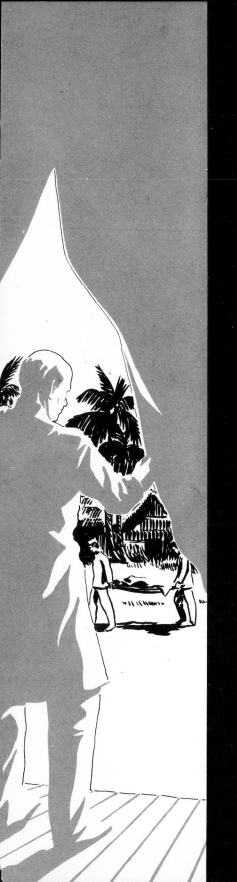

Ambassadors in White

THE STORY OF
American Tropical Medicine

CHARLES
MORROW
WILSON

New York
HENRY HOLT AND COMPANY

TO

DR. R. C. CONNOR

OF

TEXAS, PANAMA, AND POINTS NORTH

AND

DR. NEIL P. MACPHAIL

OF

SCOTLAND, GUATEMALA, AND THE AMERICAS

CONTENTS

ILLUSTRATIONS

ix

AMBASSADORS IN WHITE

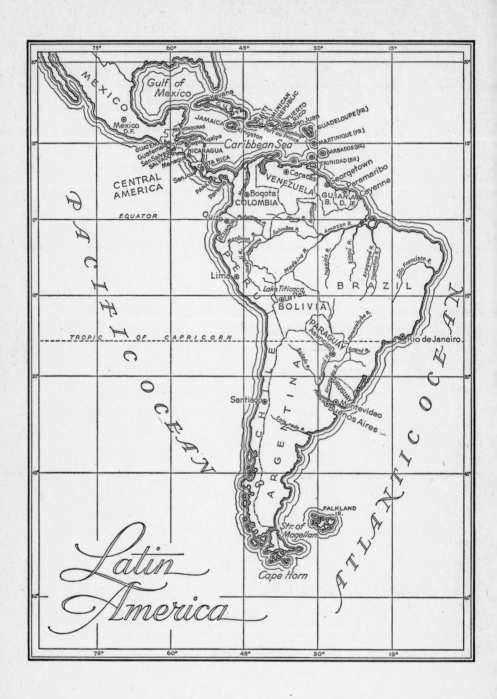

Chapter One

SICK MAN'S SOCIETY

THERE are somewhere around a hundred and twenty million people in Latin America, from the Rio Grande to Cape Horn. At this very moment it is a good bet that at least fifty million of them are sick. Sick of everything from sprue to leprosy. Sick of almost all the diseases that we in the United States encounter in our own lives, and of a multitude of savage and highly fatal diseases about which we know almost nothing.

A figure of fifty million sick men, women, and children is only an approximation, but it is reasonably close to the truth. Unfortunately, it is too huge to be understandable. You can hardly visualize what it means, what it implies. Doctors themselves, in the course of their professional work, generally think of sickness in terms of individual patients whom they are treating, and the human imagination balks at fifty million patients at once. Only gradually and partially has it begun to dawn even on the experts in the field of public health, that sickness, in Latin America, is as much a condition of life as weather or food. Even yet, we are far from understanding what fifty million sick people mean. They signify a society of sick men.

When the implications of such a society become plain to a man, the results can be dramatic. A quarter of a century ago a young doctor was beginning his medical career in a rural district of Honduras. On this particular day, a man—one of the mixed-blood Lapino farmers from the back country—brought the doctor a child, a boy whom he had carried for miles through the jungle. The boy's name, he said, was Hijo Gaitan. He was nine years old. And there was no doubt that little Hijo was very sick indeed.

Young Dr. Ricardo Aguilar could tell at a glance what was wrong. The signs were plain and familiar enough—the glassy, bloodshot eyes, the fiercely hot flesh, the pitifully bulging stomach. But because he was a scientist, and thorough, and very newly graduated from the Honduran National Faculty of Medicine, the doctor made the conventional blood test. The concentration of *Sporozoa plasmodiiae* was frighteningly high. His heart sank, but he smiled down at the boy.

"You have malaria, Hijo. It is bad malaria."

The child blinked. "Sí. Everybody has malaria, doctor—my sisters and brothers and all my cousins. . . ."

The young doctor asked cautiously, "How many brothers and sisters have you, Hijo?"

"Only two sisters . . . I had three brothers—Francisco, Juan, and Jesús. . . . They have all gone to God."

"Did they have malaria before they died?"

"Of course, señor!"

Dr. Ricardo Aguilar, twenty-six and studious, opened his medicine bag sadly. These were his people. Medicine was, and still is, his art, trade, and passion. He had come to this country district full of eagerness and determination to do a good job. But he was learning in practice that all, or most, of his people were sick. There were so many of them, he reflected, and they took their sickness so much as a matter of course. Little Hijo was not complaining. Malaria seemed an inevitable part of life to him. Dr. Aguilar frowned. He realized for the first time and with almost devastating abruptness that he lived, worked, and was himself a part of a sick man's society. . . .

That was a quarter century ago. Dr. Aguilar is still hard at work doing something about the situation which Hijo Gaitan made him realize so forcefully. Pestilence, contagion, and unnecessary death continue to sweep through the jungles and low countries and to invade the foothills, plateaus, and magnificent mountains of his part of the world. Like thousands of medical men south of the Rio Grande, he knows that the worst threats to the lives and happiness of most Latin Americans are still, as they always have been, the devastating, debilitating diseases of tropical and semitropical America.

Today at Tiquisate, in the "banana frontier" of western Guatemala, this same Ricardo Aguilar is establishing a new kind of hospital for country children of the tropics—a hospital dedicated to proving that sickness and fantastic death rates need not be the inevitable heritage of children in the Caribbean countries. That hospital itself is only one step in Dr. Aguilar's career of service to a sick man's society which, without him and men like him, might easily remain a sick man's society forever.

During his first crowded year of practice, Ricardo Aguilar also learned that Latin America in general, and particularly its rural areas, has acute and urgent need of dentists. The hundreds and hundreds of rotting and festering teeth in the mouths of his patients were proof that the great majority of his countrymen accepted the pain, infections, and health impairment resulting from poor teeth as a judgment of fate: many of his countrymen expected to be toothless by the time they were thirty or before. Usually their expectation proved to be justified.

Young Dr. Aguilar saved from his slender income money enough to study dentistry in the United States. Three years later he returned to Central America with a professional degree in dentistry to supplement his medical training. Immediately he began attending teeth along with the other ills from which his patients seemed always to be suffering.

He could not help being aware of the Latin-American need for surgery. Thousands of rural communities, hundreds of towns and smaller cities were, and alas still are, completely lacking in hospitals or even the simplest facilities for surgery. Even more fundamental was—and is—the scarcity of technical equipment and the resulting inability to solve the numerous baffling problems of standard tests and diagnosis. There are enormous hazards of infection in any operation undertaken in the tropics—far worse hazards than our own temperate climate generates. Then, too, preliminary treatment and the "building up" preliminary to surgery are far more complex in the tropics than in the United States. So extreme are all these problems that even today the average period of hospital confinement is almost twice as long in Latin America as it is farther north.

Realizing this, Ricardo Aguilar set out to make a surgeon of himself. Surgery in the American tropics is hard, man-killing work. Sometimes he had to use jungle shacks in lieu of operating rooms and siesta hammocks for operating tables. Often there was only lamplight or even moonlight instead of electricity by which to work. Frequently he had to conduct long and difficult operations without any experienced assistance. Even today, in addition to the routine problems of conventional surgery, he wrestles with the urgent, special difficulties of tropical surgery: malignant flesh ulcers about which little or nothing is yet understood. The abscessed livers which result so frequently from amoebic dysentery; the hideously swollen joints, head nodes, and other malignancies caused by tropical parasites, visible and microscopic. The struggle is unending. The future of half the world may depend upon its outcome, not in Aguilar's case alone, but in the larger whole of tropical medicine.

Ten years or less after he had begun, Aguilar was being mentioned as one of the most promising younger surgeons in all Central America. His work was leading him constantly further into the maze of problems which confront the doctor of the tropics, whether he be general practitioner, surgeon, or dentist. More than anywhere else in the world, medicine demands in the tropics the best and most effective equipment that can be bought or invented. Dr. Aguilar realized that hospitals and hospital management were central points in the attack on tropical ill-health.

Aguilar's patients and most of his fellow countrymen were far from any such realization. Twenty-five years ago most citizens of the American tropics looked on a hospital as a place where you went to die—a way station between the sickbed and the grave. Most of them preferred to stay at home until they were so sick that death appeared to them and their families as highly probable. And at home they stayed, no matter how squalid, wretched, and unsuitable the home might be. Aguilar and his colleagues, however, persevered. Hospitals began to be less of a rarity in Central America, and doctors like Ricardo Aguilar began to teach people that there was a difference between going to the hospital and dying.

Five years ago, Dr. Aguilar, somewhat plumper, somewhat older, more jovial in manner, perhaps, but no less diligent and inventive, became superintendent of a new base hospital in Tiquisate, Guatemala. It is one of the biggest, busiest, and most modern country hospitals in Central America. And it gave him an opportunity to do something he had long been planning.

Obviously, healthy children have a better chance than sick ones to become healthy adults. A child needlessly sick is a reproach to any society, a social as well as a personal tragedy. Dr. Aguilar had been thinking for years that the way to outflank the army of tropical diseases was to make sure that children get the best possible start. He never forgot little Hijo Gaitan, and all the small Gonzaleses, Martinezes, and Zomboas of the farms and jungle fringes, the little people whom he had treated in the long years of his country practice. Something had to be done for the *hijos*.

Doctoring children is no easy job anywhere. But in the tropics, which includes most of Latin America, it is a medical problem of the most intricate kind. "Ordinary" childhood diseases are frequently anything but ordinary in hot countries. Young Juans and Marias in the tropics still die regularly of such comparatively simple diseases as whooping cough, mumps, and measles. Dr. Aguilar learned from his field surveys that malaria rates were higher among children than among adults. He attended country children who were maimed and literally rotting from malarial complications. He treated innumerable cases of hookworm—an evil consequence of tropical barefootedness. He attended farm children who were being consumed alive by virulent tropical fevers. An Indian woman once walked the forty miles from her mountain pueblo to where he was holding a clinic, carrying a child already blood-splattered and dying from bacillary dysentery. He saw many a child crippled by the infections which attacked untreated scratches and the inevitable accidental cuts to which habitually naked flesh is subject. Even doctors, accustomed to suffering and death, find some things hard to forget. And for Dr. Aguilar, children held a special importance. They represented the future.

He knew the jungle-edge homes where these children lived. He knew their parents' helplessness in properly attending the sick. He treated little Alberto Raphael who was suffering from the combined infections of malaria, filariasis, and yaws—each one a malady that jeopardized the child's life. Yet Alberto's parents had not even been aware that their little son was gravely ill.

Then there were the elder Gomezes, good, hard-working country people. But their shack, like the others in which all their neighbors lived, was entirely without sanitation or the facilities necessary to attend the needs of a sick child. Like a great many of their rural neighbors the Gomezes still preferred to avoid hospitals as much and as long as possible—which meant until the time was at hand for calling the priest to administer the last rites.

So Dr. Ricardo Aguilar began to plan a children's hospital which would be attractive both to children and to country parents; an efficient, homelike hospital which would prove to all the Gomezes that hospitals can save children's lives and health. He did not have much money to begin with. For some years he had been saving royalties from his medical books and translations. Besides these, he had the friendly co-operation of a well-known banana company. And on the ground floor of the Tiquisate base hospital there was room for a child's hospital. In September, 1941, Ricardo Aguilar set out to make the best possible use of that space.

He bought attractive cribs, high chairs and miscellaneous furniture, several crates of toys, and an oversize ice-cream freezer. He directed the laying of colored tile floors and invested heavily in bathtubs and water closets. For he believes, like many other Latin Americans, that wider and better use of newfangled Norteamericano plumbing is worth more to Pan-America than any amount of fulsomely worded stuff about "cultural relations."

Having bought his equipment, Aguilar went on to secure a good dietitian and two registered nurses with long experience in child care. He laid in plenty of honey candies and sweetened quinine. Finally (and perhaps with divine assistance), the doctor came upon a native house painter who was a Walt Disney addict.

With typical Spanish-American dexterity and an inspired plagiarism which Mr. Disney would be the last to resent or begrudge, this Guatemalan house painter began producing beaming portraits of Mickey Mouses, Minnie Mouses and various other Disney masterpieces to hang above every crib, high chair and wall panel throughout the children's wards. As a final inspiration the Indian house painter spotted the bathroom floor with Donald Ducks, Plutos, and Elmer Elephants.

Late in 1941 the new Children's Hospital at the Tiquisate base was opened, with little Alberto Gomez as its first patient. Alberto is well now. Dozens of other rural children are being made well in an institution which seeks no profit and names no rates. The *salor*—colloquial for ward—is an almost instant success. Countryside parents—Indians, mixed bloods, Spaniards, and all the others—have begun to like the hospital. Sick children are finding happiness and restored health in its refuge. As many of them, that is, as the hospital can hold.

Dr. Ricardo Aguilar is happy in his newest experiment. He calls it a "step"—not a final achievement. He continues working, observing, and planning additional progress in the profession he serves so devotedly. If the term "typical doctor" is ever legitimate, Ricardo Aguilar can be described as typical of the thousands of Latin-American men of medicine who constitute a gallant and hard-working civilian army fighting Latin America's battle for health. The battle which is still far from won, the story of which is an epic, centuries long. It is also a story of profound importance for us more fortunate Americans of the north.

For generations, the people of the United States have casually thought and spoken of themselves as *the* Americans. Only recently have we taken seriously the truth that we constitute little more than one-half of the entire American people. Less than one-half, if the Canadians are to be included in the hemisphere total.

Today, with conflicting economic, political, and social interests dividing up the world according to the weight of its component ideas, *the Western Hemisphere*, not merely the United States, is America. Not the America of any imperialist dream, but the America of mankind, still the new-found land, still the community of free men determined to stand or fall by their humanity and their freedom.

When the presence of a mutual enemy made the English-speaking Americans and their neighbors to the south conscious of a set of common beliefs and interests, we were subjected to a barrage of well-meaning literature which attempted to interpret each to the other. We have assured each other of our common interest, that united we stand and divided we fall, and we have tabulated our joint assets and advantages. Unfortunately, we have ignored or glossed over the liabilities and weaknesses. Without knowledge of these, too, we cannot really know one another or reach any genuine understanding.

What we of the north have not learned or been told is a long and heartbreaking story. We have recently discovered a good deal about how Latin America lives and is gay. But why have we heard so little about how Latin America dies? How millions of our neighbors meet, every year, cruel, untimely, and unnecessary deaths? The greatest threat to Western Hemisphere solidarity is not ignorance of the manners and customs and ways of thinking of one section or another. It is *not* the penetration and mushroom spread of totalitarian doctrine. Latin America's public enemy number one is neither Nazi nor Nipponese. It is the insidious and ubiquitous column of disease. The operations of this enemy are harder to check and will continue to be far more dangerous to us of the north than anything out of *Mein Kampf.*

Add to this lamentable fact the statement of the man whose work in sanitation and preventive medicine made possible the construction of the Panama Canal, the late General William Crawford Gorgas: "If one man's labor can produce enough of the necessities to support himself and one other man, we have a certain degree of civilization and refinement. If his labor produces enough to support himself and two other men, a higher degree of civilization results. In the tropics, one man's labor applied to natural opportunities is able to support more men than the same amount of labor applied in any other part of the world. In the long run, therefore, the great civilizations of the future will be located in the tropics." [1]

That statement takes on significance when you realize that the largest and most productive part of Latin America lies in the tropics and subtropics. The problem to the south of us is not the mere political courtship of a neighbor. It is to lay the foundation of a future, a future for ourselves and for the whole world.

The comfortable belief that the heroism of a few American soldiers and the skill of United States physicians and public health officers have made Central and South America as safe as the streets of North American cities is unfortunately far from true. It is a fact that in Cuba and in the Panama Canal Zone yellow fever has been practically conquered and malaria considerably curbed. But consider a few other figures: The average life expectancy of a resident of the

[1] Footnotes for this and succeeding chapters will be found in the appendix following the text proper.

United States, as of 1940, was about sixty-two years and five months. In Latin America, according to the best statistics now available, the average life lasts between fifteen and thirty-five years less than that, depending on the locality in which it is lived. In Chile the life expectancy is about thirty-five years; in Peru, less than thirty-two; in Mexico and Uruguay, well under forty.[2]

These shocking figures are not due to the fact that most Latin Americans live in rural areas and most citizens of the United States in cities. In many countries to the south it is true that health statistics for rural areas are even more alarming than those from cities. But when you compare city with city the picture is much the same. The average yearly death rate per thousand people in the fifty largest cities of Latin America is more than twice as high as the death rate in the fifty largest cities of the United States. Our own Public Health Service gives the New York City rate, for example, as 9.8 per thousand per year. In Santiago, Chile, the comparable figure is 24.8. In Lima, Peru, the figure stands at 20.5; in Quito, Ecuador, at 21.2; in Caracas, Venezuela, at 19.4; in Mexico City, at 23.8; and in La Paz, Bolivia, at 22.4.[3]

Such figures are more than cold statistics. They mean something almost horrifying by the standards which we normally employ in thinking about ourselves. Suppose our national death rate from disease doubled in a single year? We should be talking about "plagues." We should probably be frightened. And we should promptly devote every possible resource to bringing the death rate down to where we could again regard it as normal.

Almost as important as the death rates themselves is the analysis of the causes of death. The moment the Latin-American causes of death are tabulated alongside those of the United States, a significant difference becomes apparent. To understand something of what that difference means, it is useful to look also at what were the ten principal causes of death in this country in 1900—less than half a century ago:

THE TEN PRINCIPAL CAUSES OF DEATH

In the United States in 1900	*In Latin America Today*	*In the United States Today*
Influenza-Pneumonia	Tuberculosis	Heart disease
Tuberculosis	Influenza-Pneumonia	Influenza-Pneumonia
Diarrhea-Enteritis	Malaria	Cancer
Heart disease	Diarrhea-Enteritis	Cerebral hemorrhage
Nephritis	Cancer	Nephritis
Cerebral hemorrhage	Diphtheria	Tuberculosis
Cancer	Infantile paralysis	Automobile accidents
Bronchitis	Typhoid	Diabetes
Diphtheria	Heart disease	Arteriosclerosis
Typhoid	Meningitis	Diarrhea-Enteritis [4]

What does this table mean? Above everything else it emphasizes how nearly our own medicine has come to conquering the pathogenic—or disease-causing—organisms as sources of fatality. Only three of the ten entries in that right-hand column are the result of organisms hostile to man. You cannot catch a bad heart from your neighbor at the movies or from the bite of an insect. Cancer, cerebral hemorrhage, nephritis, diabetes, arteriosclerosis—all these are failures, one way or another, of the human machine. Automobile accidents are not even that—unless you think intelligence ought to be organic. Some organism is undoubtedly at the bottom of the influenza-pneumonia group, tuberculosis is the result of a bacillary infection, and diarrhea-enteritis, which ranks tenth on our list, is also the result of various pathogenic organisms. But it begins to look as if we in the United States were well on the way to dying only when our bodies are worn out or broken by automobiles.

A single glance at the column of Latin-American causes of death will reveal how differently the cards are stacked for our southern neighbors. Eight of the ten principal sources of fatality in their countries are the result of hostile organisms, and only cancer and heart disease are not. Not until the middle column of our table comes to resemble the right-hand one will Latin-American medicine have been able to contribute to its populations the life span and freedom from infection which we are fortunate enough to enjoy today.

The left-hand column, which presents the causes of death in the United States in 1900, suggests how swiftly we have benefited, as a group, from our medical advances. In less than a single lifetime we have largely eliminated no less than three organism-borne diseases which were mighty killers forty-odd years ago. Diphtheria, typhoid, and bronchitis are no longer major sources of fatality in our own country, but the first two still are in Latin America. Indeed, a comparison of the death causes in Latin America today and in the United States four decades ago reveals a striking similarity. How comforting it would be to note this similarity and decide that in forty more years the Latin Americans will probably have caught up with where we now are, and that there is nothing to worry about.

Unfortunately, the situation is less comfortable than that. Here in the north we like to believe that we stand almost isolated from the attacks of these minute, disease-causing organisms which run riot in the south. But are we really safe? The fact that Spanish-American countries are harassed by infective diseases ought to be a matter of deep concern to us. We are sending a part at least of our vast new army to the American tropics, where our men will be exposed to these lethal viruses, bacteria, and protozoa. There is no virusproof door standing shut between us and our southern neighbors, either. The health of Latin America, just as much as its economic welfare, has become a vital problem for the United States. Our medicine and medicos have more than a goodwill job to do in this hemisphere. It is a job on which some few of them have already been working, unnoticed, for a long time. Among other things, this book attempts to tell the story of the men in white who have been our best ambassadors of goodwill to countries where most men are sick and where most sick people are without hope.

Statistics are often dull unless the reader can translate them in his imagination into living—or dead—realities. But the cold figures on some of the diseases which are decimating Latin-American countries are so appalling, turned into their reality of sick, dying, and dead people of all ages and all classes, that they deserve a close inspection. For instance, tuberculosis. To the majority of us in the United States, tuberculosis means buying some charity stamps at Christmastime and forgetting about it the rest of the year. For others, it is a more dangerous and tragic reality. But there is only *one* Spanish American country in which tuberculosis is not the thing that all of us used to call it—"the white plague."

In the year 1939, some 47.2 persons out of every hundred thousand in the United States died of tuberculosis. By no means a record to be proud of, that figure nevertheless indicates a paradise of immunity compared to the Latin-American situation. In only one southern republic, Colombia, is the tuberculosis rate lower than that of the United States. There the death rate from the disease is 46.6 per hundred thousand. But in 1938, according to estimates of the Pan American Sanitary Bureau, Mexico's rate was 55.4; El Salvador's, 61; Guatemala's, 64.3. In 1939 the rate in the Dominican Republic was 64.7; in Ecuador, 70.2; in Cuba, 82; and in Costa Rica, 83.9.

These are the Latin-American countries which are relatively free from the white plague. In the moderate group are Paraguay, with 102.4 tuberculosis deaths per hundred thousand; Argentina with 103, and Uruguay with 109, all well above twice the United States figure. The real sufferers are Panama, with 210 deaths per hundred thousand from tuberculosis; Venezuela with 243; Brazil with 250, and Chile with 276. Almost three people out of every thousand in Chile die, *each year*, of tuberculosis.[5]

In South and Central America, as elsewhere, the menace of tuberculosis has tended to increase as the concentration of population in cities increased. Add to this the fact that a large proportion of Latin-American population is Indian and you have some explanation of the terrible gravity of the disease, for the Indian, from the time of the conquistadors, has been extremely susceptible to pulmonary ailments.

To turn for a moment to the cities again, the figures suggest that the only reason more Latin Americans do not die of tuberculosis is that more of them do not yet live in metropolises. In New York City, the death rate from tuberculosis is 49 per hundred thousand, in Detroit it is 44.7, but in Santiago, Chile, it is 430; in Lima, Peru, 435, and in Guayaquil, Ecuador (1939 figures), it was 693. Particularly in Chile and Peru, tuberculosis is in a stage of infectious virulence. Dr. Aristides A. Moll, secretary of the Pan American Sanitary Bureau, says that in a certain Chilean city 50 per cent of all children of six or under were infected with tuberculosis, 80 per cent of those from six to fifteen, and in two groups between the ages of sixteen and twenty-four the percentage of infection was 85 to 90 among middle class persons and 100 among workers.[6]

Quite evidently Latin America's tuberculosis menace is not limited to any particular altitude, type of climate, or density of population. It exists at sea level in Montevideo and two miles above sea level in La Paz. It threatens the Indian, the Negro, the Spanish native, and the European. Defense against it is one of the foundation stones of any future Pan-American civilization.

Typhoid, dysentery, and other water-borne diseases are actual, not merely potential menaces in the Latin countries of this hemisphere. Malaria is as great a scourge as ever, in spite of public statements giving a contrary impression, and Latin-American malaria is no mere matter of simple chills. It is a chronic illness causing death and disability in tremendous numbers in all the lands south of Texas. Infantile paralysis is ravaging hundreds of communities which never knew it before. Trachoma, an insidious disease of the eye which frequently results in blindness, is occurring more frequently than ever, particularly in the highlands. Latin-American deaths from diseases long since controlled in the north, such as smallpox, diphtheria, and measles, are still twice as high in proportion to population as they are in the United States.

The last major epidemic of yellow fever in the United States occurred in New Orleans in 1905—several years after proof of the belief that mosquitoes were the agents for the spread of the disease. Since that epidemic in Louisiana it is fairly safe to guess that not one United States physician in a hundred has so much as seen a case of yellow fever. True. But even so, the next epidemic may be just around the corner.

In South America, large areas of the enormous Amazon basin and of southern Colombia are still reservoirs of the very yellow fever which our writers and dramatists have celebrated as long since conquered. Yellow fever is no storybook disease. Its mystery has been solved once, but it refuses to stay solved. The organisms of yellow fever attack man by way of the blood of jungle animals. The Rockefeller Foundation's researches have recently proved that it can be transmitted by other mosquitoes than the stegomyia (*Aëdes aegypti*) which Walter Reed and his colleagues made infamous and which, in the years between, medical men hopefully believed to be the only carrier. So long as jungle animals and mosquitoes remain alive in Latin America, the United States is not safe from yellow fever. Such safety as may be attained can result only from the expenditure of vast sums for sanitation and inoculation campaigns like the one which the government of Brazil (influenced by a *1,700 per cent increase* in yellow fever deaths between 1908 and 1938) is now carrying on.

Yellow fever is not the only public enemy, by any means. Typhus, a disease which few North Americans ever thought of before the recent news from the Polish ghettos, and which almost none of us associate with the Western Hemisphere, is, it is true, all but extinct in the United States. During the past year, however, alarming outbreaks of it have been reported from Mexico, Cuba, Brazil, Venezuela, and Salvador, with from a third to a half of the cases resulting in death. In Chile the disease has been on the rampage for a decade. As recently as 1933, 15,379 cases with 3,596 deaths were reported there. Fortunately for all the Americas, Chile has been able to get the better of the disease for the time being. The threat is still there.

Since 1902 smallpox has been almost unknown in the United States. It continues to threaten Latin America. Less fortunate Mexico, according to its health department, suffered 15,000 smallpox deaths as recently as 1930, as many as 5,000 in 1935 and 3,500 in 1937.[7] Yet, like most of our other nineteen neighbor republics, Mexico is doing what she can, making a brave struggle to control contagious disease. Her gross expenditures for public health administration have risen a hundredfold since 1900.

Though infinitely poorer than the United States, most Latin-American nations are much more liberal than ourselves in their financing of the defense of public health. They have to be. Since 1909, when Cuba led the world in organizing a national Ministry of Health, all Latin-American countries have established federal health services, but the work of these agencies, capable and courageous as most of them are, remains, through no fault of their own, far short of sufficient. Since most of Latin America lies in the tropics or subtropics, climatic conditions such as the human system in the United States rarely has to contend with encourage disease germs to flourish during all twelve months of the year. The unbelievable isolation of large sections of the population beyond and in the midst of vast expanses of jungle, mountain, and desert combines with scarcity of communications or public servants of any sort, lack of clinical facilities, and modern equipment, to make the control of disease in Central and South America as difficult as the carrying of water in a sieve. Racial prejudices, the scarcity of independent medical practitioners, the high percentage of illiteracy and bitter poverty throughout much of Latin America help to deliver over our less fortunate neighbors to an enemy which most of us do not even believe in.

The family with little or no income cannot choose its food for vitamin content. Records of the United States Public Health Service make it plain that in North America families with incomes of less than $2,000 per year suffer about twice as many days of sickness each year as do those with incomes of $3,000 or more. Take a fine-tooth comb and go through the population of Latin America to see how many incomes of even $2,000 you will find. North Americans simply cannot understand how small the average Latin-American income really is. The small incomes not only mean restricted food. They mean small governmental income and hence limited outlay for public health. With limited means, the governments of Central and South American nations, in spite of their energy and their recognition of the gravity of the situation confronting them, frequently meet serious difficulties even in providing purification of public water supplies. Latin America remains a chronic victim of water-borne diseases such as typhoid and amoebic dysentery. In thousands, perhaps tens of thousands, of Latin-American communities, impure drinking water remains a living danger. With the possible exception of some of the overcrowded parts of South Asia and the East Indies, South America presents drinking-water problems as serious as those of any part of the world.

Ironically but truly, Latin-American populations inhabiting what is potentially the world's greatest food-producing region suffer enormously from malnutrition and from the scores of diseases or "symptom complexes" resulting from inadequate diet. Beriberi, pellagra, and numerous other nutritional diseases are as standard to submarginal diets as vests to three-piece suits. So, very probably, are leprosy, amoebic infections, tropical ulcers, and tuberculosis. Certainly the latter four are poor man's diseases. With few exceptions, they are most virulent where poverty is most intense and where diet is least adequate.

It takes no very keen perception to notice that touring microbes, like human tourists, frequently misbehave upon arrival in the tropics. For example, Latin-American death rates from what we consider merely nuisance diseases, such as measles and chickenpox, are several times greater than in the United States. Pneumonia is more frequently fatal south of the Rio Grande than north. Influenza kills its victims more than twice as often. Malaria, lightly regarded in the United States, is a positive plague among peoples to the south. Here in the north, according to the United States Public Health Service, we have something like four million chronic cases of malaria. But the parasites which cause them are preponderantly of the mild or plain chills-and-fever order. In medical parlance, they are "benign." Not so the Latin-American variety. The greater part of Latin-American malaria is of the virulent, body-blasting types, such as tertian or estivo-autumnal. This last kind is widely known in some Spanish American countries as the *economico*, because it is so almost certainly fatal that there is no sense wasting money on doctors and drugs to treat it.

There are a hundred other examples of the ruthless intensity of Temperate Zone diseases transplanted to the tropics. This increased virulence is in at least some cases partly explainable in terms of poverty, ignorance of hygiene, and want of good nursing and adequate treatment. But there are many other factors which no man has yet explained. Speaking generally, and for one reason or another, microbes are still miles ahead of man in matters of adapting themselves to life in the tropics. The attacking enemy seems always to have the advantage. The mysterious phenomena of climate which tend to make men listless and enervated in hot countries seem to give to disease organisms added strength and inexplicable violence.

Ironically enough, the overwhelming majority of Latin-America's diseases, political as well as medical, are imported from Europe. Dr. George Cheever Shattuck of the Harvard Medical Faculty, and one of our distinguished students of diseases of the American tropics, declared: "One can say with certainty or a high degree of probability that nearly all the more deadly diseases known in the

New World since its discovery by Columbus have been imported from the Old World within historic times. This is probably true, also, of the minor epidemic diseases and of many other infectious diseases as well." [8]

So, the meningitis rate in Chile is about twenty times that of the United States. Bubonic plague, the louse-carried nemesis of medieval Europe, persists in fury through half a dozen South American nations. Latin-American death lists from scarlet fever, smallpox, lobar pneumonia, and some fifty other principal diseases, all probably imported, give a new and unpleasant interpretation to that threadbare phrase, "the white man's burden."

History tells us bluntly enough that conquest by contagious diseases, and not by Spanish or other European arms, proved the supreme tragedy of an Indian-populated Western Hemisphere. The conquistadors made their best progress when following in the wake of contagions which they themselves had brought to the New World and sent on before them. Capable scholars have estimated that no fewer than *twenty million* Central and South American Indians died of European contagions during the course of Spain's American conquests. In 1633 the chronicler, Antonio de la Calancha, noted that "for each dollar coined in Peru, ten Indians died." Between 1520 and 1820 Andean Indian populations apparently fell from a probable five million to a bare half million. The great race of the Incas was consumed in the holocaust of European disease. As smallpox swept Mexico and Yucatan, great cities vanished from the earth. Peru was ravaged by at least eight fearfully destructive epidemics; Brazil and the other Amazon countries by at least seven, the West Indies by more. Those were only the major epidemics. There must have been thousands of unrecorded local outbreaks.

Time and time again earlier historians of the New World had written of lands and people almost or entirely free of disease, of aborigines of Brazil, Cuba, Santo Domingo, and other American lands who were still without gray hair at eighty; who died of sheer old age at a hundred or even a hundred and twenty years.

But the picture changed when the white men came. Transplanted Europeans were about as helpless in combating the ruinous epidemics they brought with them as were the New World Indians. In 1584, while Central America was being decimated by typhus, Spain's governor general could do no better than command that bonfires be built in village plazas, that cannons be fired all day long to cleanse the air of evil humors, that nuns be freshly shorn, and that the populace pray to St. Rosalie. By the nineteenth century, most of Latin America was a confirmed sick man's society. Spain and much of Europe, rotten with disease, looked westward to a New World grown sparse and bleak by contagion.

Latin America is still a sick man's society. Those who first learned to want something of the Western Hemisphere made it so. We who now want Latin-American friendship and support will have to join in a declaration of war against this distinctly European heritage. The current struggle for health is the most significant of all American wars. It is no conflict of propaganda and counterpropaganda or of power politics locking horns with other power politics. We are not being shoved into this particular war. We are not being asked to send expeditionary forces or tens of billions of dollars' worth of tanks and battle planes. We are not being asked to give our shirt in order to save someone else's shirt or our own. We are not even in this war because Latin America, in her dramatic struggle for health, is demanding man power, wealth, or weapons of us. We are in it because it is our war and because our neighbors cannot hold the fort for us indefinitely.

Actually, Latin-American medical talent and governments have been putting up one of the stanchest struggles in all history, as the next chapter will indicate in detail. They are making heroic efforts today to use the best sera, vaccines and tests, the best pharmaceuticals and the most modern therapies. From their own native populations they are developing hundreds of first-class men in medicine and surgery—names to rank with our own Mayos, Murphys, Gorgases,

Reeds, Lazears, and Carters. They are making a science and a profession out of public health administration. They are educating doctors, dentists, surgeons, and sanitary engineers. The task is not too great for their spirit, but it is far beyond their present resources.

Even the most superficial survey of these resources will give some idea of how far short of adequate the Latin-American health facilities really are. Here in the United States, with about one hundred and thirty-two million people, we have some six thousand accredited public hospitals. For a total population of about one hundred and twenty million, Latin America has approximately the same number of hospitals—Brazil about 1,200, Argentina about 750, Mexico about 300, Colombia about 250, Chile has 184, and so on. But this mildly reassuring statistic is tragically misleading. In the first place, most Latin-American hospitals are neither so large nor so well endowed as ours. In the second place, the need for more beds is proportionately greater. To this point we shall return in the next chapter.

Meantime, there is the question of man power, of the men to send to the firing line of tropical disease. Here, as in the matter of the gross number of hospitals, it would appear at first glance that our neighbors are better off than we ourselves.

The science of tropical medicine is only now being born. In the United States we have schools or departments of tropical medicine in five universities—Harvard, California, South Carolina, Louisiana, and Tulane. Latin America has about twenty. Puerto Rico's Institute of Tropical Medicine and Hygiene, founded in 1917, is the oldest in the Western Hemisphere. Brazil's Oswaldo Cruz Institute, Argentina's North Argentine Mission, Panama's Gorgas Institute and Hospital, and the national medical schools in Rio de Janeiro, Montevideo, Lima, Mexico City, Havana, and Buenos Aires are among the more valuable defense posts against the still ruinous onslaught of tropical disease.

Brazil was the first nation of this hemisphere to establish a medical laboratory; only two years after the founding of Germany's first medical laboratory and seven years before the United States Public Health Service opened its first "hygiene laboratory" in New York, which was the first in the United States. Every Latin-American nation now has its National Red Cross, several of which are older than ours. Brazil and Argentina were world pioneers in founding antituberculosis leagues. South American countries had public hospitals and asylums long before we did.

But these facts, encouraging though they are, do not mean either that the problem is under control or that it shortly will be. In a society of people who are pretty largely healthy, as we are, fewer doctors, fewer clinics, fewer hospitals are required to take care of public health. Our resources of roads, railroads, and automobiles have made centralization of health facilities possible, and they have also extended the working range, so to speak, of doctors themselves. In proportion to what is needed, the medical resources of all Latin America are still fearfully inadequate. What already exists is hardly more than an earnest of what must come before disease begins to be checkmated between the tropics of Cancer and Capricorn.

South of the Rio Grande the Pan-American war for health remains a struggle against desperate odds. The same luxuriant soils, climate, and seasons which make so much of Latin America a center of luxuriance for fields and forests also help make it a generative center for disease. And disease is constantly being fed more and more human material upon which to work. It is almost possible to view the situation as a race between the speed with which tropical disease can kill and the rate at which the population can replace its staggering losses.

In Latin America as a whole, population is increasing about three times as fast as in the United States. The birth rate, always high, has finally caught up with the tragically high death rate. Between 1783 and 1883 the population of the United States gained an average of 30 per cent every ten years. During this period Latin-American populations were virtually at a standstill—largely because of uncontrollable diseases. But between 1880 and 1930, Latin-American population closely paralleled our own with an increase of about 20 per cent each decade. Between 1930 and 1940 the population of the United States added a meager 7 per cent—that of Latin America at least 20 per cent, and perhaps more. Reliable figures for the past decade are not yet available.

In 1900 there were only twelve Latin-American cities with more than a hundred thousand people. Today there are at least fifty. Dr. Aristides A. Moll, one of the ranking authorities on American population trends, estimated at the 1941 meeting of the Population Association of America that Argentina's population has grown from 5,000,000 in 1900 to 11,000,000 in 1930 and to more than 13,000,-000 at present; Brazil's from 18,000,000 in 1900 to 45,000,000 in 1930 and about 50,000,000 today; Mexico's from about 13,600,000 in 1900 to about 20,000,000 today.[9]

Though Latin-American population is now increasing rapidly, there is still plenty of room. Here in the United States we have about 36 people per square mile. Nearly nine-tenths of the land surface of Latin America has fewer than 20 to the mile. Brazil has about 14; Chile and Ecuador, 16; Venezuela, 10; Bolivia, 8; and Paraguay fewer than 6.

In terms of its known resources, most of South America is still greatly underpopulated. But in terms of public health the situation looks very different. Much of the land now standing idle and unproductive simply cannot be occupied, and for a good reason—men cannot work there and live.

Latin America's gigantic problem of disease comes down to this: hemisphere solidarity cannot be built on a sick man's society. Latin America cannot live as a contributing factor in Western Hemisphere or world civilization until it has conquered its health problems. Since the Monroe Doctrine we have considered that it was our job to help protect the southern nations from political aggressors. Today, and even more urgently, it is our job to help Latin-American nations protect themselves against the fifth column of disease.

This is no easy order. We cannot do our part merely with hand-shaking, backslapping, or noble words. We cannot do it with publicity photographs of movie stars, impersonating goodwill ambassadors, and similar childishnesses. Equally certainly, we cannot do the job with gunboats and cannon. War matériel in the form of bombers, tanks, battle fleets, and armies cannot thwart invasion by contagious or infectious disease. On the contrary, the current feat of arming a hemisphere actually invites and perpetuates the spread of disease. Today, as in centuries past, military forces are also disease-spreading forces. The ability of ships and armies to carry disease has long been known and lamented. In some parts of South America typhus is still called army fever. American historians know that both our Mexican War and our Spanish-American War poured new fuel upon the fires of yellow fever; that our Civil War contributed enormously to spreading typhoid all over the domestic landscape, and that both our Revolution and the War of 1812 distributed smallpox more generously than medals.

Today we know that spectacular increases in military and commercial travel among the American nations is helping to increase the death toll of disease, to fortify the outposts of the enemy. In Guatemala and Cuba, meccas for Caribbean travel, reported malaria rates have more than doubled during 1941. Four years ago malaria was so rare in Cuba that it appeared headed for extinction. From 1935 to 1939 in Oriente, Cuba's largest state, hospital admissions for malaria were only about one in a thousand entries.[10] As the United States Navy began expanding its Guantánamo base and importing hundreds of nonimmune workers and service personnel from the United States, malaria began to increase in the region about the bay. Hospital admissions for malaria suddenly and drastically increased.

This, like a hundred other timely items in inter-American health news, merely serves to prove that as armies and navies move, and as general migration increases, disease germs do the same. Inter-American travel is bounding higher and higher. Early opening of the Pan-American Highway may double present totals. Disease germs cannot be forced to recognize national boundary lines, and ironically, we have forged so far ahead of our southern neighbors in the suppression of general contagions that most of our people have no immunity whatever to the principal contagions to the south.

Despite much progress in preventives and vaccines, newcomers to hot countries are still easy prey to disease. According to Admiralty records, yellow fever now faces British, German, French, and Italian forces in various areas of North Africa. Malaria contagions in South China have become so acute that the United States Public Health Service has dispatched thirty of its best malaria doctors and mosquito experts to help China and democracy by leading a drive against this vicious destroyer of healthy blood. Along the Burma Road, as in many other parts of the world, disease-carrying mosquitoes remain the deadliest of all aerial foes.

In both hemispheres the intercommunication, the circulation, and the concentration of peoples provide a means of multiplication for disease. That is an item for dictators and democracies alike to ponder. The forces of disease are stealthy, corrupting, and wholly impartial. More potently than any other fifth column, they can undermine and corrupt governments and rob the common citizen of his right to live.

Dr. Ricardo Piravanos, a distinguished Argentine surgeon, recently declared that the pooled spending for a decade of some $350,-000,000 annually—approximately three dollars per capita for the population of Latin America—could produce results which would make Central and South America as healthy as North America now is.

Latin-American ability to spend three dollars per head per year on public health depends upon us in more ways than one. Most of all it depends upon trade with the United States. Better business in and with South America means better health throughout the Western Hemisphere. And better health means better opportunity and greater ability to foster and develop the ideas and ideals in defense of which the nations of the Western Hemisphere are now banded together.

Much is being done to better trade relations with the southern republics and much will undoubtedly be done to further the exchange of ideas and energies in public health. It would be impossible in a single readable volume to present every phase of the problem of tropical and subtropical medicine and public health organization. But it is the author's hope that these pages will give English-speaking Americans a picture of the gigantic problem and of the men and organizations working to meet it.

In subsequent chapters the history and record of some of those ambassadors in white who have already given their abilities, their lives, and their fortunes to solve the fatal riddles of tropical disease will be presented in the hope that the story of what they have done will give the people whom they served some sense of what remains to be done and some indication of the spirit that will point out the way to do it. Knowledge of the lives and work of these men, of the organizations, military, philanthropic and commercial, which sponsored them, and of the deep, dark mysteries which their successors will have to solve should serve better than anything else to illustrate the nature of the bond that unites us with Latin America.

Chapter Two

PAST AND PRESENT

T HE story of Latin-American medicine is a long one. It starts more than a thousand years ago, when North America was a forest wilderness, and its beginnings were in the deft hands and canny brains of the Inca, Aztec, and Maya *yerbateros,* men of medicine and magic, men who knew the depths of jungles and pampas and mountain forests where grew thousands of medicinal plants. Many of these plants have been carried over into the pharmacopoeia of civilization; most of us are familiar with some form of cocaine, cascara sagrada, quinine, Peruvian balsam, ipecac, copal, chaparro, sarsaparilla, vervain, and many others. The Aztec drug seller was an important personage in the Indian world upon which the white man descended. The historian doctor Hernandez, who was private physician to Philip II of Spain, reported that Mexican Indians used more than three thousand different plants in the treatment of human ailments. Furthermore, the rulers of the early Indian empires took a direct and personal interest in medicine and health. Prescott tells how Montezuma's botanical garden furnished almost any drug known to medicine. Health has been a preoccupation of Latin-American societies from the time of the Incas to the present, and with good reason.

Modern Latin-American medicine, however, stems from Europe rather than from the pre-Columbian yerbateros. It began five centuries ago in the medicine of Imperial Spain, France, England, Austria, Germany, Italy, and Russia, and the conquistadors brought it across the Atlantic with them. Its coming was no unmixed blessing. On the one hand, imported medical science lagged during the generations of the conquistadors. On the other, common diseases such as smallpox, scarlet fever, yellow fever, and measles themselves crossed the ocean and were listed, conveniently, as "peste." Meantime, colonization went on as best it could in spite of disease.

Spain was not only the cradle of European medicine but also the foremost European contributor to New World medicine. Salamanca University antedated Oxford. Spain had led the countries of the world in establishing schools for the deaf and the blind and in founding (at Seville and Valencia) asylums for the insane. The *Mayflower* carried no ship's doctor. But the vessels of Columbus, Cortez, Balboa, and Mendoza did.

By 1565, Gonzalo de Oviedo y Valdés, representative of Spain's king-emperor, had published under the title *De las Drogas de las Indias* an encyclopedia on healing arts and medicinal plants of the New World. In 1571, Francisco Hernandez made a scientific expedition to the Americas. What he saw of Indian medicine impressed him. A third of a century earlier, in 1538, on the island of Santo Domingo, the University of Santo Tomás had begun teaching medicine. By 1580, twenty-seven years before John Harvard was born, the University of Mexico, inaugurated in 1553, had a chair of medicine. In succeeding centuries, other schools of medicine began to appear throughout Spanish America; at Lima in 1621; at Caracas a century later; at Havana in 1728; Bogotá, 1758; in Chile in 1756; at Quito in 1787; at Buenos Aires in 1801; in Guatemala, 1805; and so on. And in the field of public health and sanitation, notable and durable work was being carried on by the Jesuits in South America and the Franciscans in Mexico long before the birth of Virginia colony.

The seventeenth century saw the introduction into Europe of quinine, probably the greatest of all natural therapeutics, the magic bark of the cinchona, long before discovered by the Quito Indians. By 1632 the Jesuit, Barnabé Cobo, was taking the miraculous malaria cure to Madrid and Rome. This discovery of quinine helped to focus European medical interest upon the New World. French and Spanish scientists came to study and record the medicinal flora of South America. In 1714 the famous Father Louis Feuillée published the first of his memorable studies of the medicinal plants of Chile and Peru.

During the eighteenth century, there had grown up in South America an indigenous science and medicine. The names of the early doctors and naturalists who were its bulwarks are practically unknown in North America, to our shame be it said, and they deserve mention here. The Abbé Giovanni Molina of Chile, who worked as a naturalist, botanist, and pharmacologist, was one of the century's great South Americans. Another was Pedro Franco Davila of Guayaquil, who became director of the Museum of Natural History at Madrid, by appointment of Charles III of Spain. His researches as a naturalist and botanist had earned this honor for him. The Brazilian, Ferreira Leal, became a renowned physician of Vienna. The Colombian, José Mutis, who died in 1808, won international renown as the botanist of the cinchona, or quinine, tree and as a great pioneer sanitarian. By 1773, indeed, Latin-American medicine had become important enough to require its own journal. The *Mercurio Volante*, founded in Mexico City in that year, was probably the first medical journal of the Western Hemisphere.[1]

Three important medical names appear in the history of eighteenth century South America. They are those of Vargas, Unanue, and Espejo.

Francísco Javier Eugenio de la Cruz y Espejo was a brilliantly meditative Indian. Born of a family of Andean medicine men whose lore came down from the unrecorded Indian centuries, this particular yerbatero became a prophet of modern medicine and modern government. He was a first citizen and patriot of Ecuador and the first national librarian of that magnificent and underestimated republic. Espejo was also a journalist—fiercely and beautifully ironical in his style and troublesomely accurate in his facts in a period when rhetoric was more popular than a strict regard for the truth. While he was attending the sick and dying, and fighting the ruthless plagues which repeatedly threatened to depopulate his country, Espejo found time to write superb descriptions of the diseases of his time (and ours) and urge the improvement of hospitals and home sanitation. Bitterly he condemned and ridiculed the medical quackeries which existed then even as now. In a very real sense Espejo was the father of Pan-Americanism. Simón Bolívar, the great liberator, sought independence and union for only the northern republics of South America. But the amazing Indian, Espejo, who wrote Spanish like a Cervantes, thought as creatively as Pasteur, and fought against odds as overwhelming as those faced by Bolívar or Jeb Stuart or Douglas MacArthur, urged and pleaded that all of South America arise and move forward as an independent and united continent.

José María Vargas was born a Spaniard, in a rural suburb of Madrid, during 1786. He studied medicine, theology, and mathematics at Cambridge University. During his twenties he came to Venezuela to join the fight-for-freedom forces of Simón Bolívar. In the course of this great struggle he became the close lifelong friend of the Great Liberator, and in due time a president of Venezuela. Still under forty, he reorganized the medical schools of the country and while earning and holding a place as the first great surgeon of Venezuela he succeeded in launching a new era of research in tropical diseases.

Vargas was a philosopher of liberalism, an enthusiastic admirer of Thomas Jefferson and of that robust young nation, the United States. He was also a superb linguist, mathematician, and theologist —as well as politician, surgeon, scientist, and liberator. Such an amazing combination of talents in one medical man seems to be characteristic of Latin-American doctors, past and present. Perhaps nowhere in the world have physicians excelled in so many different skills and arts.

José Hipólito Unanue was a small, round-faced, boyish-looking Peruvian. A great surgeon, a famous practitioner, and a superb teacher of medicine, he helped found and lead the San Fernando Medical School, which was opened in Lima in 1811. He also helped found Lima's famous Amphitheatre for the teaching of medicine. In addition, he made memorable studies of the common diseases of the Andes, of climatology, and of the development and use of vaccines. Unanue was also the faithful Boswell of other Latin-American physicians and scientists, and we owe much of what we know about South American medical history to him. His home was a perennial open house and open forum for scholars and scientists of his time and much of the scientific world eventually heard of the five-foot Peruvian who in his own day was affectionately called "The Little Flower."

Among many other medical names to achieve prominence in the lands to the south during the early nineteenth century was that of Alvares Carneiro of Brazil, who died a little more than a century ago. He was an orphan boy raised in an almshouse. During his teens a Jesuit mission sent him to Europe to study medicine. But the ship upon which he took passage was captured by pirates and Alvares was sold in Africa as a slave. He escaped, and later proceeded to Spain, studied medicine at Madrid, wandered and practiced in China, then returned to Rio de Janeiro, where he became physician to the poor and spent a busy and brilliant career in charity medicine.

The later nineteenth century saw a still greater flowering of Latin-American medical talent. Carlos Finlay, of whom more will be told later, was one outstanding figure. Utinguassú of the Rio de Janeiro Academy of Medicine was another. A third, the Brazilian, Carlos Ribas, founded the Butantan Institute in 1899 and four years later helped rid São Paulo, his home state, of yellow fever. Still later, he helped found the first child welfare service in all Latin America. And there was, too, Oswaldo Cruz, perhaps the most famous of all Brazilian medical men and certainly one of the greatest of all public health administrators.

In Mexico, Miguel Otéro spent most of his life and all of his money experimenting with human inoculation against typhus—of which he died in 1915 while treating patients. Howard Taylor Ricketts, of the United States, demonstrating the role of lice in the spread of typhus, also died of the disease while at Mexico's Institute of Hygiene, in 1910. The Mexican, Ruiz Castanedo, working with our own Hans Zinsser, developed an important antityphus vaccine. In Brazil, Rocha-Lima, Piaz, Fialho, Stanislas von Prowazek, and others have made further valuable studies of typhus. So have Weiss of Peru, Kraus of Chile, and many others from the legions of southern Americans who love medicine passionately and work fearlessly and unendingly.

The story of the heroic twenty-six-year-old Peruvian medical student, Daniel E. Carrión who in 1885 gave his own life to prove the identity of verruga peruana and Oroya fever, a ruinous disease of the Andes, is among the finest of all medical history. Young Carrión's martyrdom was in the grand tradition of medical science. He was a medical student still without license. He had listened to the controversy as to whether or not the ruthless Oroya fever and the virulent verruga warts which frequently preceded it were really the same disease. In Lima hospitals Carrión had come to believe they were. Since so many men of science doubted it, he proceeded to inoculate himself with fluid taken from one of the soft pink verruga warts on the body of a hospital patient. That was on August 27, 1885. Six weeks later, on October 5, Daniel Carrión died of Oroya fever. In the meantime he had kept a careful journal of the course of the disease.

The challenge presented by the existence of numerous lethal diseases, many of them still mysterious, continues to stimulate Latin-American medical men to heroic efforts. For example, in 1915, Robles of Guatemala described and called attention to onchocerciasis, a serious parasitic disease which frequently causes blindness. Similarly, many grave mycoses (or fungus diseases) of Latin America have been studied and to a measure conquered by medical men of many American nations: Escomel of Peru; Suarez and Meneses of Ecuador; Urueta and Velazco of Colombia; Gonzalez and Jimenez of Venezuela; Arias and Parodi of Argentina; Gatti and Delamre of Paraguay; Gonzalez, Pallares, and Palanco of Mexico, and others —names which appear suddenly and shine brightly, like torches in a black night.

Medicine is more than a matter of men, however gallant and brilliant. It is a complex, highly technical science, and nowadays its success is dependent as much upon institutions and research as upon the practice of individual men in the field. The story of this aspect of Latin-American medical history exhibits the same general characteristics that marked the account of individual doctors. There is the identical emergence of a scientific Pan-Americanism, a repeated willingness to pool findings in one country with those of another. To people familiar with the high standards of national pride separating our different Latin neighbors, this internationalism of research is significant. It suggests that the enemy is deadly and implacable, and so omnipresent that national distinctions cannot be drawn across the lines of a bitterly embattled medical profession.

As the opening chapter suggested, there are many important Central and South American medical institutions. The deliberate establishment of research institutes is a comparatively recent development in every country, but the nations of Latin America preceded us and most of the rest of the world in this important field. During 1886, when there were still barely half a dozen accredited medical laboratories in the world, Buenos Aires and Montevideo founded bacteriological institutes, even though bacteriology after the pattern of

Pasteur and Koch was still in the making. In 1887 a medical laboratory was opened at Havana. Others were established in Chile during 1892 (while Johns Hopkins was beginning to reach its stride at Baltimore), in Uruguay and Mexico in 1895; at Lima in 1903; at Guayaquil and Caracas in 1910, at La Paz in 1914.

Latin America's need for medical research is always tremendous, frequently desperate. Research centers become constantly more significant as centers of news. This is notably true of Argentina's laboratories, which include the Bacteriological Institute of the National Department of Health, the Institute of Experimental Medicine of the University of Buenos Aires, and the Buenos Aires Municipal Institutes of Physiology and of Radiology and Physiotherapy.

The Bacteriological Institute of Chile was opened at Santiago in 1929 to succeed Chile's Institute of Hygiene. This national research center provides training for bacteriologists and laboratory technicians and carries out various investigations required by Chile's public health department. The institute manufactures serums, vaccines, and biological products for Chilean use, promotes the study and prevention of typhus, rabies, anthrax, and other epidemic diseases; directs the national campaign against malnutrition; and provides training for public health workers not only in Chile but also in Bolivia, Peru, Ecuador, and Venezuela.

At Bogotá, the Lleras Institute of Medical Research, founded in 1934, has become one of the world's great centers for the study of leprosy. Mexico's new Institute of Public Health and Tropical Diseases, opened during 1939, is a fortunate dividend of Mexico's Six-Year Plan. The institute includes insect houses, greenhouses, an animal farm, and facilities for the study of bacteriology, protozoology, epidemiology, and mycology. A clinical section is undertaking studies of typhus, pinta, pneumonia, and other principal diseases. Quite significantly, this study center, too, is opening its doors to foreign students.

Since 1914 Mexico's Institute of Hygiene, an agency of the Superior Council of Health, has been an important source of serums and vaccines and a leader in Mexican defense against the fifth column of disease. The Institute of Biology of Mexico's National University carries on fruitful research in Mexican plant life, collects medicinal plants, and makes important studies of Mexican food resources.

Peru's National Institute of Hygiene and Public Health, opened at Lima during 1938, is directed by Dr. Telemaco Battistini, one of the great names in contemporary Latin-American medicine. The new institute is associated with Peru's National Institute of Vaccine and Serum Therapy, the Central Tuberculosis Dispensary, and the National Plague Service. It assists the Ministry of Public Health, supplies biological products, assigns staff members to help with the control of epidemics, co-operates with the department of medicine of the Army (Peru has the largest army in Latin America) and with the National School of Medicine.

Bolivia has its Instituto Medico Sucre, established in 1896, and the National Institute of Bacteriology, opened at La Paz in 1911. Brazil's São Paulo Institute of Hygiene, housed in buildings provided by the Rockefeller Foundation, is another important center for study of communicable diseases and a haven for many distinguished scientists of Brazil and neighboring nations. Colombia's National Institute of Hygiene at Bogotá continues studies in tropical and cosmopolitan diseases. In Paraguay the National Institute of Parasitology at Asunción also promotes valuable research. Brazil's Oswaldo Cruz Institute and the Butantan Institute are with good reason world renowned and revered.

In 1929 the Gorgas Memorial Institute of Panama was opened for the continuing study of tropical diseases. The buildings which the institute occupies were donated by the Republic of Panama and the institution is supported by contributions from the United States and other American governments. Associated with the institute are the Gorgas Hospital and the Gorgas Laboratory. At Montevideo the International American Institute for the Protection of Childhood is a superb instance of inter-American co-operation in administration of public health and social service. There is room for many more of its kind.

Even this listing of Latin-American strongholds or outposts of medical research is not complete. There are numerous other important institutions, any one of which could provide the subject matter for a book, or for several books. But enough have been mentioned to show that research on medical problems is not going by default in Central and South America. All told, though, those excellent laboratories and technical centers do not add up to enough. They are doing tremendous work, but they are up against fearful odds. The health problem which confronts and threatens the southern republics is not lack of interest or energy. It is basically a lack of sufficient means. The tragic economic quandary of Latin America's sick poor is still unsolved.

Consider, for instance, the matter of hospitals. As the first chapter suggested, in actual numbers and in proportion to population, Latin-American hospitals compare favorably enough with those of the United States. And in length of service these same hospitals of Central and South America were pioneers in our hemisphere. The health problem does not remain unsolved simply because the Latin-American attack on it is too recent to have achieved its full effect. Far from it, the first hospital in the United States was opened at Philadelphia during 1751. Elsewhere in the British colonies at that time there was nothing better than pesthouses. The second hospital in the United States was opened in New York in 1791—eight years after the Revolution. To the southward, however, we discover that Santo Domingo had a hospital before 1503; Puerto Rico as early as 1511; Panama in 1521; Cuba in 1522; Mexico by 1524; Guatemala in 1529; Peru in 1540; Brazil in 1543; Bolivia in 1550; Chile in 1552; Paraguay in 1557; Colombia in 1564; Ecuador in 1565; Argentina in 1576; Venezuela in 1590.[2]

As a group, the public hospitals of Latin America antedate our own by nearly three centuries. Spain was a pioneer in the building and maintenance of hospitals—both military and civil. Spain's rulers insisted that hospitals be founded in the New World as an essential part of Spanish imperialism. In 1541 Charles V decreed that hospitals for Indians be built in principal cities of Mexico. Repeatedly the emperors of Spain ordered the building of hospitals and asylums in preference to convents and monasteries. In 1800, when there were barely a dozen hospitals in all the United States, Lima alone had hospitals totaling 900 beds for the use of its 60,000 people.

On the face of it, this looks like a splendid record, an excellent foundation for medical work in a part of the world where it is most important. Ironically enough, Latin America's supply of hospitals is still acutely inadequate. Why?

The answer to that question lies in weighing the existing facilities against the actual needs of the situation instead of against the statistics of some other part of the world.

Ten hospital beds per thousand people in our own nation is a ratio long sought—and not yet attained—by medical leaders in the United States. Some of our states have already passed the goal. Massachusetts already has 13.2 hospital beds per thousand citizens; New York has 12; Colorado has 12.7. Other states, particularly in the South, are notoriously lacking in hospital beds. Arkansas and North Carolina have only 4.9 per thousand inhabitants; Alabama, 4.4; Mississippi, 4.5; and South Carolina, 4.2.[3] Undoubtedly the establishment of adequate hospital facilities for Negroes would improve the present disgraceful ratios of these southern states.

To turn to Central and South America, it is probable (in the absence of precise statistics) that the combined hospital facilities of all Latin America would result in an average of less than two beds per thousand people; in some of the countries there is less than one bed per thousand.

Latin-American population is increasing about three times as rapidly as ours, despite almost incessant contagions, and in spite of sick rates and death rates vastly greater than our own. Each year, therefore, the ratio of available beds to population will become less favorable unless something is done about it. Nor is that all. Hospital beds in Spanish American hospitals can serve, individually, a much smaller number of patients per year because the average periods of hospital confinement in Latin America are much longer than those current in the United States. In Chile the average stay is about 18 days per patient. In Buenos Aires and Lima it is 25, roughly twice the contemporary average in New York or Chicago.[4]

Although the population of Latin America as a whole is much less urbanized than our own, the great majority of the hospitals are in capitals and principal cities. Millions of rural and village people are completely without hospital accommodations. For example, Peru has an estimated 12,000 hospital beds—about 1.4 per thousand people for the entire nation, but in Lima, the capital, there are 9 hospital beds per thousand. The hospital capacity of Buenos Aires compares favorably with that of any city in the world. But about 40,000 of the total of 60,000 beds in all Argentina are in Buenos Aires and its suburbs. The five largest cities of Argentina have between 4 and 6 hospital beds per thousand people; Santiago de Chile has 9; Bogotá, Havana, Caracas and Montevideo, about 6 each; the larger cities of Mexico, about 4.

But thousands of Latin-American cities and towns have no hospital resources at all. This is true, for example, of half the 250 towns and cities of São Paulo, the richest and most densely peopled Brazilian state. In Colombia a recent President's Message declared that fewer than one-third of the towns and cities of Colombia have hospital accommodations of any kind. In Cuba a former Secretary of Health recently stated that nine-tenths of all Cuban hospitals are badly in need of repairs or of new equipment. In 1940 the Health Department of Chile reported that 53 per cent of all Chilean hospitals are lacking in obstetrical wards, 75 per cent lack surgical wards, 76 per cent have no children's wards, and 40 per cent lack X-ray services.

In Argentina, a former administration leader points out that, although Argentina's hospital facilities are probably the most adequate

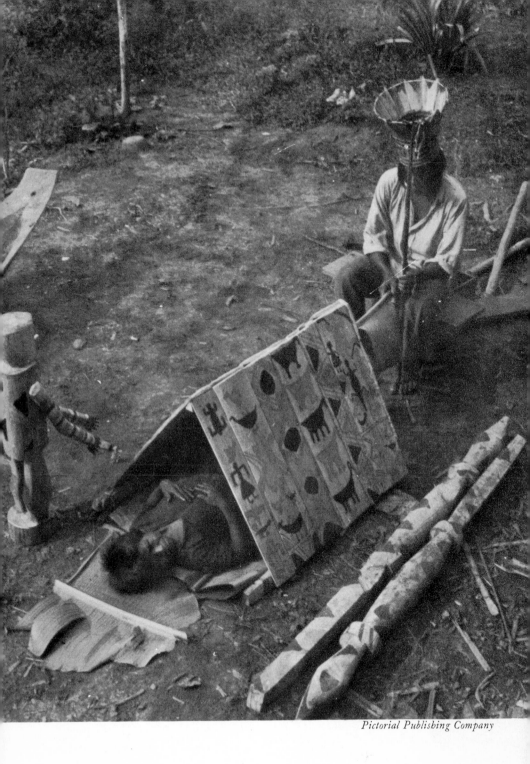

Bolivian Indian medicine man watches over the sick.

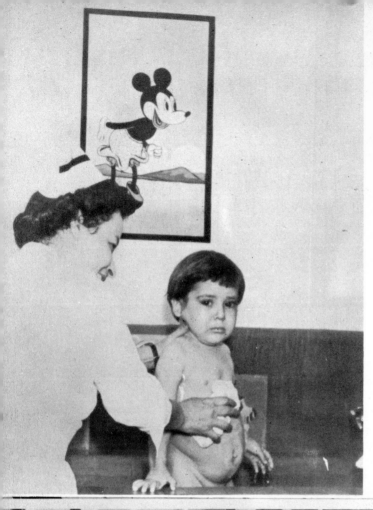

In Dr. Aguilar's new children's ward at Tiqui sate, Guatemala.

Dinner time in Dr. Aguilar's ward for sick children.

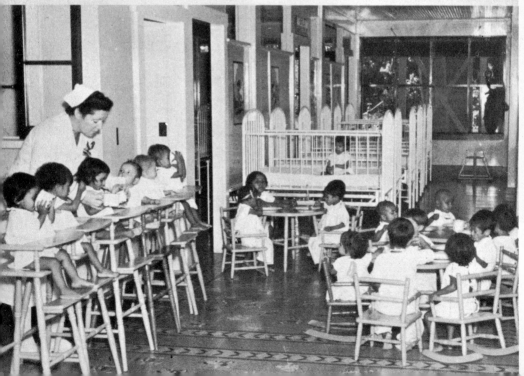

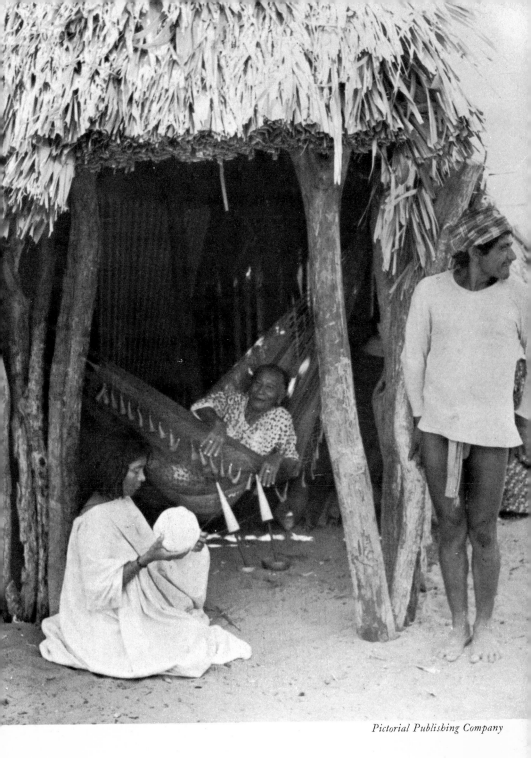

Sick bed in the upper Amazon country.

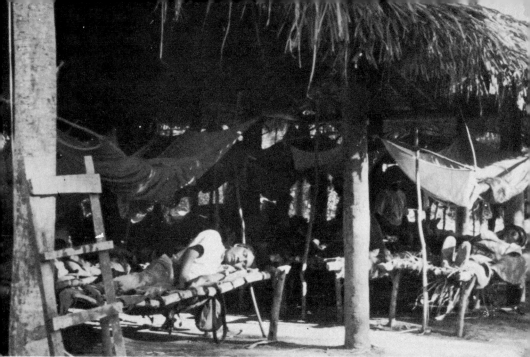

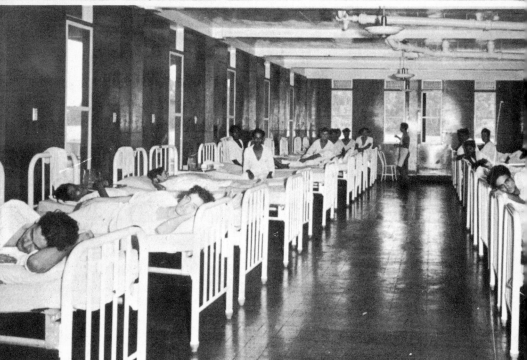

Pictorial Publishing Company
(Upper) In Paraguay temporary army hospitals were improvised for
Chaco war soldiers.

By Iris Woolcock
(Lower) Workman's ward in a new United Fruit Company hospital
at Golfito, Costa Rica.

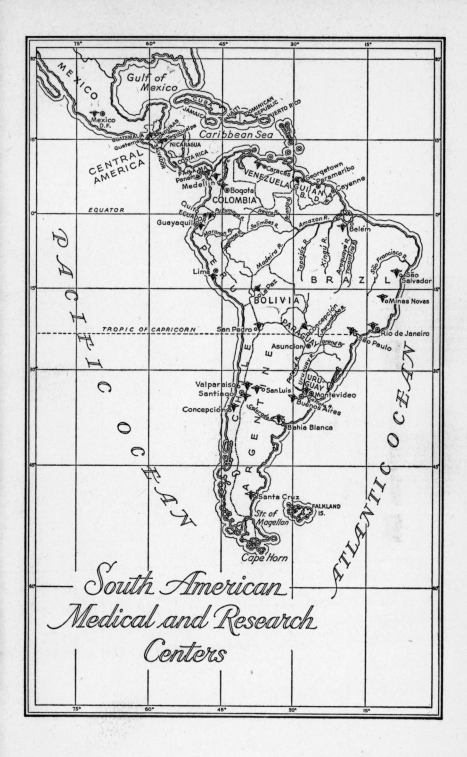

South American
Medical and Research
Centers

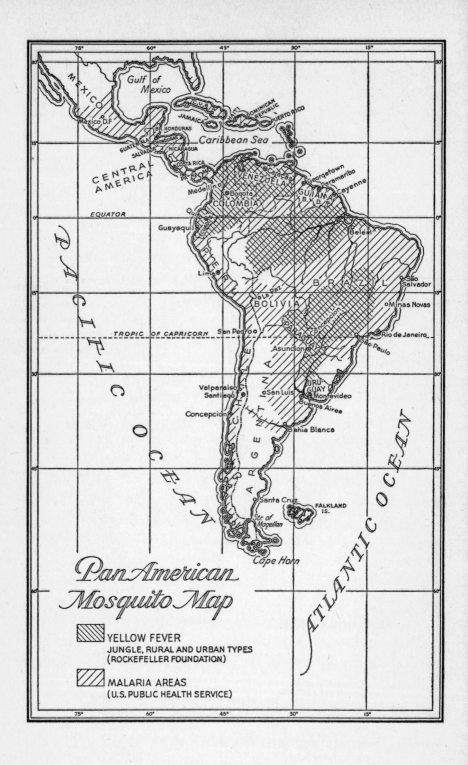

Pan American Mosquito Map

▨ YELLOW FEVER
JUNGLE, RURAL AND URBAN TYPES
(ROCKEFELLER FOUNDATION)

▧ MALARIA AREAS
(U.S. PUBLIC HEALTH SERVICE)

in all South America, actual hospital accommodations are available for only 4,300 of that nation's estimated 140,000 tuberculosis sufferers; 14,000 of its 54,000 insanity cases; 200 of its 3,300 cancer patients; 250 of its 2,500 registered lepers; 225 of its 8,500 deaf and dumb; and 325 of its 6,000 blind.[5]

In calling attention to this deficiency, it should be clear that there is no intention of belittling the great medical work being done by the other American republics or of underestimating the awareness of authorities in those nations of the seriousness of their problem. Men of science in Latin America are neither stupid nor lazy, but the greatest physician in the world cannot carry on his work without the tools or funds for essential equipment, and without adequate supporting staffs. These things our Latin-American neighbors still lack, and their lack of them is largely the result of the absence of economic integration in the Western Hemisphere. We are now, almost at the eleventh hour, trying to offset a generations-old mistake in hemisphere policy.

Economic problems in South and Central America reach even deeper, medically as well as otherwise, than the lack of tools and equipment. They create a set of circumstances with which, for the most part, we of North America do not have to contend. For one thing, as has been suggested, South American and Central American population is principally rural. Lack of local civic organization creates a dependence on federal government and the church. This dependence is plainly illustrated by the very different nature of Latin-American hospitalization. The Latin American has always been, and still is, inclined to regard a hospital as a place of charity and refuge, a shelter wherein the sick and the distressed are welcome. This is a traditional attitude, the outgrowth of those early days when a shrewdly calculating empire, working with a powerful and canny missionary church, set out somewhat frantically to defend a 7,000-mile line of frontiers which were being decimated by contagions. Hospital refuge and medication, in so far as they could be provided, became an essential service of an on-the-scene church and a faraway seat of empire.

In Latin-American medicine today the result of this situation is both a liability and an asset. It costs a great deal to support such a tradition but it is one way of reaching a sick people who without its free help would probably simply crawl away to die. Hundreds of United States hospitals are, as their patients have good reason to know, quite unashamedly profit-making institutions. Thousands more are supported wholly or in part by their patients' fees. We of the north are accustomed to enter a hospital with a checkbook in one hand—or a friend to vouch for the checkbook if we happen to be unconscious—and a toothbrush in the other. The Latin may or may not bring a toothbrush with him. The chances are, however, a thousand to one that he will not bring either checkbook or wallet and that he will receive treatment without being asked where they are. He is a sick man and he knows that it is the hospital's business to treat the sick.

Given this willingness of the Latin American to trust himself to an institution which he regards as part of his life, like the rituals of his faith, it is obvious what development of the power of the hospital could do for public health. Yet the resources to develop that power by extending the reach of hospital, clinic and sanitarium are in themselves undeveloped, partly because of the very health problems which their use might eliminate and even more because we of the north have paid too little attention to the economy of South and Central America and have permitted our sister republics to become dependent upon Europe, a dependence instituted for the benefit, not of the Western Hemisphere, but of Europe.

Now that European markets are cut off, the Latin-American nations are trying their best to find in home sources the means, the tools, and the talents for carrying on the essential struggle for health. In spite of their efforts, they are still far short of being able to create health standards comparable to those of the United States. If with our natural interest in the Latin countries—an interest as vital and compelling as a man's interest in his own leg—we had been one-fiftieth as active in their midst as have some of our present enemies, the health problems south of Texas would be much less serious than they are today.

Meantime, not everybody has been so shortsighted as we. For half a century, at least, German business houses have made a point of studying and contributing to the study of Latin-American disease. And not for philanthropic reasons, in most cases. For the same half century, German firms have been the leading peddlers of medicine, good and bad, to the people of South and Central America. German manufacturers are largely responsible for making those regions a salesman's paradise for proprietary medicines, quack remedies, nostrums, and bogus cures for everything from housemaid's knee to heart disease. In the course of accomplishing this end the Germans took pains to capture Latin-American markets for legitimate medicines and pharmaceuticals. Even during the war years of 1939, 1940, and 1941 the German position has been maintained.

Actually the Nazis have been making use of their drug trade with South America to provide a source of revenue for propaganda and fifth column activity. They have found it possible to do this because of the great value and slight bulk of most essential pharmaceuticals, making such products extremely likely subjects for smuggling. Some drugs have been shipped in on vessels which have run the British blockade but still more have been flown in on planes of a commercial Italian air line, which until very recently maintained scheduled service between bases in West Africa and Natal, Brazil. It is possible for one large transport plane to carry more than $250,000 worth of drugs.

So far as anyone is officially aware, commercial air lines of Axis powers no longer visit Latin America. Nevertheless, the Nazis are well intrenched and cannot be easily dislodged. Sterling Products Corporation, an American drug export house, estimates that at the beginning of 1942 Nazi firms and individuals in South America had stored there some $30,000,000 worth of pharmaceuticals and drugs—enough for two years' trade.

While the fact of Axis domination of Latin-American trade in drugs is not directly connected with Western Hemisphere health problems—German drugs, in themselves, are excellent—it should be borne in mind that the drug trade is capable of being used as an entering wedge for other trade from North America which might provide a better economic balance than now prevails in the lands to the south. Without economic balance the problem of Latin-American health will never be solved, and we of the north will inevitably suffer because of it.

This survey of the Latin-American medical and health crisis, past and present, has necessarily been almost misleadingly brief. It will barely make a start toward filling the vacuum of knowledge and information about hemisphere medicine that persists north of the Rio Grande. Indeed, the whole published literature on the subject, in any language, is pitifully brief and inconclusive. Medical history as a whole is a neglected chapter in human annals, even today, and nowhere more so than in the field lying right at our own southern door. It will be a long while before the situation is very different.

The time has come, though, to advance the case for what medicine and sanitation are actually able to accomplish for our Latin-American neighbors and, not so indirectly, for ourselves as well. A few instances out of the more recent past make dramatic reading and dramatic object lessons for a future policy. Not all the battles have been defeats, even on this front. The stories of Gorgas, Finlay, Reed, Deeks, and the others who appear in subsequent chapters embody the problems of hemisphere medicine, and recount how certain of those problems have been already solved. In the last analysis, the war on disease is a story of men, of men dying or not dying as other men have failed or succeeded.

Chapter Three

DITCHES, BIG AND LITTLE

THERE'S a ditty they sometimes sing down in the tropics. It goes to the familiar tune of "The Prisoner's Song," and the words run like this:

If I had a thousand dollars,
    I'd go to the boss and I'd say:
"I'll be leavin' the tropics tomorrow—
    There's no ship a-sailin' today."

Many a newcomer feels just that way about the tropics, and the state of mind is not a new one. Four centuries ago the conquistadors found great difficulty in recruiting the members of their expeditions into the hot lands of the New World. The black-green depths of the jungle, the heat, the sweat, the torrential rains, the unfamiliar fauna and flora all combined to oppress the spirits of even the most plunder-hungry *hidalgo*.

The beauty of the lands between Cancer and Capricorn has often been described: the crowded, year-round luxuriance of jungle and bushland, the gorgeous flowers and birds, the rivers winding mysteriously back into towering fastnesses of trees, and all the rest. But after a time this fabulous luxuriance grows wearisome to the eye of the Temperate Zone migrant who has come to live in the midst of it.

He finds himself beginning to be appalled by the very fertility of everything he sees, by the incessant fecundity that multiplies out of all familiar proportion every type of life, vegetable and animal. There is too much of everything. The recent arrival begins to feel, consciously or unconsciously, a certain menace in so much and such intemperate life as is spawned in the tropics. He feels hemmed in, almost suffocated.

Such an impression is not neurotic. The unnatural sterility of city buildings and pavements is more familiar to many a North American who has come to the tropics than this new, crowded luxuriance around him. Even the farmer and the countryman from the Temperate Zone is frequently subject to the same reaction. He, too, is accustomed to a long period of natural sterility in the course of each year. Northern winters bring death, or a dormant appearance of death, to the vegetation with which he is familiar. Even the lushness of summer he understands to be temporary; the frost will presently change green to brown, and winter will come to kill and sterilize the abundance of summer life.

The tropics, on the other hand, have no real winter. Their vegetation is not destroyed or checked by heavy frosts or prolonged freezing. In the tropics and warmer subtropics, which include the greater part of all Latin America, life multiplies interminably. Usually the newcomer becomes aware of his inability to recognize even a fraction of the visible life-forms about him. In due course he begins to be conscious that there is an even richer profusion of life which he cannot see. He notices how swiftly decay consumes anything, animal or vegetable, that has died. He learns that even trivial scratches and abrasions will fester and become infected unless he takes prompt and thorough precautions. Quite inescapably, subvisible lives also populate the bright green hills and the black-green valleys, and even more densely than all the visible ones.

The insects and bacteria of these lands of eternal summer make a constantly greater impression on the transplanted northerner. No matter how reasonable he tries to be about it he usually passes through a phase of fearing them. From time to time he has object lessons in what these minute and deadly organisms can do to human beings. He sees men, women, children attacked by them in a hundred ways—the sores of hookworm, the nodes and abscesses of yaws, the bulging, splenetic abdomens of malarial children and adults, and the other malignancies of tropical disease at its worst and most obvious. He comes to learn, also, how limited is the ability of even the ablest doctors to cope with these omnipresent bacteria.

If he sticks it out until he is acclimated, the tropical newcomer learns not to think too much about these perils. If he is wise, he comes to believe passionately in the necessity of sanitation. Not the kind of sanitation he knew at home, the checking up on water supply, forcing restaurant keepers to sterilize dishes, and compelling filling stations to keep their restrooms clean. He becomes an advocate of sanitation on the grand scale, sanitation from the ground up, a concerted, far-reaching campaign against swamps, mosquitoes, municipal and domestic filth, flies, and the thousand and one uncleanlinesses which menace his own health and that of everybody else.

What sanitation can do in the war on tropic disease is far from hypothetical. A case history exists, and its record is open to anyone to read. The story of William Crawford Gorgas and the "Gorgas gangs" in Havana and the Canal Zone is the blueprint for tropical sanitation. It illustrates both what happens when there is no concerted effort toward sanitation and what major improvements follow when funds, equipment, and personnel of the right kind and necessary quantity are available. Fortunately for us, too, the role played by the United States in this drama of sanitation is one that we can point to with pride. Our sanitarians have demonstrated to Latin Americans that the United States is not always a blundering "colossus of the North."

Our adventure in tropical sanitation began with the Spanish-American War. However confused that struggle may seem to us today, it had one aftermath of immense importance to the future of our hemisphere. It introduced North Americans to the problems of the tropics. The introduction was a rude one. Yellow fever had proved a more potent enemy than the Spanish, and we had lost thousands of men to an opponent too small to see or shoot at. Blundering and bumbling though our army may have been in its military campaigns, it realized immediately that something would have to be done about yellow fever. We could not garrison the islands we had won unless some way was found to force an armistice on "yellow-jack" as well as on the Spanish.

The war ended in 1898 with the Treaty of Paris, as every schoolboy does not know, and in December of that year an army major named Gorgas was appointed health officer of the city of Havana. His job was to clean up the place and call a halt to the epidemic spread of yellow fever. It was no easy assignment. Walter Reed and his Army Medical Board had not yet presented their epic proof of the way in which yellow fever is transmitted. Gorgas had no certainty about how to approach his problem.

True enough, when our army occupied Havana, Cuba contained one man who held the key to the whole enigma. Dr. Carlos Finlay, whose story will be told later, had been asserting for seventeen years that yellow fever was transmitted by the mosquito, but almost nobody believed Finlay or bothered to check up on his contention. He had been snubbed by United States medicine with the same obstinate blindness which had greeted his predecessor of fifty years earlier, Dr. J. C. Nott.

Dr. Nott, a South Carolinian who practiced medicine in Mobile, Alabama, had contended that yellow fever could not be explained in terms of an air-borne "miasm" and that there must be a traceable agent of transmission. He had even suggested that insects such as mosquitoes might be responsible. But when Gorgas went to Havana, nobody remembered Nott and few paid any attention to Carlos Finlay.

Major Gorgas knew that he was up against a job that would take time. Effective sanitation presupposes that the sanitary engineer knows what he is doing, and in 1898 there was no such certainty on which to base an attack on yellow fever. He had to learn by a process of trial and error what conditions to overcome. Furthermore, sanitation is best effected in an area with adequate resources upon which to draw. Havana was impoverished, partly by the very epidemic that was raging when Gorgas arrived. So were twenty other New World cities. The Major was aware of the close relation between disease and economics. Yellowjack had taken hundreds of thousands of lives in the New World alone. People were mortally afraid of it, and because they did not know how it spread, each new outbreak resulted in ineffective but incessant quarantines which held up the flow of goods throughout Central and South America. Billions of dollars in trade were being lost.

Not in Latin America alone. Only ten years before Gorgas came to Havana, the trade of the whole Mississippi basin had come to a standstill because of a fierce outbreak of the disease. Time and again in the past yellow fever had blockaded the great ports of the United States. This new epidemic was only another in a long series. People expected that there would always be yellow fever. Throughout half the hemisphere men without proof of immunity to the terrible disease were regarded as poor employment risks. Immunity could be proved only by surviving an attack of the plague itself or by having been exposed for at least ten years without contracting it.

William Crawford Gorgas, as a later chapter will demonstrate, was the right man to send to Havana. He was the acknowledged yellow fever expert of the United States Army. He had fought the pestilence before, over and over. He did not, however, know how it was transmitted. He was only certain that the cleaner and more insect-free a city the lower the disease incidence was likely to be. When his colleague, Walter Reed, another major in the Army Medical Corps and the chairman of the army's Yellow Fever Board, invited him to Camp Lazear to see a demonstration of the fact that mosquitoes alone were responsible for transmitting yellow fever,

Gorgas was too good a doctor and too wise a man not to go. But he went to Camp Lazear a skeptic. He came away convinced that Reed and his staff were right.

When Gorgas finally accepted the theory of mosquito transmission of yellow fever he accepted it without reservation. Understanding now that cleanliness was not enough, he supplemented the cleanup of Havana with an intensive warfare against all mosquitoes. He divided the city of a quarter million people into twenty sanitation districts and ordered that all sufferers from yellow fever be taken to the same hospital—Las Animas—for treament and observation. He directed that the hospital be screened and completely cleared of mosquitoes. Next, Gorgas "gangs" proceeded to fumigate the home of each yellow fever patient and all adjacent homes, closing windows and doors, plugging cracks and crevices, and burning sulphur, placed in Dutch ovens and fired with sprinklings of alcohol.

For interior surfaces sulphur smoke is one of the most effective of all insecticides. But in the wet air of Havana sulphur fumes tarnished fabrics and metals. When they had to, the Gorgas men used pyrethrum powder instead. Pyrethrum deadens mosquitoes for a time, so that they can be picked up and burned. The sanitary squads also fumigated thousands of homes by using one part of camphor to three of carbolic acid and vaporizing the mixture with a spirit lamp.

The cigar factories and tobacco storehouses of Havana proved almost impregnable strongholds for mosquitoes. The value of the tobacco was marred or destroyed by fumigation. Dr. Gorgas and Joseph Le Prince, his sanitation engineer, solved that problem by having all tobacco storages "smoked out" with smudge fires generated by burning unusable stems and scraps of tobacco.

Next the Gorgas gangs attacked the places in which mosquitoes were known to breed. The larval stage of this disease-carrying insect, normally lasting eight or nine days, must be spent in water, and the yellow fever mosquito (*Aëdes aegypti*) usually breeds in comparatively clean water. A sluggish and a rather fragile insect, it rarely travels more than a few hundred yards from its place of birth.

In Havana at the turn of the century, water supplies came principally from cisterns, tanks, and rain barrels. Dr. Gorgas placed a chief inspector in charge of each of the twenty sanitary districts. The inspector visited each dwelling in his district at least once a month, made a careful inspection and prepared a written report upon the fact or possibility of mosquito breeding within the premises. Meanwhile the military government proclaimed it a "sanitary nuisance" for any householder to have mosquito larvae on or about his premises. The health officer had authority to impose a fine for each nuisance; the fine to be collected by Cuban courts and deposited to the Cuban National Treasury. The health officer also had authority to remit the fine when and if the nuisance was abated. Under Gorgas, more than 95 per cent of all fines were remitted. During the final nine months of 1901, about 2,500 fines were levied, and only fifty, averaging five dollars each, were actually paid.

Gorgas also recruited squads of carpenters, who went through the city covering water barrels and other receptacles with screening and placing spigots at the bottom of each barrel as a substitute for the customary dippers. Most Cuban households used earthen jars on stands to hold drinking water. It was the inspector's duty to visit each water stand and instruct the housekeeper to empty the drinking water at least once a day and each time to wash the container.

Each sanitary inspector was accompanied on his rounds by a force of five workmen. These workmen carried oil to pour on all pools or puddles they came upon. They also cleaned or drained all gutters, water spouts, and tile drains.

Rapidly and provably the toll of yellow fever began to fall. In Havana between 1870 and 1874 deaths from yellow fever had ranged from 515 to 1,244 per year. Beginning in 1874 losses from yellowjack became more serious; 1,425 in 1874; 1,619 in 1876; 1,444 in 1879. Havana's average of yellow fever deaths between 1880 and 1890 was about 400 per year. During 1895 the toll climbed to 553. During 1896 it spurted to 1,282. Four years later, after the American sanitary work had begun, it was down to 310. In 1901 it was down to 18, lowest recorded for Havana up to that time. It was destined to go still lower.[1]

Cuban government statistics show that yellow fever had existed in Havana continuously since 1762, when the city was first besieged and captured by British troops. Two years of vigorous work in sanitation by the Gorgas gangs reduced yellow fever death tolls by about 90 per cent. Five more years made deaths from yellow fever negligible and found Havana approximately as healthful as any city of similar size in the United States.

Shortly after the proved success of Gorgas's sanitation work in Havana, the government of the United States considered reviving the construction of an Isthmian canal in Panama, a gigantic undertaking at which the French had already failed. What Gorgas had learned from his experience in Cuba prompted him to suggest that similar measures adopted in Panama might result in success. He pointed out to the surgeon general the enormous casualties from tropical diseases suffered by workers of the French Canal Company, directed by Ferdinand de Lesseps whose success with Suez had helped him not at all in his Central American venture. The surgeon general agreed, and promptly recommended that Gorgas be appointed sanitation officer of the Isthmus of Panama.

During the autumn of 1903, the United States secured a concession for building the Panama Canal. A year earlier Gorgas had been relieved from Cuban duty and returned to the United States to make preliminary surveys of the sanitation problems in Panama. Early in 1903, Gorgas was sent to the Egyptian Medical Congress as the representative of the United States Army Medical Department.

In Egypt he visited the site of the newly completed Suez Canal. But he saw no sanitation problems or challenges comparable to those of Panama. At Suez, de Lesseps and his French associates had paid little heed to employee health. The route of the Suez Canal is through dry, sandy desert, which at the time of the canal's construction was free of mosquito-borne diseases. The proposed route of the Panama Canal was through low and swampy jungle alternating with rugged mountains; a land of excessive rainfall and an alarming frequency of yellow fever, malaria, and many other tropical diseases.

In Egypt, Gorgas discovered that the town of Ismailia, about halfway across the Isthmus of Suez, had become a pesthole of malaria. While the canal was under construction there had been no convenient supply of drinking water. Fresh water was carried by camel-back from the nearest branch of the Nile. That required hiring as many as 1,600 camels and camel drivers. Annoyed at that expense and inconvenience, de Lesseps ordered the reopening of the ancient canal of the Israelites, which leads up from the Nile through the land of Goshen, to within a few miles of the present Suez. The French engineers extended the ancient waterway to join the new construction and built a small fresh-water canal to parallel the entire route of the Suez.

Arabs used the fresh water to irrigate farms. Malarial mosquitoes used it as a breeding ground and accordingly Ismailia and other towns of the Isthmus suffered outbreaks of malaria. Sir Ronald Ross, one of England's greatest and most practical students of tropical diseases and tropical sanitation, was employed to advise the French Canal Company how to overcome the plague. Sir Ronald's work was immediately effective and he, like Gorgas, soon became celebrated in the history of tropical sanitation.

William Gorgas returned from Cairo to find the Panama Canal still something of a pipe dream. Pending further organization, he went to the Hygiene Congress at Paris, again representing the Medical Department of the United States Army, and spent some months gathering information at the Paris offices of the work-weary French Panama Canal Company. Meanwhile the Congress of the

United States had authorized President Theodore Roosevelt to appoint the Isthmian Canal Commission. Of the seven commissioners five were engineers and none were doctors. The American Medical Association protested. Poor sanitation—far more than poor engineering or finance—had beaten the French. The President refused the American Medical Association request, but did order Gorgas to accompany the commission to Panama as "sanitary adviser." The Alabaman promptly requested three assistants—Dr. John W. Ross, of the United States Navy; Major Lewis A. La Garde, a surgeon of the United States Army, and Major Cassius E. Gillette of the Army Engineers. This committee proceeded to Panama in company with six of the seven commissioners. At the port of Colon they noticed that a large cargo of coffins was being unloaded at the pier and that, rather significantly, six of the coffins were huge, ornate and bronze, with much elegance and many ornaments. The six commissioners were visibly impressed. The port doctor appeared and explained that there should have been seven of the high-class caskets, but since only six Canal Commissioners had come to Panama, the six de luxe coffins would no doubt be sufficient. . . .

Gorgas's sanitation committee was the first to get to work. It took over from the weary French concessionaires and moved into the humble frame building known as "De Lesseps' Palace." They crossed the Isthmus to attend a dinner, and returned to the Atlantic coast to sleep. In April, 1904, William Gorgas was formally appointed chief sanitary officer for the Isthmus. During May of the same year, the United States took over all Canal Zone property. In June, Gorgas began his sanitation work, with an appropriation of $50,000, not a vast sum when you consider the unprecedented size of the job in hand.

Necessary supplies were distressingly scarce. During the first year as sanitation director few of Gorgas's requisitions for men and materials were honored. But the "Gorgas gangs" again took up the fight against yellow fever, which was even more prevalent than normal throughout the region. From the first it was evident that unless yellow fever was conquered there was going to be no Panama Canal. The French had already found that out. During each year that it had been working, the French Canal Company had lost more than one-third of all its white personnel. Even an army in combat cannot afford losses like that.

Gorgas and his men looked the situation over carefully. This was no second Havana; the "strip," or Zone, was fifty miles long and ten miles wide—a total area of 500 square miles. And what miles! They included the noisome swamps of innumerable jungle streams and the tangled dark waters of the Chagres River, which was also a widow's cruse of mosquitoes. Of course, *Aëdes aegypti*, the mosquito carrying yellow fever, was a slow traveler, was most dangerous within town or city areas where she had a chance to bite infected human beings, and could probably be controlled without cleaning out the whole Isthmus. Even so, the hearts of Gorgas and his men must have sunk as they surveyed the mosquito resources of the Zone. And as it was to prove in the end, there can be no halfway sanitation when it comes to the tropics.

Meantime, the sanitarians decided to begin at the principal foci of yellow fever infection. There were two of them—the cities of Colon and Panama, located one at each end of the projected canal. Gorgas and his men gave both places the same kind of going-over that Havana had received a few years before. After a month of grueling work, in the course of which they fumigated every single building in Panama City, that unfortunate port continued to be a pesthole of yellow fever. The sanitarians sighed and went back over the city a second time, repeating the job with even more thoroughness. Still the yellow fever persisted. For the third time they subjected the whole city to a barrage of sulphur and pyrethrum fumes. By then they had consumed about 300 tons of sulphur and 120 tons of insect powder. Apparently this latter figure represented the entire annual output of pyrethrum in the United States.

Herculean as the job had been, it did not get visible results. All through the first half of 1905, as nonimmune North American workers continued to pour into the Isthmus, the yellow fever rate continued to skyrocket. The situation was disastrous, and the shadow of the fate that had overtaken the French began to fall across the engineers' blueprints. Laborers were panic-stricken. Work on the canal first began to lag, and then stopped entirely. The governor, the chief engineer, and the Executive Committee of the commission were at their wits' end. They had watched the Gorgas gangs pouring pyrethrum and sulphur fumes into every shack in Panama without getting anywhere. Very probably the whole enterprise looked silly to them. The politicians on the commission didn't even believe that anything so trivial as a mosquito could be responsible for a scourge such as yellowjack. They issued an urgent recommendation that Gorgas and his associates be dismissed and men of "more practical views" appointed.

They sent their petition to the wrong address. Theodore Roosevelt was a veteran Rough Rider, and he knew something about Cuba and what Gorgas and his men had done there. If anybody could stop yellow fever on the Isthmus, the army major from Alabama was the man to do it. The President dismissed the recommendation instead of the major, and ordered the commission to give Gorgas and his men every possible assistance.

The tide began to turn. Month by month the incidence of yellow fever along the route of the canal kept dropping. By November of 1905 it was apparent that the plague was beaten. It was a victory in the nick of time, but it did not wholly satisfy the sanitarians themselves.

What haunted Gorgas was that, except for the antimosquito campaigns, at the end of two years of sanitation work in Panama he could not see that the medical methods of the United States were in any way superior to those which the ill-fated French Company had relied upon so disastrously. True, yellow fever was checkmated, but without a fight against the mosquito Gorgas could see no reason why the death rate among American workers should have been lower than 250 per thousand workmen *each year,* to say nothing of the sickness ratio, which would have been appalling. He once said that, without his mosquito campaigns, "the reputation of Dr. Carter, Dr. Ross, Mr. Le Prince [the chief sanitary engineer] and myself, as sanitary officials, would have been irretrievably ruined. We took a tremendous risk and came very near failing." [2]

That failure would have had incalculable historical consequences for the United States, Latin America, and the whole world. The American taste for adventure might have brought down from the north a continuing supply of young workmen completely lacking in immunity. Deaths among them would presently have grown to such an appalling number that Congress, deluged with constituent protests, might again have abandoned the canal which others had repeatedly projected and abandoned for almost five centuries. Thanks to the elimination of the yellow fever mosquito, the canal and its builders prospered. But the margin of safety had been frighteningly narrow, and other problems almost equally grave demanded swift solution.

Yellow fever was not the only scourge. The Sanitation Department soon found that it had to launch a widespread drive against malaria, a drive which shortly became world famous for its effectiveness. Unlike *Aëdes aegypti,* the usual carrier of yellow fever, the *Anopheles,* which transmits malaria, is generally a rural insect. Like the *Aëdes,* it prefers to breed in clear fresh water in which grass and algae are plentiful. Along the banks of the small mountain streams of Panama, grass and algae are abundant and in their abundance protect the larvae from fish—those other, involuntary sanitarians.

Gorgas and his men promptly manned the two dozen sanitation districts of the Zone and another at Puerto Bello, in Panama territory about twenty miles north of Colon. Puerto Bello had been the northern terminus of Spain's royal highway across the Isthmus. Four stone forts had made the port the strongest of Spain's New World outposts and nature had made it the most nearly ideal seaport within the

American tropics. But it was also nature which canceled that blessing by making the old fortress one of the most virulent strongholds of pestilence in all the New World. That was still the case when the North American canal builders chose Puerto Bello as their principal quarry for canal materials.

Gorgas placed a sanitary inspector in charge of each of the twenty-five sanitation districts. To each he assigned a force of between twenty and a hundred laborers. Though the original strip covered five miles on each side of the canal, initial sanitation work was confined to one-mile strips fronting the actual building site, areas in which most of the working population of the Zone was located. The first step was to cut away brush and undergrowth within two hundred yards of all dwellings, to drain the standing water, and to trim all grass more than a foot in height. There was sound horse sense behind this rough-and-ready landscape gardening.

Before opening his great war against malaria Dr. Gorgas had made a careful study of the life of the *Anopheles* mosquito. He knew that it was a sluggish, frail insect, easily destroyed by wind or sunlight; an insect that sought shrubbery, grass, and foliage for protection from sun and rain. He believed, therefore, that clearing grass and shrubbery from the vicinity of human habitation would serve to limit the activity of the malaria carrier.

Drainage of the open water was no easy task. In the tropics, ordinary open ditches soon become clogged with grass and vegetation. Without active attention they become ideal breeding grounds for mosquitoes. Thus open ditches must be cleaned frequently—two or three times a month. The cost of such primitive drainage was prohibitive. With the assistance of Joseph Le Prince, Gorgas directed the construction of cement-lined drainage ditches and ordered that earthen ditches be filled with stone to discourage the propagation of mosquito larvae or else treated with arsenic solutions to kill the protective vegetation. Gorgas gangs also began using, for killing, grass burners fueled by crude oil atomized by air pressure. On wider stretches they used horse-drawn mowers. Everywhere they laid tile for subsoil drainage.

It required a great many little ditches to make "the Big Ditch" a reality. Policing a hundred square miles of tropical Isthmus against malaria required over 1,700 miles of ditches; 947 miles of open ditch, 95 miles of concrete ditch, and almost 200 miles each of rock-filled ditch and subsoil tile. Meanwhile the "oilers," searching continuously for puddles and mire, distributed water-diluted crude oil from cans carried on their backs and squirted by means of hand pumps. At the outset the hundred square miles under treatment required about 50,000 gallons of oil each month.

The great reservoir of Gatun Lake, formed by damming the Chagres River, was proving one of the most serious mosquito problems. Since it was a man-made lake, its creation did not consider the natural forces which, left to themselves, keep mosquito population somewhat under control. Dr. Samuel Darling, laboratory director for the Gorgas staff, developed a "larvicide" which dissolved in water and killed the mosquito larvae. The solution was a mixture of carbolic acid, resin, and alkali, and it did wonders.

Introduction of wire screening to every dwelling within the Canal Zone was the next step in sanitation. In 1906, the Canal Strip had several thousand buildings located in thirty different towns and settlements. Most of them were unscreened. Assisted by the Canal Commission architect, the sanitation department undertook to make all buildings mosquitoproof by means of copper screening. Each inspector assigned a workman to make continuous inspection of all screens. It was not long, however, before some areas of the zone ceased to need such protection. Within two years there were virtually no mosquitoes to keep out.

Wherever mosquitoes persisted (principally in laborers' barracks) sanitation workers armed with "traps" made of glass test tubes (containing deposits of chloroform in cotton) made the rounds, catching mosquitoes by hand. This was laborious and costly, but it was effective. The cycle of the malarial organism is such that ten days must intervene between the time the female *Anopheles* bites a malaria sufferer and the time when her subsequent stings are infected and able to retransmit the disease. Few *Anopheles* could escape Gorgas's persistent mosquito catchers for ten successive days.

In spite of these precautions, the marines who subsequently landed and pitched tents on top of Diablo hill did not immediately have the situation under control. They were promptly mowed down by malaria. Their open tents could not be screened, and as any visitor to the tropics—or any camper, for that matter—knows, mosquito bars rarely protect the sleeper entirely from mosquitoes. Moreover, the Gorgas gangs soon discovered that, when driven by the wind, malaria-carrying mosquitoes often travel a mile or more from their birthplaces.

In an attempt to locate out-of-the-way mosquito breeding places the ingenious Joseph Le Prince established a routine of mosquito trapping. He directed his workmen to collect large numbers of anopheles, place them in screened cages, and then spray them with a solution of aniline blue dye. The next step was to set up an open tent within the locality being examined, place some tempting, live human bait in the tent, and cover it with a fine-screen mosquito bar to keep off unrecognizable mosquitoes. At the proper moment the research workers would liberate the blue-dyed mosquitoes from all the suspicious locations within the area. Once the test insects were in the air the curtains would be drawn and the human bait exposed. Shortly before dawn the tent would be carefully closed and all the mosquitoes within it caught and examined. When Blue-stained mosquitoes were proof of the direction and distance the mosquitoes could travel under various conditions.

Gorgas, who had a keen eye for human nature, observed: "The job of acting as bait for the mosquitoes during these investigations was a position much sought after by our Negro employees. They were paid by the hour the same wages that the day laborers received. To be paid full wages for sleeping in a comfortable bed struck the Jamaican as being as near complete bliss as anything in this world." [3]

The Canal Zone experiment in tropical sanitation made another lesson plain. The elimination of sources of infection must be accompanied by the development of hospitals and field clinic services. In the Philippines, in the first years of the twentieth century, the constant sick rate of the United States Army had been about ninety men out of every thousand. In Cuba it had been several times that. When they began their gigantic undertaking in Panama, Gorgas and his assistants had anticipated that eventually the Isthmus would show a constant sick rate of at least 50 out of every thousand workers. But even in 1913, while the maximum force of 58,000 men was working on the canal, the constant sick rate was actually only 22 per thousand. But no matter what the rate, sick men would inevitably require buildings and medical facilities for their care.

The Canal Zone hospital system proved a masterly achievement. Dr. John W. Ross was directly in charge of the work. With the support of Gorgas, Ross placed maximum emphasis upon good hospital equipment and spent comparatively little on buildings. He asked for—and got—the best possible medical talent from the United States, energetic young doctors with good medical educations and the ability to adapt themselves readily to a new and exacting environment. At its peak the Canal Zone medical staff consisted of 102 physicians and 130 registered nurses.

Gorgas's French predecessors had already built two base hospitals—Ancon, on a mountainside near Panama City, and Colon Hospital, at the northern terminus of the canal. The major and his assistants proceeded to divide the entire Canal Zone into twenty-five medical districts, generally coincident with the sanitation districts. In eighteen of the districts they built small hospitals of from twenty to a hundred beds. To extend the facilities they built about forty "subdistrict" infirmaries of from five to fifteen beds each. These were called "rest camps" and used as receiving points for the district hospitals. Thus the Canal Zone as a whole was equipped with about sixty hospitals. There were railway hospital cars to carry the sick and wounded from district hospitals to the base hospitals at Colon and Ancon. At these points ambulances met the "sick trains."

A district physician supervised each local hospital and the care of the sick within his prescribed area, attending not only the canal employees, but their families as well. Canal employees received medical treatment without cost and families or dependents received medical treatment at minimum charge. At first many canal workers (particularly the Negroes) were fearful of hospitals, but capable physicians and kindly attendants soon overcame their fears.

Each medical district was also provided with one or more dispensaries directed by a qualified pharmacist. These dispensaries furnished medicine to anyone who applied, and usually without charge. All the dispensaries issued quinine free to anyone requesting it. Dr. Gorgas was convinced that free medication for the tropical public had more than sound philanthropy to recommend it. It kept the district physician accurately informed as to the character of all sickness occurring within a given district and provided authentic information on pathological conditions, endemic and epidemic. As a result, field sanitation workers could be promptly directed to the scene of an outbreak and epidemics snuffed before they could get started.

District physicians supervised all hotels, restaurants, and other public places of the Canal Zone. Sanitary inspectors were charged with the care and supervision of all cemeteries. No burials were allowed in any but inspected cemeteries. Official registers of deaths provided valuable statistics and health information.

The immediate purpose of the field sanitation and hospital system of the Canal Zone was not only to cure malaria patients but to treat all human malaria carriers, since the disease cannot be perpetuated without human agents. Gorgas and his men believed that, if all Canal Zone residents could be persuaded to take five grains of quinine every day, human carriers of malaria might soon vanish. Accordingly, each district physician appointed a special quinine dispenser who traveled through his district every day, offering free quinine to all workers. Of course, it was necessary to add a few extra ingredients in order to make the quinine as attractive as possible. The dispenser distributed brightly colored quinine tonics, also quinine pills, capsules and tablets, and saw to it that they were placed upon the tables of all hotels and eating houses operated by the Canal Commission.

Explanation and persuasion were effective substitutes for compulsion. William Gorgas was a wise man. He knew that the healthy American cannot be forced to swallow pills and powders. Yet at the height of canal construction more than 42,000 doses of quinine were being consumed daily by the 58,000 workers. As might have been expected, malaria began to show a decline.

At Taboga, down in Panama Bay, Gorgas built a convalescent hospital for sufferers from the more severe forms of malaria. The convalescent treatment was designed to rid the patient's blood of malarial parasites and so prevent his becoming a carrier. The Taboga treatment was to continue large doses of quinine for ten days after the cessation of fever. Gorgas was aware of the difficulties:

"A certain number of men, when they were given their daily dose of quinine in the dispensary, would manage to throw their tablets out of the window. The old turkey gobbler who was a pet of the hospital seemed to like the stimulating effect of the quinine and gobbled up all the tablets he could find. He became so dissipated in this way that he finally developed quinine amblyopia. This amblyopia is a species of blindness that is sometimes caused by too much quinine. The doctor finally had to confine his old gobbler and keep him away from quinine tablets until he recovered his sight." [4]

Ancon Hospital, the Canal Zone medical center, had been built by the French on the slope of Ancon Mountain, north of Panama City, in 1882. Under the De Lesseps Company, Ancon was a well-managed 700-bed hospital. The French Canal Company let most of the canal work by contract. Patients were not employees of the company, but of one or more of the thirty-five or forty subcontractors. Under French direction each contractor was required to pay one dollar a day for the hospitalization of each sick employee. The result was that most invalids never saw a hospital bed. The contractors were there to make profit, not to cure the sick.

Under French direction Ancon Hospital, in spite of its excellence in other ways, was a pesthole of yellow fever. A canal worker hospitalized for a broken leg might die there of yellow fever. When the United States took over, Gorgas and his men faced the task of "sanitizing" their principal sanitation center. During June, 1904, Major La Garde became superintendent of Ancon Hospital. He promptly directed that its bed capacity be doubled, that all buildings be thoroughly screened, and that modern plumbing and electric lights replace the privies, kerosene lamps, and candles used by the French. Orderlies were stationed to make certain that all outside doors were kept closed. Grounds were policed for rubbish. All standing water, shrubbery, and tall grass were removed. In due course Ancon became a center of health for a million square miles of American tropics. It was re-equipped with X ray, modern surgical facilities, and a carefully selected staff. Dr. Alfred B. Herrick was appointed chief surgeon; Dr. W. E. Deeks, of Canada, whose story comes later in this book, became director of clinic; and Dr. Samuel Darling, laboratory director.

As the fame of Ancon spread, hundreds of private patients applied for entry. They came from as far south as Chile and as far north as Mexico, and their coming proved a point that is of prime importance today: in tropical countries good will and good health go together. And though fees at Ancon were moderate, the admission of foreign patients soon began to produce revenues of a quarter million dollars a year. A department for ear, eye, nose, and throat treatment was added; then a department for the insane, which also accepted patients for the Panamanian government. Expansion made it necessary to add, first, a laundry, then a modern, efficient dairy; then a 400-

acre farm to provide livestock, poultry, and vegetables. By 1913, Ancon Hospital was sheltering 775 canal employees and 665 pay patients who received ward accommodations at an average price of one dollar a day. To supplement all this, the Canal Commission established a convalescent center in the bay, twelve miles south of Panama City, on Taboga Island, once a stronghold of buccaneers. On a nearer peninsula a well-equipped and much-needed leper colony came into being.

Having established sanitation and therapeutic centers, Gorgas looked still further ahead. Panama was a crossroads for contagion from all the Americas and, with the opening of the canal, from most of the world. Ships brought infected insects and infected crews and passengers to its ports. The Sanitation Department inaugurated port quarantine, proceeded to fumigate all ships with yellow fever cases aboard, and to detain all passengers or crew members of such ships for an observation period of six days. Such measures were essential if the value of all the intensive work the Gorgas gangs had done was not to be undermined. In its beginning the great canal venture was surrounded by yellow fever infection—Guayaquil in Ecuador, Corinto in Nicaragua; Cartegena, Colombia; Puerto Cabello, and even Caracas were strongholds of the disease. So were Veracruz, Mexico; Progreso, capital of Yucatan, many areas of Cuba, and even our own port of New Orleans.

Between 1904 and 1914 the sanitation of the Canal Zone grew into one of the really great achievements in the brief history of preventive medicine. Yellow fever, fiercely epidemic during 1905, was quelled within two years and virtually eradicated before the close of the decade. During 1906, no less than 821 of every thousand canal employees entering Canal Zone hospitals had been admitted because of malaria. By 1913, malaria admissions were down to 76 per thousand—an average decline of about 91 per cent.

Here is the official table for the Canal Zone malaria rate: [5]

1906 .... 821 per 1,000
1907 .... 426 "   1,000
1908 .... 282 "   1,000
1909 .... 215 "   1,000
1910 .... 187 "   1,000
1911 .... 184 "   1,000
1912 .... 110 "   1,000
1913 .... 76 "   1,000

The French Panama Canal Company was active for eight years—from 1881 to 1889. There is good evidence that the death rate among its workers was in the vicinity of two hundred and fifty per thousand each year, and that the constant sick rate was at least three hundred and thirty-three per thousand. Health records of the United States Army showed a constant sick rate of about six hundred men per thousand during the final two months of the Santiago campaign of the Spanish-American War.

During the ten years which it took the United States government to build the Panama Canal our total working force averaged 39,000 men. A constant sick rate of one-third would have produced an average of thirteen thousand sick employees in hospitals every day of the decade. With William Gorgas directing sanitation of the Canal Zone, the actual sick list averaged nine hundred per day for the ten-year period, a grand total of about 3,285,000 days of sickness. If the sick rate suffered during the de Lesseps canal-building venture had been continued under United States operation, days of sickness would have totaled not less than 42,705,000. Thus the saving of nearly 40,000,000 days of sickness can be credited to the work and direction of Dr. Gorgas and his men.

Under Gorgas's control the care of sick canal workers cost the United States about one dollar a day for each patient. In hospital bills alone rigorous sanitation of the 100 square miles of Isthmus strip probably saved the United States around $40,000,000.

But this figure represents only a small part of the actual saving.

The United States paid salaries or wages to the sick. These, added to that depreciation of morale and productive ability invariably resulting from widespread sickness, produced savings which probably equaled a third or even a half of the total cost of building the canal.

During the ten years of construction an average of six hundred and sixty-three workers died each year of accident or disease. Had sanitary conditions remained as they were prior to 1904, and had the death rate of the French Canal Company's working personnel been continued under American direction, deaths from disease incident to the completion of the Panama Canal would have been at least 78,000. William Gorgas could rightly claim that the work of his Sanitary Department saved no fewer than 71,000 human lives which might have been lost in the building of the Panama Canal.

For science and for the Americas the world's greatest drama of sanitation proved enormously profitable. Today, as in 1913 when the canal was opened to trade, the actual death rate of the district is lower than that of New York, or Chicago, or any other one of the ten largest cities of the Americas. The Isthmus of Panama has become an island of good health in a vast sea of recurring pestilence. Within one decade, capable sanitation changed one of the least healthy regions of the Western Hemisphere to one of the most healthful.

The sanitation of the Canal Zone was the climax to four centuries of Temperate Zone enterprise in the tropics. The great colonizing nations of Europe had been quick to assume that tropical lands were not for major settlement by white men; that the white race could not live and thrive in the tropics, nor leave behind a healthy progeny.

Millions of us still hold this view. Yet there is ample evidence that before the spread and infiltration of disease, when what are now the Temperate Zones were made uninhabitable by the inhospitalities of ice-laden air, almost the entire population of the world had its home in the tropics.

Tropical climates are great producers of life and their very productivity, multiplying as it did the lower as well as the higher types of living matter, resulted in an overdevelopment of pathogenic organisms. Man, in the tropics, began to be attacked with a violence which he had no immunity to counteract. For relatively primitive man there was only one way out—migration to climatic zones which would reduce the vitality of the attacking organisms without reducing his own.

The temperate regions, however, did not immediately and without modification produce an ideal home any more than the tropics do today. Dr. Gorgas, whose work speaks for itself, stated the case clearly: "The greatest sanitarian that the human race ever produced was probably the individual who discovered fire, and next in importance, the individual who first wore some kind of clothing. These two discoveries enabled man to overcome the hitherto insurmountable sanitary obstacle of the temperate regions, namely, cold. With the application of these two sanitary discoveries, the human race was enabled to migrate from the tropics and continue healthy development in the temperate regions.

"At the present time, we have just reversed the process; we have just made sanitary discoveries which will enable man to return from the temperate regions to which he was forced to migrate long ages ago, and again live and develop in his natural home, the tropics. . . .

"The practical application of these great discoveries has just been demonstrated during the construction of the Panama Canal. . . . The conditions were such at Panama that they attracted the attention of the whole world, and probably the general knowledge that the white man can live and thrive in the tropics will date in future times from the construction of this great work. . . .

"The discovery of the Americas was a great epoch in the history of the white man, and threw large areas of fertile and healthy country open to his settlement. The demonstration made at Panama that he can live a healthy life in the tropics will be an equally important milestone in the history of the race, and will throw just as large an area of the earth's surface open to man's settlement, and a very much more productive area." [6]

In his formal annual report to the surgeon general of the United States Army Gorgas once wrote:

"I do not believe that posterity will consider the commercial and physical success of the Canal the greatest good it has conferred upon mankind. I hope that as time passes our descendants will see that the greatest good the Canal has brought has been the opportunity it gave for demonstration that the white man can live and work in the tropics, and maintain his health at as high a point as he can, doing the same work, in the temperate zone. That this has been demonstrated, none can gainsay." [7]

So, the occupation of Cuba was a noteworthy overture to the greater adventure in Panama. Both attainments are of even greater significance today than they were at the time of their actual occurrence. The challenge and the importance of hemisphere sanitation appears in its true light only today, when the twenty-one American nations are beginning to merge into an essential New World commonwealth.

Chapter Four

CARLOS FINLAY OF CUBA

I F you look up the name of Carlos Finlay in the latest edition of the *Encyclopedia Britannica,* the chances are that you will not find it. There is no mention of him in volume 9—EXTRACTI to GAMB, and none in volume 23—VASE to ZYGO—where the account of yellow fever is to be found. A persevering researcher will find his name in the index volume, however, and turning to the reference given there, discover an article on preventive medicine. It contains one of the shortest mentions ever allocated to human greatness:

In 1882 Carlos Finlay implicated the responsible mosquito.

Even so, that isn't exactly correct. The year was 1881, the forty-ninth year of the obscure life of a man who was to remain almost unknown even after he had pointed the way to saving millions of lives, present and to come. Famous or forgotten, Carlos Finlay has his true memorial in the men, women, and children who would have been killed by yellow fever, who might still be dying today, if it were not for his intuitive genius.

Those two words, "yellow fever," do not mean much to the modern North American who reads them. He is more likely to respond emphatically to other disease names like "black death" or even "leprosy." There is, at the moment, no more yellow fever in the United States, and even the memory of it has died out. When this same edition of the *Britannica* went to press, its editors were able to say: "No case has been reported in the entire Western Hemisphere for many months." The same favorable report, as a subsequent chapter will make clear, is no longer possible, and it may be that before long the disease will have broken out of bounds and be on the attack again. But even if that happens, the work of Carlos Finlay will provide a starting point for the counterattack.

White men in the tropics called it "yellowjack" in the years when it was slaughtering whole populations, and Spanish Americans had an even less pleasant phrase: "el vomito negro." For four centuries it was widespread and a wholesale killer; the mortality rates averaged 50 per cent of the people who got it, and one outbreak in Rio de Janeiro in 1898 showed the appalling figure of 94.5 per cent. Any man who had contracted the disease and survived it could command far better wages than a nonimmune person. Fear, death, and economic disaster rode with yellow fever when it was on the march, and it was on the march over and over again in the history of the Western Hemisphere, as a glance at the epidemic table at the end of this book will make abundantly plain.

To say that yellow fever has been the most powerful pathogenic factor affecting the history of the Western world is probably not extreme. It is, or has been, endemic in more than half of our own hemisphere—in most of the West Indies Islands and tropical South America and probably in almost all of Central America and Mexico. Its violence has threatened American cities as far north as Montreal and Quebec and as far south as Buenos Aires and Montevideo.

For centuries the countries of the Caribbean have been isolated and impoverished by it. A huge proportion of what is carelessly considered Latin-American "backwardness" is readily attributable to the influence of yellowjack. During almost four centuries this frightful pestilence was prevalent in the chief ports of Cuba, Mexico, Brazil, and many other South American lands. During the epidemic of 1878 it took more than 13,000 lives in our own Mississippi Valley. In 1664 at St. Lucia 1,411 of the regiment of 1,500 British soldiers died of it. In the Windward and Leeward Islands, with an estimated population of about 12,000, a yellow fever epidemic in 1794 caused more than 6,000 deaths. During 1802 half of Santo Domingo's population of 40,000 died of it; six years earlier, two-thirds of the people of Guadeloupe perished during a single year. During 1804 there were about 53,000 yellow fever deaths in the seaports of Spain and more than a quarter million cases. By 1870 New York City had suffered twenty-three recorded epidemics and Philadelphia had had twenty-five.[1]

Yellow fever begins like most other fevers, but its victims soon take on a characteristic look, which once seen is not likely to be forgotten: their faces flushed, their eyes suffused, their lips and tongue a bright red. At this stage the fever is frighteningly high. Then, two days or so later, comes the phase which gives the disease its name. The temperature falls below normal and the victim's pulse slows down to feebleness. His skin grows cold and takes on a yellow, jaundiced tint. The evidences of internal bleeding become apparent in his vomiting, which begins early in the attack and which, at this stage, becomes black with blood. There are other manifestations even less pleasant. From this phase the victim may rally to recovery. Or he may not.

Such was the disease that had been ravaging the tropical and subtropical Americas for centuries before the birth of Carlos Finlay. In all those years little progress had been made in treating the disease, and none at all in discovering how it was spread. Its presence in the lands to the south of us was a menace which stood fairly astride any hopeful future for the hot countries.

It was highly appropriate that the life of the man who was to bring about the defeat of yellow fever should combine many of the elements which have distinguished American tropical medicine throughout its history. No one people or nationality, no single background of culture appears to be enough for the problem. All kinds of strands have to be brought together by the fates, and so it was in the case of Carlos Finlay.

His grandfather, Edward Finlay, was a native of Whitehaven, a seaport and market town in Cumberland, England, which John Paul Jones had harried in the winter of 1777-1778. (The New World was thus drawn rather forcefully to the attention of the Finlays long before Carlos!) Not long thereafter, Finlay married a Mary Wilson of Glasgow, Scotland; no less than fifteen children were born to the couple in the years that followed. Carlos Finlay's father, also named Edward, was the fourth of nine sons.

Whether it was the family memory of John Paul Jones or, more probably, the fever of adventure and the passion for freedom which were so much a part of the times, young Edward Finlay was not long in casting in his lot with the New World. He had studied medicine at the University of Edinburgh and then gone to Rouen to continue his training. In 1821, Simón Bolívar, in distant Venezuela, was fighting to liberate his country. Edward Finlay joined the British contingent which went to volunteer under Bolívar. His ship was wrecked in a Caribbean hurricane, and the young Scotch-English doctor barely escaped with his life. After a series of adventures, both numerous and painful, he landed in Trinidad in 1826.

The next five years were busy ones for Edward Finlay. He became admitted to medical practice in Port-of-Spain, and in a short time was considered one of the ranking West Indian surgeons. He founded a hospital. And he married. The bride, Eliza de Barrès, was a French girl. Scotch, English, and French blood, and a background of Western Hemisphere medicine—all these strands were thus woven together. There were to be still others.

In 1831 the Finlays moved to Cuba. They settled near Camagüey, the largest interior city on the island. It lies midway between the north and south coasts and is the center of a rich agricultural district. And Camagüey is an old city—older than most of our own. Founded in 1515, it had three full centuries behind it when the Finlays arrived. This was no frontier outpost, but a center of much that was best and most traditional in Latin-American culture.

Dr. Edward Finlay lost no time in finding a place for himself. He established his medical position by taking a degree of *Cirujano Latino,* or Latin surgeon, and later an M.D. from the University of Havana. He also acquired a coffee plantation near Alquizar. Most important of all, in 1833 he and Eliza had a son whom they christened Juan Carlos.

Carlos's father was properly ambitious for him. He wanted the boy to follow in his own footsteps, and perhaps to become, as he had, the greatest doctor in Havana. So little Carlos spent his first eleven years largely on the acres of the coffee farm at Alquizar, but before he was twelve his father sent him to France to secure the best Continental schooling. It was a tragic adventure for the boy. No sooner had he landed than he contracted a throat ailment which left him a stutterer for the rest of his life. He came home, but the damage was done.

When Carlos was fifteen, Dr. Finlay tried again. He sent his son abroad for the second time, and once more the venture ended disastrously. After studying at Mainz on the Rhine, in London, and at the Lycée in Rouen, the boy contracted typhoid. This second illness forced him home once again and put an end to his father's plan to give him a European medical education. Still, he had acquired much that the Old World had to offer, and his determination to go on with medicine was unshaken. He turned his eyes to the north and determined to study at the Jefferson Medical College in Philadelphia.[2]

The strands were beginning to multiply, and to knit themselves into their ultimate pattern. At Philadelphia young Carlos met the man who was to teach him the things that made his life work possible—the famous John Kearsley Mitchell. It was Dr. Mitchell's thesis to his pupils at Jefferson that nothing ever absolved the scientist or the doctor from the obligation of close observation of the actual facts. He warned them against accepting traditional authority blindly; they must investigate and decide for themselves. In the case of Carlos Finlay, that teaching was to bear special fruit and to justify itself many times over.

Meantime, the young Cuban had formed a close friendship with the slightly older son of his favorite teacher, S. Weir Mitchell, who was just beginning his own teaching career. As Dr. Mitchell himself was later to admit, this association came near to being less happy— at least for the history of tropical medicine: "I endeavored in vain to persuade Finlay, who was my first student, to settle in New York, where then there were many Spaniards and many Cubans. Fortunately he made up his mind not to take my advice." [3]

In 1856 Carlos Juan (who had been christened Juan Carlos but elected to reverse the order) returned to Havana and accompanied his father upon a year's medical excursion to Lima, Peru. Back in Havana, he passed his incorporation examinations at the university and practiced medicine for three years. Then, at thirty-one, he went to Paris to "follow" the clinics in general medicine and eye diseases. Handsome, bearded, and thirty-two, he returned to Havana to practice. Later, during October, 1865, he married Adele Shine, an Irish girl of his own age from Port-of-Spain, Trinidad.

The bride, an orphan who had been educated at the Ursuline Convent of Cork, Ireland, was intensely religious and filled with misgivings and fears about a world which seemed to her to be unrepentantly wicked. But she proved a splendid wife for a brilliant, and not particularly prosperous husband. She sympathized with his ingratiating but unprofitable instinct for openhanded charity. She helped in his homemade laboratory, counted and squeezed pesos and pennies to make their slender income support a home, and somehow found time to play the violin, sing, write poetry, and even supplement the family income by giving music lessons.

Meanwhile the dreamy and philanthropic Carlos had begun to demonstrate his powers of observation and deduction. During

1867 and 1868 Havana was visited by a death-dealing epidemic of cholera. For many exhausting months young Dr. Finlay tended the sick and the dying and studied the dead. He became convinced that cholera was transmitted by drinking water. He gave instructions that the drinking water of his own household be carefully boiled. None of his family took cholera.

The young doctor made another significant observation. At Cerro, a Havana suburb, cholera had appeared on only one side of the street. That side of this particular street was occupied by the wealthier families. Yet cholera, reputedly a disease of poverty, was spreading like fire among the well-to-do.

Finlay began searching for an explanation. Within a few hours he had found a clue. The water supply for one side of the main street of Cerro came down an open canal which passed through a row of back gardens (As a contrast to modern practices of hygiene, in several of these gardens the homeowners maintained private swimming pools fed by the same canal, which also supplied household water.) Finlay learned that a Chinese laundryman had died of cholera near the junction of the canal and the Almendares River. He fixed upon this spot as the probable point of infection. Sure that he was right, he wrote a letter to Havana's principal newspaper, *Diario de la Marina,* in which he explained the situation. Cuba's censor refused to permit publication of the letter. Cubans continued to die of cholera.[4]

The year 1868 saw the beginning of Cuba's ten-year revolution, when rebels under Carlos Manuel de Cespedes tried to win the island's independence from Spain. During this tumultuous period, Carlos Finlay moved his family to the comparative tranquillity of Trinidad. By 1870, however, he was again in Havana with his family and a diminishing load of luggage. The latter included a somewhat primitive microscope acquired years before in Philadelphia. The patient doctor resumed his practice.

Finlay was a man of science, in an era when medicine was, in practice, comparatively unscientific and he was also a broad-minded thinker in a generation of almost universal bigotry and ignorance. His viewpoint had been influenced by the many strands of his own background—his English and French ancestry, Spanish-Cuban upbringing, and his schooling in the Rhineland, in Paris, and in the United States. He was intensely interested in national viewpoints and literatures. Though deeply Catholic, he usually avoided discussion of religion. Graciously contemptuous of money, he studied medicine fervently, regarding his service to it as a kind of priesthood. Even with the development of his practice he remained poor.

Remembering John Mitchell's teaching, Carlos Finlay regarded research as the personal obligation of every physician. In all Havana there were few if any scientists and no commercial laboratories, so the doctor built a laboratory for himself. He studied continuously in many fields of science—chemistry, meteorology, physics, and even history. He worked early and late and slept little. He was a man who reveled in humor and who cherished conversation for its own sake, but primarily he was a worker—a worker who worked himself unsparingly.

But he was no mere drudge. Like a true Cuban, Finlay loved cigarettes. Less like a Cuban, he keenly enjoyed good wine. He dressed immaculately and carefully, usually in white. As carefully, he supervised the upbringing of his family. He insisted, to the point of painfulness, that his three sons be orderly and precise in their manner, their diet, and their hygiene. Like most Cubans, he delighted in baseball and encouraged his three boys to play the game. It is not surprising that his home life was happy and that his sons grew up to be successful men who loved and understood him.

During his school days in France he had learned fencing, but in his thirties he found that it strained his heart and gave it up. Chess and cards took its place. During the Franco-Prussian War he invented a game of his own. It involved cavalry, infantry and artillery, all moved about on a kind of chessboard. His son Carlos has suggested that the doctor's devotion to such games was an important factor in the development of an ability to piece together information and make of it something not evident in any of its parts. It was certainly this ability, whatever its origin, which led after a long and heartbreaking study to the discovery of the source and the preparation of a cure for yellow fever.

It was yellow fever that became the touchstone for Carlos Finlay's greatness. As we have already seen, the challenge it offered to medical research was inescapable. For more than three hundred years the vast and still unexplored fields of tropical medicine were measured by the extent of yellow fever. Carlos Finlay knew that "el vomito negro" was the principal scourge of hot countries; all other tropical maladies, however formidable, seemed insignificant by comparison. It seemed to him that discovery of its causes and the establishment of practical measures for its prevention were a first obligation on tropical medicine. But there was not much to build on in the way of previous research and knowledge.

When Carlos Finlay turned his inquiring mind upon it, yellow fever was one of the most baffling mysteries in all the mysterious world of medicine. Its literature was a welter of confusion and contradiction. Only a few of its characteristics were beyond dispute. It was recognized as a disease of the lowlands and one that rarely occurred in epidemic form at altitudes above 4,000 feet. Plainly, it was most prevalent in the region lying between thirty degrees north and thirty degrees south latitude. Medical men agreed that in temperate climates it was usually a "summer disease," tending to vanish after the coming of frost, also that it was most frequently a malady of ocean fronts and seaports.

Beyond these established bits of evidence the medical world was in confused indecision. Disagreement which was far from scientific was general. During the 1880's, for instance, La Roche and Bérenger-Féraud, writing about the disease, declined to step into the controversy by expressing an opinion as to whether it was contagious. They simply stated with engaging candor that man's existing knowledge of it was negligible; that for two centuries medicine had learned virtually nothing of one of the worst plagues of mankind.[5]

Dr. George M. Sternberg, in 1890, pointed out that the disease is contracted in infected localities and not by direct contact with the sick; that patients derive the disease from infected houses.

On a given street adjacent houses harbored cases even though the occupants lived behind locked doors. Contamination of localities appeared to be influenced by travel routes. Accredited medical texts, however, taught that yellow fever was spread by *fomites*, objects and articles of clothing which had been in physical contact with sufferers, by excreta from infected persons, or by "miasms"—vapors given off by infected bodies or localities.

Racial predisposition was another foremost subject of argument. For a long time Negroes were believed to be immune. Although this theory was eventually discredited by the occurrence of severe epidemics in darkest Africa, La Roche, using medical records of the British Army, proved that in British West Indian possessions where both white and colored troops were on duty, yellow fever mortality among white troops was approximately ten times that among Negroes.[6] More recent investigations in Africa confirm the Negro's susceptibility to yellow fever but characterize the majority of occurrences among Negroes as "mild, silent or unrecognizable forms" which may show a natural racial resistance to malaria as well as yellow fever on the part of Negroes.

The yellow race, too, apparently showed racial resistance to the disease. Carlos Finlay noticed the rarity of yellow fever among the Chinese workers in the West Indies, and Cuban records showed no yellow fever occurrence among Chinese immigrants. On the other hand, many Chinese and other Orientals fell victim to yellow fever in Guiana and in Brazil. That Indians are highly susceptible to the scourge has never been denied, but the contention that yellow fever is preponderantly an adults' disease was blasted by Juan Guiteras of Cuba, who pointed out that although it occurs in children it is usually so mild that it is rarely accurately diagnosed.

Carlos Finlay believed yellow fever was indigenous to the Americas; and that the disease was widespread in the American tropics before the time of Columbus, that it was later transported to West Coast Africa by ships engaged in the slave trade and by other ships traveling to various parts of the world.

In part he based this belief upon the writings of the Spanish historians who recorded the voyages of Columbus and the earliest expeditions to Spanish America. There is no conclusive record that Columbus's first voyage encountered any unknown malignant diseases. Columbus's second expedition, composed of about 1,500 men, "fell sick from fevers shortly after their arrival in November, 1493." [7] But these fevers did not produce many deaths. Finlay, studying the records, judged the sickness to be malaria. Bérenger-Féraud expressed the same opinion.

On March 19, 1494, Columbus and his followers fought the battle of Vega Real against 100,000 Indians, "after which a disease broke out not only among his men, but also among the neighboring natives, with a loss of a third of their number." Finlay believed that that disease was yellow fever, for at the time there were probably only four other diseases of man (plague, typhus, smallpox, and cholera) capable of inflicting such high mortality in so short a time and any of the latter four diseases would certainly have been recognized by Europeans. Finlay further believed that Columbus's attackers, principally Caribs from the Spanish Main, brought the disease to the Spaniards. But Antonio de Herrera, historian of the Conquest, blamed the food: "The lack of food in Hispaniola (the Castillians have to eat most nasty stuffs), and the suffering of the Indians from lack of planting caused in them much illness. They became very yellow appearing, saffron colored, this lasting for many days." [8]

The yellow plague of the New World terrified the Spaniards and for good reason. Lores, who arrived at Hispaniola in 1502 with 2,000 men, lost half his force through sickness within a few weeks. News from the tropical mainlands was no better. Seven years later

Alonso de Hojeda, at New Andalucia, lost 260 of his followers from various ailments. During 1514 most of the 1,500 members of the Panama expedition of Pedrarias de Avilas died of a malignant "yellowing" disease.

Records indicate that those who were fortunate enough to survive an attack became immune to the disease thereafter. Finlay contended that this apparent immunization of older colonists, as contrasted to the prompt infection of newcomers, was another first-rate bit of evidence that the disease they suffered from was yellow fever.

But Panama, particularly the Darien coast and Nombre de Dios, became a focus of the New World pestilence. Carlos Finlay quoted the following paragraph written in 1537 by Bishop Francisco Marroquin to Emperor Charles V of Spain:

Likewise your Majesty should order that the people come to this new Spain or to Puerto de Cavallos and not to that of Nombre de Dios which is the sepulchre of all; and so that people from all sides do not excuse themselves from coming, it is necessary for your Majesty to provide the ports with hospitals, doctors and pharmacies; likewise in Peru, where there are so many interests, 10,000 pesos could be well employed, and please God let your Majesty spend 20,000 in Nombre de Dios, Panama and Puerto Viego where I aver that 4,000 have died, more on the roads and beaches and some have hung themselves from hunger. I really believe that your Majesty has not been well informed of this, so I do so now. For the love of God please provide New Spain with these necessities; in this part of Veracruz 500 people die each year and also in great numbers in the roads and inns.[9]

More than four hundred years ago royal Spain was learning that sick men cannot be conquerors.

Like many other scholars, Carlos Finlay found Mexico a particularly rich source of early New World history. In that country, centuries before the coming of white men, Indians wrote hieroglyphic histories which they continued and enlarged for many decades after the arrival of the conquistadors. During the first period of Spanish conquest, Spanish historians collected information from natives and others familiar with Nahuatl, Mexico's original language.

Early Mexican picture writing, ending about 1513, tells little of diseases, but records years of famine and of extremely high death rates. Immediately following the first conquest by the Spaniards these records tell of two years of famine and five years of epidemics. During the two decades following 1521, when Spain's conquest of Mexico was well in progress, Spanish writers such as Luis Molina, Bernardino de Sahagun, Diego Duran, and Torquemada wrote extensively, at least in part from native Indian sources. These historians knew Nahuatl and they also knew in intimate detail the habits and lives of native Mexicans.

Finlay could find no indications of yellow fever in early accounts of the *Tierra Fria*, or Central Mexican Plateau. But he discovered that, in Nahuatl picture writing, the year 1454 (almost half a century before Columbus) was represented by two men and a woman vomiting. Presumably this indicated some widespread sickness like yellow fever in which nausea is a prominent feature. It is interesting to note, however, that the hieroglyphics were found at altitudes normally beyond the yellow fever range.

During the half century following the arrival of the Spaniards, Nahuatl records tell of the appearance of many diseases of white men, such as smallpox (in 1520); typhus (in 1526 and repeatedly thereafter); measles (in 1531); mumps (in 1560). White men were bringing a dark cloud of disease to a not altogether bright new world.

Herrera wrote of Mexico's *Tierra Caliente* (Hot Land) in the area of Veracruz:

Of the disease called "cocoliztle" and from which the coast of the north is depopulated . . . I have already said that the city of Veracruz is sickly, and all the coast of the north being a hot country, where all diseases are more fatal because the heat of the region adds itself to the natural heat and does not allow the sick man to recuperate because the hot air prevents him, and children are not raised because with any kind of disorder a fever supervenes.

For this reason the coast is found depopulated and the reason why it had so many people at the time of Montezuma is that although it had the same diseases . . . prevalent and in some years more than others as is the case now, Montezuma was accustomed, in view of the mortality and lack of population in these lands, to draw from Mexico and from other pueblos, where there were many people, 8,000 families, and this number of 8,000 families they called "zexiquipil" and sent them to people where there had been a great "cocoliztle" (epidemic) and gave them houses and lands and made them free of tribute for many years, and thus he returned to repeople the coast whenever there was need without making lack in the pueblos whence he drew them. . . .[10]

Both Finlay and Bérenger-Féraud believed that the Veracruz area was actually a pre-Columbian focus of yellow fever and that the repopulation efforts of Emperor Montezuma merely served to introduce recurrent supplies of nonimmunes into the area and thus perpetuate the ravages of the disease.

In the course of his lifelong studies, Finlay also considered the Mayas, another great pre-Columbian Indian civilization centered in Yucatan, Campeche, and Guatemala. Large areas of these regions are ideal breeding grounds for *Aëdes aegypti* mosquitoes. Since much of the land is dry, it has for centuries been necessary to store water supplies in pools and ponds. For centuries, too, populations of the Mayan lands have been comparatively dense, supplying an abundance of human hosts.

Prior to the Spanish conquest, Mayan culture was probably the most highly developed anywhere within the Western Hemisphere. Mayan hieroglyphics were more advanced and more specific than the Mexican. Many of their records remain as inscriptions upon rocks, monuments, and structure ruins.

The Mayan day was the *Kin*. These days were grouped in periods called the *tun*—or 360 days. The *Katun* consisted of 20 *tuns*. Mayan documents included official papers, titles to land and local histories of respective communities. The latter tell of a great pestilence which occurred in Katun 4 ahau, perhaps 1482 or 1483 A.D. That particular pestilence may have been smallpox. But Bishop Crescencio Carrillo y Ancona, of Yucatan, who was a collector of rare Mayan documents and a recognized authority on Mayan literature, found in the Mayan Chilam-Balam books the statement: "There was black vomit which began to occasion death among us in 1648." [11]

Carlos Finlay corresponded with Bishop Carrillo in the hope of finding further testimony that yellow fever had been known to the Yucatan area before the Spanish invasion. The bishop presented a brilliant array of proof that the pre-Columbian pestilence described in Mayan records was in truth yellow fever. He pointed out that the Spanish settlement of Yucatan (begun in 1517) had continued until 1648 without records of serious epidemic. From this he concluded that the disease called *cocoliztle*, widespread in lowland Mexico, had not been common in Yucatan. His conviction that the epidemic of black vomit of 1648 was in truth yellow fever was based upon the impressive descriptions of the Yucatan historian, Fray Diego Lopez de Cogolludo, who had himself suffered from the disease. Cogolludo's description of the epidemic is masterly journalism as well as excellent clinical description:

. . . At the beginning of June the scourge of the *"peste"* commenced in the town of Campeche and in a few days became so severe that the place was completely ravaged. . . . The roads to Campeche were guarded for fear that contagion should spread, but if the Lord guards not the city what shall human efforts avail. With the fear of Divine Justice the month of July passed until towards the end a few persons began to sicken, dying very soon; but the disease was not considered as epidemic until the month of August.

With such a violence and rapidity were the people attacked, big and small, rich and poor, that in less than eight days the whole population of the city were sick at the same time and many citizens of the highest rank and authority died. . . . While the city was thus afflicted by this calamity *never before seen since the country was conquered by the Spanish nation*, permission was asked that the image of Our Lady of Itzamal might be brought . . .

It is impossible to say what the disease was, for the physicians did not recognize it. In most of the cases the patients were taken with a most severe and intense headache with pains in all the bones of their bodies, so violent that their limbs felt as if turned asunder or squeezed in a press. A few moments after the pains, there came a very intense fever which in most cases produced delirium, though not in all.

This was followed by vomiting of blood, as if putrified, and of all such cases very few survived. Some were attacked with discharges from the bowels of a bilious humor (humor-colics) which being corrupt occasioned dysentery without vomiting, while others made violent efforts to vomit without being able to discharge anything, and many suffered the fever and pains in the bones without any of the other symptoms, and in the majority the fever seems to remit completely on the third day; they would say they felt no pains whatever, the delirium would cease, the patients conversing in their full senses, but they were unable to eat or drink anything; they would continue thus one or several days and while still talking and saying they were quite well, they expired.

A great number did not pass the third day, the majority died on the fifth and very few reached the seventh, excepting those who survived. . . . The most robust and healthy of the men were violently attacked and died soonest. . . . Some cases occurred in which the patients passed the fever in a sleep until they recovered, having had no one to administer remedies to them. . . .

In houses of large families there was scarcely anyone to attend the sick or to fetch the sacraments for them. This spiritual difficulty was remedied by the charity of the priests . . . who went about the streets both day and night carrying with them the Holy Viaticum and the Holy Oils and visited the houses to administer the same to such as required them. . . . When the laity began to improve, the disease broke out among the priests. Of eight members of the Jesuits' College, six died. . . . Of our own Order (Franciscans) twenty died in the city. . . . The disease continued over the whole country during the space of two years. . . . Few that lived in this land or visited it in the course of these two years escaped being sick soon, and it rarely happened that anyone died of the sickness attacked after having recovered from the first. All remained pale as ghosts, without hair, many lost their eyebrows. . . .[12]

After long and painstaking study of these early records, Carlos Finlay concluded that at least three epidemics of yellow fever had swept over the land of the Mayas prior to the Spanish conquest. He likewise became convinced that the pre-Columbian Americas had suffered many other virulent maladies about which regrettably little is known. For example, Friar Don Diego de Landa, a missionary in Yucatan during the first generation of Spanish occupation, wrote:

Various calamities were experienced in Yucatan before the Conquest; hurricanes, pestilences, wars, etc. . . . There came over all the land certain pestilential diseases which lasted 24 hours and after they ceased the patients would swell and break out full of worms, and from this pestilence a great number died and a great part of the crops could not be gathered; after the epidemic had ceased they had a period of 16 good years during which the quarrels and dissensions [of the Mayas] were renewed, so that 150,000 men were killed in wars, after which they were quieted, made peace and rested during 20 years, when they were attacked by a pestilence of large boils which rotted their body . . . so that their limbs would drop off in pieces in the course of four or five days. . . .

Eagerly, Finlay gathered up these threads of information, realizing their significance in the study of indigenous American diseases which may play enormously important roles in the development of others imported from Europe and Africa. He discovered that during the sixteenth century French writers had reported a disease called *coup de barre*, reputedly common among Indians of the West Indies; that later, in 1648, when a *peste* overcame the French colonies of Martinique and Guadeloupe, its symptoms, as recorded by Du Tertre and other historians, appeared identical with reliable descriptions of epidemic yellow fever. Finlay noted Pezuela's statement that during 1649 Cuba had been attacked by an "unknown and horrible epidemic imported from the American continent. One-third of its population were devoured from May to October by the putrid fever which destroyed those attacked in three days." [13] There was reason to believe that this malady also was yellow fever. More than a century and a half later Cuba was again stricken by the same pestilence, reportedly imported from Mexico. For almost two hundred years thereafter, having been opened to world trade, Cuba had remained a focus of chronic yellow fever.

In 1872 Carlos Finlay presented to the Havana Academy of Sciences a summary of his first thirteen years of investigation of the causes of yellow fever—an ingenious explanation of the "climate theory" of yellow fever transmission. That was an interesting trail leading nowhere, but some of its records and experiments have been of value to medical research both past and present.

Seven years later Spain's Governor General in Cuba appointed Finlay to represent Cuba in scientific co-operation with members of the first American Yellow Fever Commission being sent to Havana by the United States government. Dr. Stanford E. Chaillé was president of the commission, Drs. Sternberg, Guiteras, and Finlay would be Chaillé's assistants, and a medical student, Rudolph Matas, was appointed clerk. The commission arrived in Cuba during August, 1879, and promptly began work on an elaborate, noteworthy, and extremely confusing report. Chaillé and his assistants worked with microscopes, and they worked with human blood. Quite significantly they concluded that "the poison of yellow fever spreads, multiplies, and is endowed with the functions of reproduction which is limited to living organisms." [14]

A great many attractive fables have been devised to explain just why Carlos Finlay chose the mosquito as the probable carrier of yellow fever. Finlay's own records suggest that his selection of the mosquito as the carrier of yellow fever resulted in part from a misunderstanding.

On leaving Cuba, the commission presented Dr. Finlay with a collection of photomicrographs prepared by Dr. Sternberg. In studying these the observing Cuban noted that red blood globules are discharged unbroken into the hemorrhages of yellow fever. He pondered this fact. He began to picture the spread of the disease in terms of man-made vaccination, then noted in his work journal:

. . . Assimilating the disease to smallpox and to vaccination (interesting though somewhat inaccurate scientifically) it occurred to me that in order to inoculate yellow fever it would be necessary to pick out the inoculable material from within the blood vessels of a yellow fever patient and to carry it likewise into the interior of a blood vessel of the person who was to be inoculated. All of which conditions the mosquito satisfied most admirably through its bite, in a manner which it would be almost impossible for us to imitate, with the comparatively coarse instruments which the most skillful worker could produce. . . .[15]

Finlay had also followed Van Tieghem's pioneer study of the *Puccinia graminis,* a parasitic fungus which attacks grain, leaving its winter spores on the dead plants, and spreading by means of a complex cycle of reproduction which involves several different plant hosts. The Cuban scientist inferred a possible corollary between the fungus enemy of European grain crops and the unknown organism of yellow fever. This was a far cry from the millrun of medical deductions. But it proved to be a significant idea.

In his address at the Washington International Sanitary Conference of February, 1881, which Finlay attended as special delegate for Cuba, he suggested that propagation of yellow fever requires three things: the presence of a previous case of yellow fever within certain limits of time; the presence of a person liable to contract the disease; and the presence of an agent "entirely independent, for its existence, both of the disease and of the sick man, but which is necessary in order that the disease shall be conveyed from the yellow fever patient to a healthy individual." [16]

Such an hypothesis was entirely unsupported in the medical literature of Finlay's day. Later in the year the great Dr. Patrick Manson published his discovery of the indirect transmission of filaria by the mosquito. But in August of 1881 (still ahead of Sir Patrick's publication), Carlos Finlay, speaking to the Academy of Sciences of Havana, named the *Culex* mosquito, now called *Aëdes aegypti*, as the transmission agent of yellow fever and announced for the first time in history the transmission of a disease by an insect vector.

Between February and August, Finlay had been studying mosquitoes, examining them with the aged two-prong microscope he had brought home from Philadelphia, and recording handwritten volumes of findings. The *Culex*, he found, was one of the more common species of house mosquitoes, the one most likely to ferry blood and to bite both the sick and the healthy. In the course of this research, Carlos Finlay even had to teach himself the technique of adroit mosquito catching. He used test tubes cushioned with cotton. He learned the breeding habits and life cycles and the varying characteristics of many species. He recorded the findings and fed his prisoner mosquitoes on fresh blood—of people, horses, rabbits, and mice. He dissected mosquitoes and wrote pioneer reports on mosquito anatomy. He learned that some mosquitoes live seventy days or longer. One of his journals contains the entry:

I had not reached the more advanced views concerning the development of the germ in the salivary glands of the infected mosquito.

By the same train of thought I was led to the conclusion that yellow fever could be stamped out from an infected locality either by suppressing the *Culex* mosquito (*Stegomyia*) or by preventing the approach of nonimmunes to the said locality until the last of the infected insects had died.[17]

He told his findings to medical men who did not believe. Cuban listeners were at least gracious. Most North Americans were rude. But the great Cuban worked on. He devised a back-yard laboratory in which he studied mosquitoes by day, and wrote his findings at night. He heard himself described as the mosquito doctor. He heard himself described as "touched." But it made no difference to him; he worked on through eighteen unbelieving years.

Also, Finlay steadfastly contended that commerce outbound from the Americas served to carry the mosquito vector of yellow fever to other continents: "The vector mosquito was distributed by vessels, especially by the old sailing vessels, breeding aboard them en route, and no matter in what seaport it first existed in permanence, it would ultimately be distributed from that port to all others (climatic conditions allowing) to which the vessel of the first part went. Ultimately, when interlocking commerce of ships had continued long enough this mosquito would be found in all ports in which were found the conditions of temperature and breeding places necessary for its propagation and existence." [18]

This is commonplace knowledge today. But it was written by Carlos Finlay nearly twenty years before North American medical men had conceded that the mosquito could possibly be responsible for the spreading of yellowjack.

Men of science knew practically nothing about mosquitoes. For years, and without assistance, Carlos Finlay had striven to learn the salient facts of mosquito life.

For twenty trying years, however, from 1880 to 1900, the date of the renowned Camp Lazear experiments of Walter Reed and the Army Yellow Fever Board, almost all the medical world continued to doubt Finlay of Cuba, even as yellow fever continued to ravage the earth with desolation and death. But the Cuban was neither cowed nor discouraged. Time and time again he presented his deductions and records to medical groups and scientific societies throughout his own country, the United States, and Europe. His busy practice and his always slender purse suffered the consequences. But he fought on, presenting the clinical features of his experimental cases, presenting statistics of his trial inoculations, and outlining methods of public sanitation whereby the scourge could be halted.

Still the medical world suggested that Cuba's Finlay was "touched." Various medical men with whom he worked, to whom he gave freely of hospitality and hints of his laboratory work, remained in the ranks of the doubters. Superb in theory, Finlay's proof was weak. Writers of medical texts shunned what they called his "fantastics." The few believers were Cubans and for the most part they were laymen. The exception was the ever-loyal, almost worshipful Dr. Claudio Delgado of Havana, Finlay's loyal disciple. Havana Jesuits, who had taken part in some of Finlay's earlier experiments, also accepted his theory.

Years before the final proof, even years before his own mosquito hypothesis, Finlay had predicted that the plague would be long continuing and that a successful fight against it would be prerequisite for American survival in the tropics. While the medical world generally continued to ridicule his theory, Finlay persevered in trying to find a way to fight yellow fever by immunization. He did noteworthy work in the development of a preventive serum, first reporting it to the Havana Academy of Medicine in 1892—eight years before Walter Reed arrived in Cuba and nearly forty years before North American medical talent had centered its research effort upon a suitable vaccine. Finlay proposed that nonimmune people be inoculated by means of blister serum from an active case of the disease. During 1893 he used such serum for an experimental inoculation of thirteen Spanish artillerymen then in garrison at Havana. Though yellow fever had swept through the garrison many times, none of the thirteen inoculated soldiers had contracted the disease as late as 1895. After that time the Cuban revolution closed Spain's military hospitals to civilians and Finlay was unable to follow his subjects further.

In 1899, after nineteen years of being doubted and discredited, Carlos Finlay received his first recorded support from men of medicine. A pair of famous British physicians, Drs. H. E. Durham and Myers, stopped by Havana on their way to study the yellow fever epidemics of Brazil. They met Finlay and listened. The following year, September 8, 1900, they jointly published in the *British*

Medical Journal an article expressing confidence in the soundness of Finlay's mosquito research.[19]

A year earlier Surgeon General Wyman of the United States Army had assigned Drs. Wasdin and Gedding, two surgeons from the Marine Hospital Service, to make a study of yellow fever etiology. Solemnly Wasdin and Gedding had reported that the *Bacillus icteroides* of Sanarelli is the cause of yellow fever, that the bacillus is found only in yellow fever, and that yellow fever sufferers are infected through the respiratory tract.[20] Within a few months Sternberg succeeded Wyman as surgeon general. He promptly rejected the Wasdin-Gedding report and named a commission of army doctors to study the "acute infectious diseases of Cuba." This was the genesis of the renowned Army Yellow Fever Board. Dr. Walter Reed, of Virginia, of whom more later, was its surgeon and Drs. James Carroll, Aristides Agramonte, and Jesse Lazear were assistant surgeons.

The board voted to give first attention to the etiology and prophylaxis of yellow fever. A yellow fever epidemic was then raging in the Cuban town of Marianao. The board proceeded to that place and set to work with the help of three local physicians, Drs. Nicasio Silverio, Manuel Herrera, and Eduardo Angles, and another, an American physician, Dr. Roger P. Ames, all of whom assisted in clinical diagnosis.

As the following chapter will tell in greater detail, the Army Yellow Fever Board opened its work with a blood analysis of yellow fever patients—checking blood vessels for the alleged *Bacillus icteroides*. Their study resulted in complete contradiction of the Wasdin-Gedding report.

Apparently, the attack on yellow fever was back at the very starting point. The board did not know what caused the disease, or how the cause, whatever it was, got from one person to another. The only thing left to do was to track down all the leads available, however implausible they might sound. It was at this point, and probably very much in this spirit, that Walter Reed and his associates turned to Finlay. As a letter now in the possession of Dr. Carlos E. Finlay, son of the great Cuban, suggests, even Walter Reed was going to take no chance on another blind alley. But he had evidently been reading some of the British medical reports, particularly those of Ronald Ross on malaria, and was interested in the idea of an insect carrier of the disease:

Camp Columbia, Marianao
Oct. 7th., 1900

Dr. Carlos Finlay,
Havana.

My dear Doctor:

I am very sorry that neither Dr. Carroll nor myself can call at your residence this afternoon, as agreed by Dr. C. & yourself, on his visit of yesterday. I shall hope to pay my respects very soon. In the meantime I have taken the liberty of sending my Driver for the British Med. Journal containing Durham and Meyer's note [paper], and for any other articles or publications of yours concerning the Mosquito & Yellow Fever. I have found amongst Dr. Lazear's books your copy of the Anales de la Real Acad. Vol. 18, and am now reading your article. I will take the best of care of any journals or books loaned & will promptly return them.

With best wishes,
Sincerely yours,
Walter Reed.
Maj. & Surg. U.S.A.[21]

And so it was that Walter Reed and his associates became acquainted with Finlay of Havana, but only *after* they had become acquainted with some of Finlay's published work. Carlos Finlay's son describes the meeting more specifically:

Reed then paid a visit to my father who, with characteristic frankness, put at his disposal all of the data he had at hand and gave him samples of the eggs of the *Aedes* mosquito, which he considered responsible for yellow fever transmission. The mosquitoes developed from these eggs were utilized in the experiments of the commission, and a sample, sent to the etomologist of the Department of Agriculture in Washington, was identified by M. L. A. Howard as *Culex fasciatus Fabr.* Regarding the experimental cases previously reported by Finlay, the commission, without entering into their discussion, concluded that he had not been able to produce a real attack of yellow fever within the habitual period of incubation of the disease." [22]

In the manner of a devoted scientist Finlay gave all his findings to medicine and to mankind. Walter Reed and the Army Yellow Fever Board were the fortunate instruments of transmission. The board's extremely arbitrary declaration that in previous experimental cases Finlay had not been able to produce yellow fever was apparently not very charitable. For actually, Walter Reed and his associates accepted Finlay's work in its entirety and used it in their own. It was distinctly unfortunate for American medicine generally that Finlay's pioneer work should not have been accepted more graciously or more justly. Carlos Finlay's son makes this comment:

The brilliant achievements of the commission received the warmest praise from Finlay. He was the first to recognize and applaud their work without the slightest mental reserve. Unfortunately, this attitude was not reciprocated and it was sad to see the members of the commission trying again and again to belittle the value of his experimental cases, practically ignoring his whole work on the subject and tending to attach to themselves the exclusive glory of the discovery. [23]

At the outbreak of the Spanish-American War, Carlos Finlay had been on a vacation with his family at Tampa, Florida. Though sixty-five he immediately offered his services to Surgeon General Sternberg of the United States Army. The surgeon general promptly accepted him, named him an assistant surgeon, and directed him to report at Santiago de Cuba.

Finlay arrived at that picturesque citadel just as American forces took over. At once he went to work at a camp hospital for yellow fever and malaria. In August, 1899, when the United States established the provisional government of Cuba, Carlos Finlay was named chairman of the Yellow Fever Board whose members included Dr. Diego Tamayo, Henry R. Carter, then of the United States Marine Hospital Service, William C. Gorgas of the Army Medical Corps, and John G. Davis, who was acting as chief sanitary officer of Havana. Gorgas, in particular, became Finlay's friend and the two discussed at great length Finlay's theory of mosquito transmission which Gorgas, at that time, amiably and respectfully disbelieved.

Meanwhile Finlay was also closely associated with Walter Reed and the United States Army Yellow Fever Board's highly publicized experiments in Havana and Camp Lazear. From his own amateurish laboratory Finlay supplied the eggs and later the mosquitoes used in these experiments. And when William Gorgas became chief sanitary officer of Havana Carlos Finlay served as his adviser.

In 1902, as the throngs of North Americans took leave of Cuba, Carlos Finlay became chairman of the Cuban Commission of Hygiene and later the same year a member of the National Board of Health named by the provisional government. Estrada Palma, first president of the Republic of Cuba, promptly named Finlay as chief sanitary officer of Cuba, a position which the doctor held until 1909 when, at seventy-six, he was officially retired on pension.

Actually Finlay of Cuba made his early seventies his years of greatest accomplishment. In this period he founded a National Sanitary Board, drafted a superb volume of sanitary regulations, directed Cuba's first independent warfare against mosquito-borne diseases, tuberculosis, tetanus, infantile paralysis, typhoid, and other principal contagions, and instituted nation-wide vaccination against smallpox.

All these were important in sanitation. More important, they were also significant accomplishments in human relations and diplomatic persuasion.

In Cuba, as elsewhere, diseases are a part of the casual patterns of everyday life. Tetanus, for example, had resulted principally from the traditional use of cobwebs as a dressing for the newborn's navel. Finlay perfected an approved antiseptic dressing and was able to enforce popular use of it. Glanders was, commonly, the result of stabling horses and mules in occupied dwellings. Carlos Finlay devised and directed a successful educational program to persuade the poor people to stable their animals outside their homes. He launched a widespread and effective campaign against the spread of typhoid by pollution of drinking water. He directed Cuba's defense against invasions of bubonic plague from Europe and of smallpox and yellow fever from the United States.

During 1905 yellow fever again invaded Cuba, this time from New Orleans. Using the sanitation tactics so skillfully effected by William Gorgas, Finlay and his associates managed to avert another Havana epidemic. When the Estrada Palma government was overthrown other outbreaks of yellow fever occurred in rural areas of the island. At the time of Finlay's retirement—in 1909—these were easily under control.

Study of the *Selected Papers of Carlos Finlay* shows the range of his research. In the field of Cuba's imported diseases he published researches and clinical observations dealing with goiter, trichinosis, and relapsing fever. In the sector of distinctly tropical diseases he wrote of filariasis, beriberi, leprosy, and abscess of the liver. His researches in epidemic diseases dealt principally with cholera. In the field of hygiene and sanitary medicine he contributed notable papers on the control of leprosy, on tuberculosis, and on sanitary statistics. He wrote, too, of the prevention of tetanus in newborn babies and published a classic study of the necessity for physical exercise in tropical lands.

In general medicine, Finlay studied and reported on hernia, anesthesia, electrotherapy, and diseases of the heart. He investigated and reported on eye diseases in the American tropics. He wrote a notable essay on "Scientific Truth," which he delivered as a "discourse" on receiving the degree of Officier of France's Legion of Honor, and another Emersonian discourse presented when he was awarded the Kingsley medal of the Liverpool School of Tropical Medicine.

After an enormously busy half century in medicine Carlos Finlay could not endure the enforced idleness of retirement. His health and enthusiasms began to fail. Juan Guiteras, his loyal friend and co-worker through thirty tiring years, became physician to the great man. Finlay was failing. His speech impediment of earlier years became an ungovernable stutter. A facial palsy constantly harassed him. In August, 1915, after six faltering years of old age, he died at his Havana home. His doctor son, Carlos E. Finlay, describes the last hours of one of the most amazing careers in the history of American medicine:

His end came quite suddenly. That morning I visited him and in our talk I noticed in his conversation some vaguery and some hallucinations. That afternoon at about six o'clock, I was suddenly called to him and found him lying in bed in his last throes. On returning to his room after a cold bath, of which he was very fond, he had fainted. He was breathing, but his pulse was extremely faint. . . . My mother was at his bedside reciting with great fortitude the prayers for the dying, having placed a crucifix in his hands, which she every now and again placed on his lips. A hypodermic of caffein and another of ether failed to revive him, and a priest, who had been sent for, arrived just in time to give him the last rites of his Church and grant him the Papal Benediction.[24]

Although the general public has been slow to understand what a great place Carlos Finlay won for himself in the history of research and preventive medicine, the oversight has been largely confined to the United States and Great Britain. But even in those countries the men who knew have been proud to honor his memory. His own alma mater, Jefferson Medical College, granted him a posthumous LL.D. and named him an Honorary Fellow of the Philadelphia College of Physicians. The Liverpool School of Tropical Medicine also awarded him posthumous honors. France, even during his life, had recognized him for what he was and had made him an Officer of the French Legion of Honor and awarded him the Breant Prize.

But it is in his own country that Finlay has been best remembered, as is only natural, and his greatness most truly appraised. In the court of the Public Health Department's building at Havana you will see an heroic bust of Carlos Juan Finlay. Cuba twice proposed him for the Nobel Prize. Fifteen years ago the Finlay Institute of Havana was founded to do research work in tropical disease and preventive medicine, and in 1928 the Republic of Cuba created the Finlay Order of Merit to recognize outstanding service to public health and charities in that country. Even streets, in Havana and Camagüey, have been named for him.

Wherever the importance of tropical medicine is understood his memory is green. In Panama, the laboratory of the Santo Tomas Hospital was named Laboratorio Carlos Finlay. The Pan American Medical Congress has designated his birthday, December 3rd, as the official Day of American Medicine. In Paris, in 1933, a special session of the Academy of Medicine was dedicated to his memory, and in Madrid, in 1935, the International Congress of History passed a resolution recognizing Finlay's priority in the discovery of the mosquito transmission of yellow fever. That last honor would have meant much to him if he had received it twenty-five years earlier.

So, without assistance, without modern laboratory equipment or endowment, without recognition or just credit, indeed without so much as a friendly nod from his medical brethren of the north, Carlos Finlay, a poor practitioner of Havana, a physician who rarely remembered to charge for his services, not only discovered the origin and transmission of the worst scourge of the Americas but led the way toward its prevention and eradication. For thirty years other medical men and research workers followed the way he had marked out, in quest of a vaccine against yellow fever: Theiler, Sellards, Lloyd, Kitchen, Duval, Monteiro, Chagas, Aragao, Davis, and many others. In Africa and South America heroes of medicine, such as Stokes, Young, Lewis, Haynes, and Noguchi, gave their lives in the century-old struggle to save mankind from yellowjack.

In New York after more than thirty laboratory workers had accidentally contracted the ruinous virus, the Yellow Fever Institute of New York, co-operating with the International Health Board of the Rockefeller Foundation, carried on the work so brilliantly pioneered by Carlos Finlay. During 1921 the Rockefeller Foundation began vaccination against yellow fever for all workers in its International Health Division.

Though reasonably successful, the usefulness of this vaccine was severely limited by scarcity of human serum. Other researchers, including Lloyd, Theiler, and Ricci, developed a more practical formula which substituted tissue virus taken from cultures produced from the blood of immunized monkeys.[25] Improvement followed improvement. Finally the Rockefeller researchers overcame the need of immune serum for the vaccination. Theiler and Smith reported production of a yellow fever virus modified by prolonged culture in a medium of chick embryo tissue as a vaccine. With consequent improvement the latter has become workable vaccine against yellow fever and is now used to protect millions of North Americans, Central Americans, and South Americans from an historically infamous plague which still lingers in many areas south of the Rio Grande, a scourge which might, unless controlled, again sweep across boundaries into the United States.

The great work of Carlos Finlay lives on and continues to bear fruit.

Chapter Five

REED OF VIRGINIA

I N Arlington Cemetery there is a knoll that overlooks the Potomac River and the nation's capital. On that knoll stands a shaft of dark granite five feet high; the bronze tablet on it reads simply:

> Walter Reed, M.D. of the University of Virginia
> A.M. of Harvard University
> LL.D. of the University of Michigan
> Professor of Bacteriology, Army Medical School
> and
> Columbian University, Washington, D. C.
> "He gave to man control over that dreadful scourge,
> Yellow Fever."

A memorial as unpretentious as the man it commemorates, a doctor who was a pioneer among our ambassadors in white and who proved himself one of the greatest of them. If the statement that Reed gave to man control over yellow fever is not quite so valid as it seemed when the monument was erected, the great Virginia doctor's achievement in pointing the way toward saving thousands of lives in every part of the world is not at all belittled by the fact that what he pointed out was the beginning and not the end of the way.

There seems almost to be a pattern in the story of yellow fever. It is a parable in the lesson that all men are brothers and that no one man is sufficient in himself to conquer our bitterest enemies of disease and death. First there was Finlay of Cuba, already introduced to the reader, the intuitive genius who understood the way in which yellow fever must be transmitted but who lacked the driving force to prove his point, and perhaps also the opportunity. After Finlay came Walter Reed, an obscure army doctor who was great enough to understand Finlay's work and able enough to prove it. Yet even Reed's work would have been insufficient to mark the doom of yellow fever had it not been for William C. Gorgas's ability to apply his genius to the practical problem of stopping yellow fever and malaria before they got started. But that is getting ahead of the story.

At the beginning of the century, few people realized that there was a story. There was only a disease and an impractical Cuban and some almost unknown United States Army doctors and privates. It had been played up in the papers but, as few knew what the problem was, few could be interested in the seed of its solution. The war was our first since the Civil War, and in spite of its flag-waving publicity it was proving a comitragedy for the men engaged in it. They were dying like flies, not from bullets but from disease. The swamps of Cuba were more dangerous than San Juan Hill and were taking a greater toll of lives. Even when the fighting was over, the mosquitoes were as unconquered as ever, as dangerous, and as numerous. They failed to evacuate Cuba when the Spanish Army packed up its troubles and, licking its wounds, went home.

The Spanish-American War was, above everything else, a politicians' war. "Pull" was its watchword. On every side army surgeons had been relegated to unimportant posts and friends-who-knew-a-friend were elbowing their way to leadership. Volunteers were dying of needless disease and unpardonable neglect. On every side the Medical Corps was being roundly damned.

In spite of politics and incompetence, in spite of the fact that few of the thinking citizens of the United States supported the war and that most of them did not hesitate to condemn the prosecution of it as imperialistic aggression, it was our first adventure in Latin-American amity. Cuba's liberation was not its chief accomplishment. Those who opposed meddling with Spain's management of her colonies did not foresee what might be the result of the very action they condemned. The American eye for a job to do, however, went with the Caribbean thrust of 1898-1900 and the job which the eye found and which the hand set out to do was the apparently hopeless one of eliminating yellow fever from the American tropics.

Walter Reed's first connection with the appalling medical problems left in the wake of the Spanish-American War was as chairman of a committee appointed by the Army to study the typhoid ravaging the camps throughout the nation's eastern seaboard. In association with Dr. W. C. Vaughn, of the University of Michigan, and Dr. E. O. Shakespeare, of Philadelphia, Reed spent a busy year investigating training camp typhoid and eventually published a report—*Report of the Origin and Spread of Typhoid Fever in the United States Military Camps during the Spanish American War*—which, although not published until long after the death of its compilers, has become something of a medical classic. In this report Majors Reed and Shakespeare contended that infected water was not an important factor in the spread of typhoid; that flies unquestionably act as carriers of the disease; that the development of typhoid was characterized by series of epidemics in companies; that the infection was probably spread, to an additional measure, by blowing dust.

The study was painstaking, fearless, and little noticed. His typhoid report finished, Walter Reed returned to Washington and began to concentrate his thinking on yellow fever, which he preferred to call by its Spanish name—*el vomito negro*—the black vomit.

Until the great Philadelphia epidemic of 1793, men had been inclined to regard the black vomit as a divine punishment. Then con-

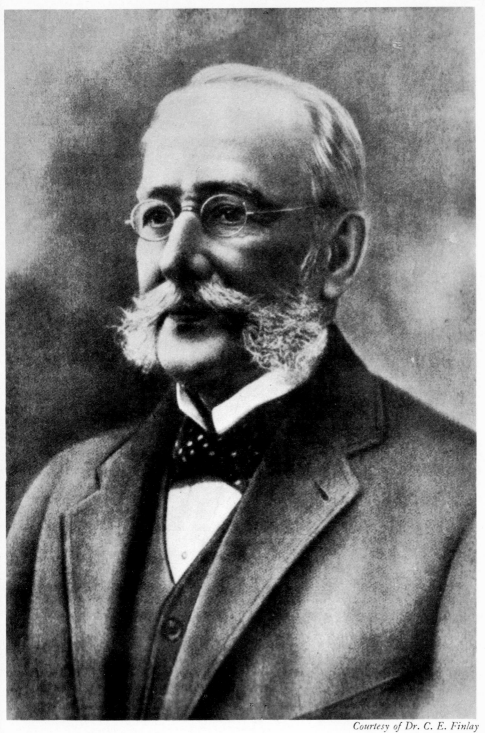

Dr. Carlos Finlay of Cuba.

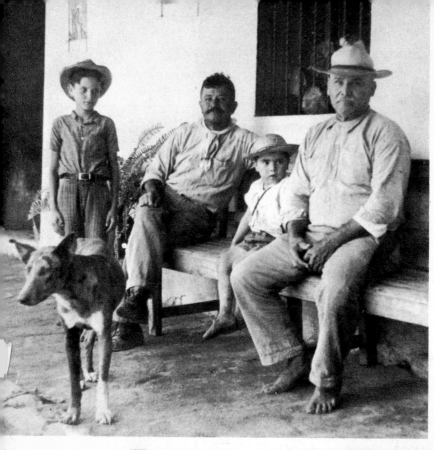

By Iris Woolcock

In Latin Ameri
as elsewhere, g
farmers must
healthy.

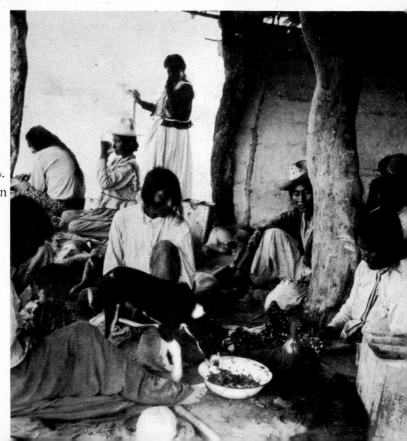

Pictorial Publishing Co.

South American
Indian home.

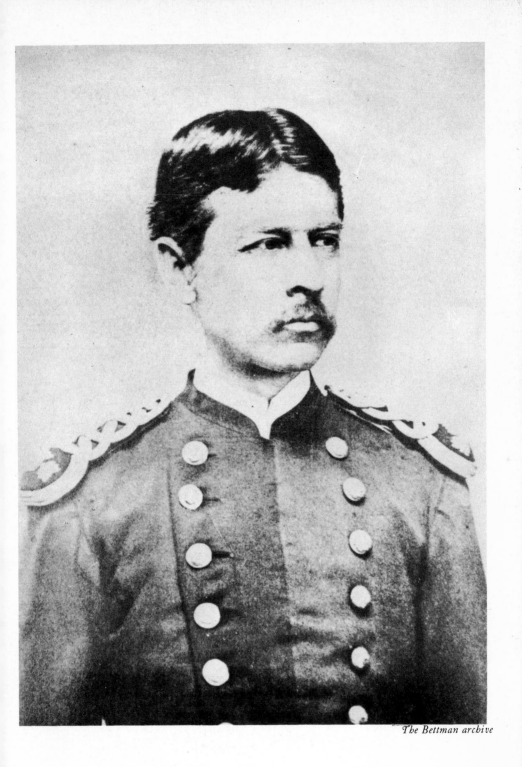

Dr. Walter Reed of Virginia.

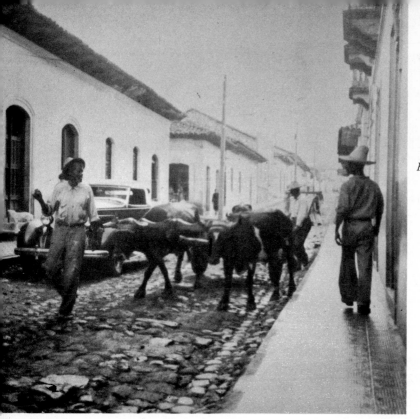

By C. M. Wilson
Street scene,
Tegucigalpa,
Honduras.

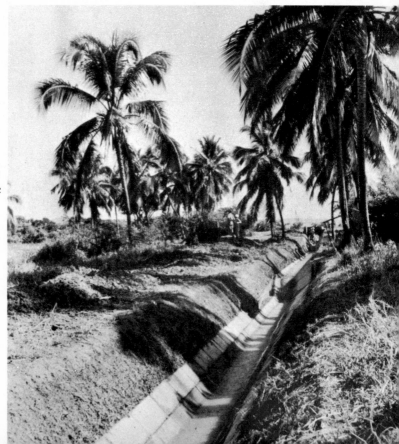

Permission of The Rocke-
feller Foundation Review
Malarial drainage
ditch.

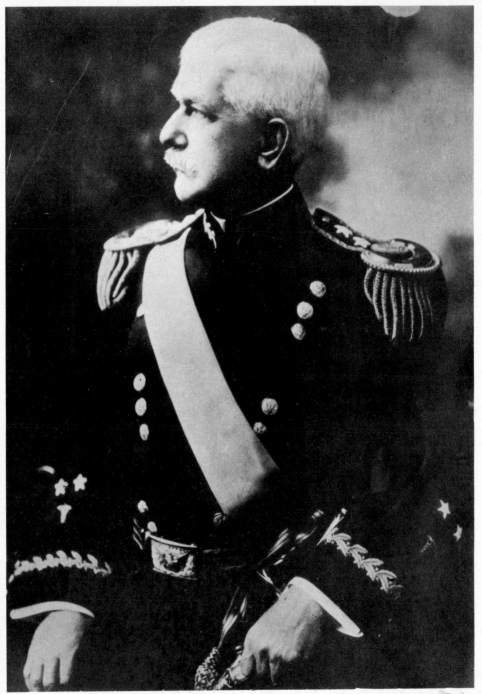

Dr. William Crawford Gorgas.

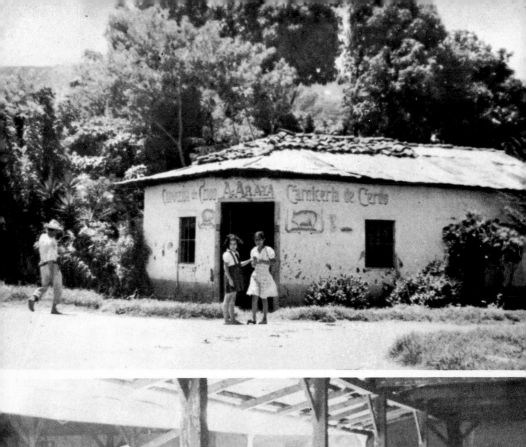

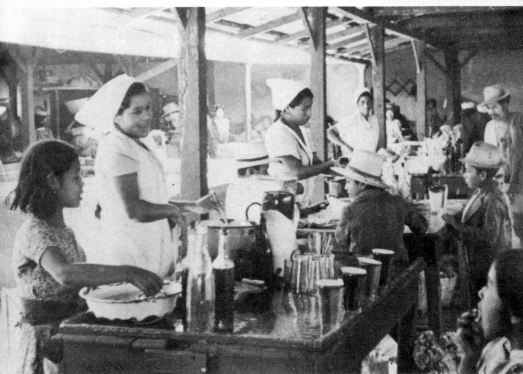

By Iris Woolcock
(Upper) Village butcher shop, Latin American style.

By Iris Woolcock
(Lower) Guatemalan version of the *Yanqui* soda fountain.

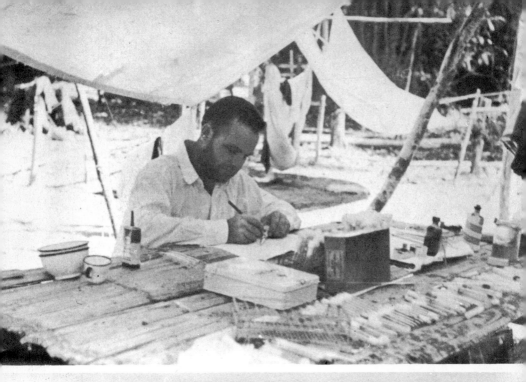

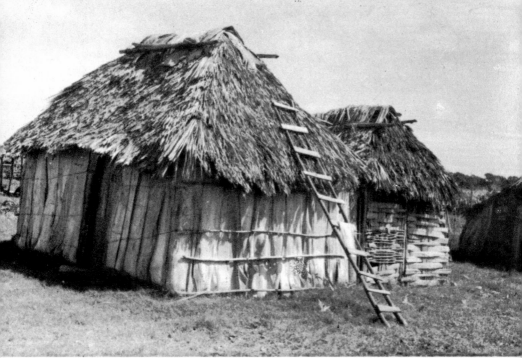

(Upper) Yellow fever expedition in Colombia.

(Lower) Haitian homes built of palms.

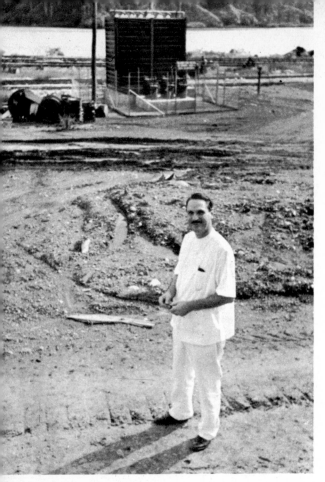

By Iris Woolcock
Dr. Edward Irving Salisbury — Ambassador in White.

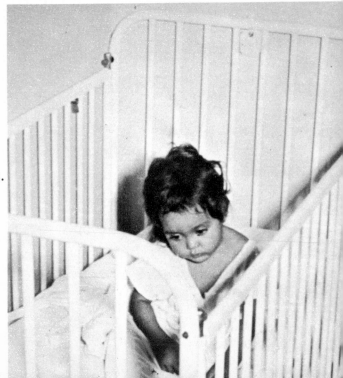

By Iris Woolcock
Sick child of the tropics.

flicting theories began to appear. Some contended that the malady was imported from the West Indies; others that it was a "spontaneous generation" from heat, filth, and moisture. One medical camp held that it was contagious, the other that it was not.

Dr. J. M. Clements, of Louisville, attributed what he called yellow fever "poison" to some order of fungus indigenous to the tropics. A St. Louis physician described it as a principle of fermentation. Dr. P. Stille, of Mobile, attributed the disease to influence of the Gulf Stream. Another physician of the early eighties held that the disease resulted from a subtle poison which exploded in the air. Dr. Warren Stone described it as a wave, or cycle, disease, a theory which, as a supplement to others, is not entirely abandoned today.

Many other rational men attributed the disease to a specific germ. Dr. L. S. Tracy, of New York, observed: ". . . the germs seem to require an appropriate nidus in which to germinate and develop. The germ are portable and may be conveyed in baggage or merchandise . . . for hundreds or thousands of miles."

At the outbreak of the Spanish-American War, man's ignorance of this lethal disease was appalling. Except by Carlos Finlay in Havana, nothing was learned of the yellow plague during the century that saw the actual birth of scientific medicine.

The ability of insects to carry disease was widely recognized, but the actual diseases they carried and their manner of passing them from host to victim was seldom clear. For centuries men of medicine had blamed flies and other winged creatures for the spreading of virtually every infectious or contagious disease known, including leprosy, tuberculosis, black plague, malaria, cholera, anthrax, and a hundred others.

Perhaps the first scientific proof of insect transmission of diseases was established about 1880 by Sir Patrick Manson, who demonstrated beyond reasonable question that the mosquito acts as intermediary host and is thus directly instrumental in the production of elephantiasis scroti and other maladies.

In 1898 the theory of mosquito transmission of disease was respected if not accepted. Koch and Laveran, working independently, had contributed to the incrimination of the mosquito as sole carrier of malaria. By 1894, Major Ronald Ross, of the British Army in India, had identified the anopheles mosquito, dissected it and found in it the unmistakable zygotes of malaria parasites. By 1899 an expedition sent to Sierra Leone by the Liverpool School of Tropical Medicine had confirmed Ross's experiments in India, and the true story of malaria was becoming known throughout the world. But the vital analogy between yellow fever and malaria had not been recognized.

While the Spanish-American War was running its ambiguous course, Surgeon General Sternberg designated Dr. Walter Reed and Dr. James Carroll, a brilliant self-made Canadian bacteriologist, to study, confirm, or disprove the contention of the Italian Giuseppe Sanarelli, who claimed that he had discovered the specific cause of yellow fever in the form of a bacillus which he named *Bacillus icteroides*.

Drs. Reed and Carroll promptly noted that Sanarelli's bacillus was no more than a rather common variety of the hog-cholera bacillus.

Early in 1900 yellow fever appeared among United States troops stationed at Havana. The surgeon general promptly appointed that Yellow Fever Board which was destined to be better known than his own name. Dr. Walter Reed was chairman and director; Dr. James Carroll directed its bacteriological investigations; Dr. Jesse W. Lazear led its mosquito research; Dr. Aristides Agramonte had charge of autopsies and pathological research. Of the four, only Agramonte was immune to yellow fever. In childhood he had proved tough enough to survive an attack. Reed, Carroll, and Lazear, all nonimmunes, were quite evidently risking their lives.

Walter Reed was forty-nine. His skin was sun-browned and leathery. His blackish brown hair, not yet showing a trace of gray, supported its customary frond trailing toward the left brow. Clean shaven during most of his life, he had begun work on a mustache.

James Carroll, second in command, was forty-six, black-haired and growing bald in front. He was tall, rather frail in appearance, strong featured and, like Reed, wore upon his upper lip the heavy badge of his time. His rimless glasses were hooked rather precariously behind his huge ears and his habitual expression was one of great gentleness and infinite curiosity. Quite legitimately, Carroll spoke with a still noticeable British accent. He was English born, a native of Woolwich and schooled in England. When he was fifteen his family had migrated to Canada where he grew to manhood as a frontier farmer and worked his way into medicine. Carroll was married and the father of five children. In voting to risk his life in conquest of yellowjack it was plain that he had much to lose.

Jesse W. Lazear of Baltimore was the third member of the commission. In 1900 he was thirty-four and well established in medical research. Eleven years earlier he had been graduated from Johns Hopkins. Then he had studied medicine at Columbia University, receiving his M.D. in 1892. After two years of internship at Bellevue Hospital, in New York, he studied for a year at the Pasteur Institute in Paris, then returned to become bacteriologist to Johns Hopkins Hospital.

Professionally, Lazear was the ideal man to undertake the experimental study of yellow fever. At Bellevue he had begun investigation of malaria parasites. He had left Johns Hopkins and his beginning family and proceeded to Cuba early in 1900. There he had been observing yellow fever, performing autopsies, and taking blood cultures.

Lazear was handsome and black-haired. With him the mustache was encouraged to extend itself in whiskers. He was slow-spoken, timid, and extravagantly modest. He worked doggedly, almost fiercely, claimed little, loved his profession and his family. A second son had been born to the Lazears since the young father's arrival in Cuba, a child whom Jesse Lazear was never to see.

The fourth and youngest member of the board was the handsome, thirty-two-year-old Cuban, Aristides Agramonte, son of the illustrious insurgent General Eduardo Agramonte who was killed in battle when Aristides was only four. The general's bereaved family found refuge in the United States. Aristides was raised in New York, attended the public schools of that city, and like Lazear, studied medicine at Columbia. Early in 1898, Agramonte joined the United States Army Medical Corps and was promptly sent to Cuba for duty. Late in the year he was ordered to Havana to study the bacteriology of yellow fever. During May, 1901, he was made director of the Army Laboratory of the Division of Cuba.

Agramonte knew yellow fever and he knew Cuba. At the barracks of Pinar del Rio, he diagnosed an epidemic of yellowjack in open contradiction to medical officers who had termed the contagion "pernicious malaria." Agramonte ridiculed their ignorance. He was in line for appointment as professor of bacteriology and experimental pathology at the University of Havana; he was a Cuban returning to his native land; a brilliant and charming Cuban who neither respected nor feared the pompousness of United States medicine.

These were the four men who were about to make history. On the first day of summer Drs. Reed and Carroll sailed from New York en route to Havana. By early July the Yellow Fever Board was assembled and at work. On the last day of July, Walter Reed made his first yellow fever autopsy in Cuba. During the same month yellow fever had appeared in an army guardhouse—a single cell occupied by nine prisoners. One contracted yellow fever and died in the post hospital twelve days later. The eight other prisoners in the one-room guardhouse did not take the disease. One slept in the bed vacated by the sick man. But he remained in good health.

Walter Reed pondered: As these nine prisoners had been kept under strict military guard, it was impossible that the individual attacked could have acquired his infection in the town of Pinar del Rio, although Lazear had shown that yellow fever existed there. The sick man simply could not have been there. He was, so far as could be ascertained, exposed to no source of infection to which his companions had not been equally exposed, and yet he alone acquired the disease. It was conjectured at the time that perhaps some insect . . . such as the mosquito, had entered through the cell window, bitten this particular prisoner, and then passed out again.[1] . . .

He had heard of the comments of a pair of English physicians, on the ideas which Carlos Finlay's work had given them. He wrote Finlay, as already indicated, asking for more information. He was perhaps a little cold, afraid of showing too much interest in a suggestion that might turn out to be nonsense. His coldness was met by Finlay—with generous enthusiasm. The Cuban, more interested in results than in credit for them, offered the American commission his notes, his help, his materials, and the use of his laboratory. Reed may have been cold but he was far from mulish. It was not long before he realized that the clue to the solution of the yellow fever problem had for twenty years been in existence in Carlos Finlay's shrewd but unresolved work. Finlay, with that same imaginative inference which gave to the ancient Greeks scientific knowledge far in advance of their time, believed that the mosquito was the disseminating agent in yellow fever.

Walter Reed was Virginia born, a Methodist preacher's son. The family was English, descended from Sir Christopher Reed, of Steeplechase Castle on Tyne. Walter's father, the Reverend Lemuel Sutton Reed, suffered the misfortune of having been born outside the Old Dominion—in North Carolina. But a ministerial career of more than forty years spent in Virginia helped somewhat to expiate the misfortune of his birth. Pharaba White was Walter Reed's mother, Parson Reed's first wife, and the daughter of a Carolina plantation owner.

In Virginia, five children were born to Lemuel and Pharaba Reed. Laura, the daughter, grew up to marry J. W. Blincoe, of the Virginia Blincoes. The four male Reeds were James, Thomas, Christopher, and Walter; the last and youngest born in Gloucester County, September 13, 1851.

When Walter was five, Parson Reed and his family were "called" to Farmville, picturesque tobacco capital of Prince Edward County. The Reed children were entered in an extremely respectable private school kept by a Mrs. Booker. Little Walter Reed may have been somewhat misplaced in so proper a school. At six, according to his brother Christopher, Walter had learned to chew tobacco and spit, to make the rounds of the Farmville tobacco warehouses, sampling a chew of each stock.

Walter was ten when the Civil War began. The Reverend Lemuel Reed stayed with his church and charges. For a time Prince Edward County waited as a somewhat accidental oasis of peace, until Sheridan's Raiders began to sweep the countryside, pillaging, burning, and stealing.

One summer day a Rebel courier rode into Farmville to give warning of the approach of the Raiders. Parson Lem Reed sent his two younger sons to hide the Reed horses. Walter and Christopher tethered the horses within a bushy bend of a near-by river and, confident that the hiding place was secure, shucked their clothes and went swimming. While the boys were in the river, a posse of Raiders appeared and captured them. When the horses had been appropriated the Yankees released the naked hostages, to the accompaniment of a comment from Walter that an army of horse thieves is "a damned sorry kind of establishment."

When the Civil War ended, Virginia was a place of death, of poverty, and a gallant but far from confident determination to rise from its own ashes. When Walter Reed's mother died the Reverend Lemuel moved his family, his library, and his ministry to Charlottesville. The four older children were approaching college age. Walter, then fifteen, attended two semesters of private school kept by a Mr. Abbott, who thought Walter a good student of history and literature but a poor scientist.

The next year Walter entered the University of Virginia. But James, Thomas, and Christopher had preceded him, and the Reverend Lemuel Reed was poor. Walter, rather tall, handsome, sensitive featured and cavalierish, withdrew from college on the condition that he might study at home for the medical examination. He had asked the university's medical faculty if he could be granted the degree of Doctor of Medicine, provided he could pass the prescribed examination. The faculty said yes, considering it a promise they would never be asked to keep.

After nine months of study, Walter reported for the traditionally terrifying examination. He passed third highest in a class of about forty. Dean Maupin, presenting Virginia's diplomas, commented that Walter Reed was the youngest student ever graduated from the medical school at Charlottesville, and one of the very few who had been able to complete the exacting course in one year. Many had tried. Men in their thirties had broken down under attempts to "stand exam" within a year, but here a boy of seventeen had easily managed one of the most difficult medical examinations known to the United States of 1869.

At the unripe age of seventeen, therefore, Walter Reed became a doctor, without attending medical school or visiting a patient. The following year he journeyed to New York with his brother Christopher, who practiced law while Walter entered Bellevue Hospital Medical College and went on to earn another degree of Doctor of Medicine within one year.

Properly graduated from Bellevue, Walter Reed spent a year as intern at Kings County Hospital and at Randalls Island Clinic. Then he became a "public health physician," or charity doctor for New York slums. He worked hard and conscientiously and sometimes the spirit of his earnestness was, if we are to believe his brother Christopher, overcome by intense dejection.

Reed was capable and charming. His high forehead was pleasantly freckled. His large blue eyes were curious and young. His neatly combed hair was a glistening black. Only twenty-two, he could have been mistaken for seventeen. He was, however, already a good doctor. His charity work attracted the attention of Dr. Joseph C.

Hutchinson, a ranking physician and surgeon of Brooklyn. Dr. Hutchinson recommended Reed's appointment as one of the five medical inspectors of the Brooklyn Board of Health; salary $65 per month and free office space.

The Brooklyn of 1870 was in far more acute need of medical inspectors than of the private physicians among whom Reed hoped to be numbered. One day Christopher Reed found his younger brother unusually depressed. He inquired the reasons and Walter answered:

. . . today an elegant rig with coachman and footman stopped in front of my office, and a finely dressed gentleman came in, introducing himself as Dr. ——, and saying that he wished to report the death of a child. He was so grossly ignorant that he could not use medical nomenclature correctly or even state symptoms.

I then asked him if he didn't think it was such a disease (using the Latin term) and he answered "yes" repeating the words backward. Yet this man has the leading practice in this part of Brooklyn, although he is a first-class quack. I am disgusted. . . .[2]

In June, 1873, while on a visit to his father in Murfreesboro, North Carolina, the young doctor had the good fortune to meet a young lady named Emilie Lawrence, daughter of a successful Murfreesboro planter. After his return to Brooklyn, Walter wrote to Emilie:

Brooklyn, July 18, 1874

. . . I have made up my mind to make a strenuous effort to enter the Medical Corps of the U. S. Army. . . . The Board of Health are requiring more work of the inspectors every day, and to such a degree that the idea of a private practice cannot be thought of. . . . These great cities have lost the fascination which formerly held me so fast. Four years ago I would have remained here though the heavens fall. . . . But since then a few springs have come and gone, and though no gray hairs adorn my head, I have become a little wiser, I have carefully noted the success or failure of those around me and I have watched them in their sorrows and joys. Yet during this time I have been unable to discover the great advantage of living in the metropolitan cities, except it be in "wear and tear."

I have still a third reason. Having entered my profession about five years earlier than is the custom, I have experienced all the troubles of a youthful aspirant for honors. As long as my success depended upon actual knowledge and experience, I managed to overcome all obstacles, but the moment that I entered upon the race of life, I at once found out the disadvantages of a youthful appearance. *It is a remarkable fact that a man's success during the first decade depends more upon his beard than his brains!* And inasmuch as I could boast of none of the former, and but an infinitesimal quantity of the latter, I found "Jordan to be a hard road to travel!" [3]

A few weeks later Reed again wrote to Emilie:

Brooklyn, Aug. 12, 1874

One thing I will not permit to forsake me is my courage. . . . I went over to New York . . . and had a long talk with the recorder of the examining board. To my utter astonishment he informed me that candidates must stand an examination in Latin, Greek, mathematics and history in addition to medical subjects. Horror of horrors! Imagine me conjugating an irregular verb or telling what x plus y equals, or what year Rome was founded or the Battle of Marathon fought! Why, the thing is impossible! I shall utterly fail. Add to this each applicant is examined five hours each day for six successive days—thirty hours questioning and, to cap the climax, there are more than 500 applicants for less than 30 vacancies. The very thought of it makes me dizzy. Think of my condition and pity me.[4]

Within another month Reed was knocked out by overwork and anxiety. But when examination week finally came, he was on hand, and he was again an honor man. June of 1875 found him assistant surgeon with the rank of first lieutenant in the United States Army Medical Corps on duty at Willets Point, New York Harbor, and, to his way of thinking no less of a distinction, engaged to Emilie Lawrence.

On the fifteenth of the following September, Reed wrote of the passing of his twenty-fifth birthday:

Willets Point, Sept. 15, 1875

Alas, my 25th birthday has passed and what have I to show for it! What good deeds have I done that merit approbation! How negligent and wayward I have been! What golden moments of opportunity have come and gone, all unheeded. As I look back over my past life tonight but few thoughts occur to me such as cause my bosom to swell with honest pride.[5]

Perhaps this somewhat callow humility was for Emilie's benefit. At least it had no adverse effect upon her. When he again visited Murfreesboro it was to plan for their marriage. During the spring of 1876, however, after the wedding arrangements had been made and the invitations sent out, the Surgeon General's Office ordered Reed to proceed at once to Arizona. Although this surgeon general apparently expected the young officer to put off his marriage, Reed did nothing of the sort. He simply moved up his wedding date to April 25, 1876, and two weeks later set out to his command alone.

Emilie followed her husband during the next October, traveled by train to San Francisco, encountering blizzards, a railroad wreck, and other mishaps. The newlyweds met at San Diego, where Reed waited with a four-mule army ambulance, painted white, a driver, a surgery case, and several rifles. It was a twenty-day wagon trip through the desert to Fort Lowell, Arizona.

The bone-jolting route lay through a series of outposts, or stations, one-house hamlets separated by incredibly rough roads, untrustworthy Indians, and infinite discomforts. Emilie was twenty and game. Rifles swung from the ambulance ceiling, cooking utensils, food supplies, and extra clothes were packed ingeniously. Emilie topped the load with a little white dog named Undina.

In a letter to his sister-in-law, Mrs. N. F. Harrell, Reed described the journey:

. . . On the back seat was Emilie, the dog Undina; under the back seat, medicine, lunch basket, bag of cooking utensils. Under front seat, mess chest, tableware, provisions and clothes baskets containing everything from hairpins to pair of shoes. Suspended from various points of the roof were two hats, a sword, an umbrella, a pair of E's shoes, a carbine, a pistol, a belt full of cartridges and 2 canteens filled with water.

. . . Underneath the driver's seat in front were my private case of instruments, weighing 50 pounds, a sack of grain and the driver's rations for 10 days; on the seat behind, my trunk and bedding consisting of a mattress, blanket, etc., done up in a canvas. . . . If there was anything on top I did not see it. I have a lurking idea, however, that the driver concealed several chairs and boxes in odd places about the vehicle. I forgot to say that beside the driver was a corporal on the seat with him, a very light man weighing just two hundred pounds. . . .

Thus equipped, after bidding goodbye to our Lowell friends, we started for Camp Apache, external temperature 110 degrees. As Undina had never before ridden in a vehicle, she straightway set up a terrific barking, which she kept up until she was so hoarse she couldn't hear herself, then stopped. . . . Perhaps you have never taken what is called a flying lunch. If not, let me tell you, you have missed a great deal of fun. Mind you, everything connected with the meal is done with the ambulance in full progress—and the road is very rough and rocky . . . the feat of getting anything into your mouth becomes a matter of considerable uncertainty. . . .[6]

In the early West, army paydays came every second month. Beginning with payday it was traditional for common soldiers to spend a few days, or even a week, happily and often belligerently drunk, while officers indulged in prolonged bouts with whisky-and-soda. On the whole, the United States Army of 1877 was nothing to boast of. Its personnel languished and died of needless sickness. Its leadership was notoriously political. Too frequently common soldiers were brutally abused by officers who were frequently small-caliber politicians in gold braid.

At Camp Apache, in the farthest wilds of Arizona, the Reeds remained for four years close to each other, to nature, and to hard work. In 1877 their first child was born, a son named Walter Lawrence.

Life at the army post was both colorful and grim. Walter Reed,

still handsome, black-haired and boyish, made the best of it. When
their son was born, a "high private in the rear rank" became cus-
todian of the Reed household. "On one occasion he served the soup
in the cream pitcher, on another day on lifting the lid of the soup
toureen what should I find but half-a-dozen peach dumplings re-
posing therein. . . . A few days later when I attempted to fill my
glass with water and found instead boiled potatoes in the pitcher,
I may have betrayed some momentary surprise, but I think
not. . . ." [7]

Walter Reed was sole physician for Camp Apache and for hundreds of square miles of adjacent God-forsaken frontier. He attended the military sick. He stuffed his saddlebags with instruments
and medicine and rode through desolate countrysides, attending to
the needs of the widely separated and poverty-stricken inhabitants.
He set broken bones, he delivered babies, tended diphtheria cases,
struggled with typhoid and many other maladies which tyrannized
the pioneers. He also doctored sick Indians. One day he returned to
Camp Apache with an Indian child swung to his saddle, a little girl
four or five years who had been severely burned in an open fire
and abandoned by her Apache family to die. Walter Reed took the
child into his home, nursed her to recovery and kept her for some
years as a companion to his own children, until she ran away and
disappeared into the desert from which she had come.

As the years went on, Reed came to be known as "the Indian
doctor." Indians frequently showed their gratitude to him with gifts
of venison. "If no one was in the house to receive it, they would
walk in stealthily and lay it on Mrs. Reed's dressing table, or
perhaps take a picture from the wall and hang the venison in its
stead." [8]

After four years in Arizona, Walter Reed was promoted to the
rank of captain. During 1891, a great and important change came
in his life. He was given a brief assignment to Fort McHenry,
Baltimore, Maryland. He became acquainted with Johns Hopkins

Hospital and had an opportunity to study physiology. It was too good to last. Soon the Reeds were again shunted to the West—to Fort Omaha. There in Nebraska, the captain found a fresh opportunity to indulge his taste for helping his fellow men, but his medical studies languished. He did his best among the "grangers," newly settled dryland farmers who toiled and suffered, hoped and died while waiting for rain. After five years in western Nebraska, during which time his daughter, Emilie Lawrence, was born, he was sent to Mount Vernon Barracks near Mobile, Alabama. One more Southerner eagerly discovered the South. Although he was busy and happy in Alabama, he was glad to be transferred again to Baltimore as attending surgeon and examiner of recruits.

It was a fortunate assignment for Reed and for the nation; indeed, for all the Americas. Johns Hopkins Hospital was allowing visiting physicians an opportunity to study clinical medicine, surgery, and laboratory methods. Walter Reed took up the study of pathology and bacteriology. It was meat and drink to him to be among men of real caliber, to be accepted by them. The great Dr. William Welch became his particular friend and leader. The science of bacteriology was emerging from its swaddling clothes with the help of the many great medical men who were assembled at the university. Abbott and Flexner were studying diphtheria, a toxin of which had newly been discovered; Councilman and Lafleur were working on amoebic dysentery; Clement and Welch were on the track of the hog-cholera bacillus, so easily and frequently confused with the bacillus of yellow fever. There was plenty of stimulus and plenty of opportunity. Reed studied and learned with the rest of them. As an initial subject, he chose the lymphoid nodules which afflict the livers of typhoid sufferers . . .

This year at Johns Hopkins was the turning point in Reed's life. From then on he was not simply an army doctor. He was a man of science, a man of wisdom and imagination. Although he again was ordered to North Dakota for another two years of garrison duty, it must have been clear to him where he was really going. During

1893 he was returned for duty in the Surgeon General's Office at Washington. The United States Army Medical School was being established and Walter Reed was to be its professor of bacteriology and clinical microscopy, as well as curator of the army medical museum. He was promoted to the grade of surgeon with the military rank of major.

After eighteen years in garrisons, and fifteen changes of station, Walter Reed at forty-two found himself a scientist in his own right. His gay spirit was unconquered. His hair was still black. His Virginia drawl lingered. His features and bearing were amazingly young.

This was the man who found his great opportunity in the work of the Army Yellow Fever Board in Havana from 1900 to 1902. The opportunity came in the homemade laboratory of Carlos Finlay. There Walter Reed became acquainted at first hand with the suspected mosquito, *Stegomyia fasciata* (now called *Aëdes aegypti*).

Reed observed the distinguishing characteristics of this particular genus: the silvery stripe on the lateral surface of the thorax and the white stripes at the base of the tarsal joints. He reflected on its special mode of existence—its preference for breeding places in clean, standing water, and realized that water of this kind was to be found principally in towns. The female, he found, laid her eggs at night—twenty-five to seventy to the "raft." The eggs were jet black and unusually tough. Freezing, even, did not easily destroy them. Stored in a dry box for three months they would still hatch.[9]

Reed, Carroll, Lazear, and Agramonte agreed that practical tests with human subjects was the next necessary step in proving Finlay's mosquito-transmission theory. That meant serious responsibility and serious risk. The four doctors agreed that members of the commission should not hesitate to take as much risk with their own lives as they asked of others. They resolved that each person subjected to the experiment should be a volunteer and fully informed of his risk.

Late in July, without forewarning and for no clearly convincing reason, Walter Reed was recalled to Washington. During his absence, Jesse Lazear was elected to begin experiments. He acquired a collection of yellow fever-infected stegomyia mosquitoes hatched from eggs furnished by Carlos Finlay. He imprisoned them and allowed them to bite himself and several other subjects. At first there were no results. Then Dr. Lazear applied another infected mosquito to Dr. James Carroll's arm. The experiment was immediately successful. Within four days the meditative James Carroll was writhing with yellow fever.

By September 13th, Carroll's recovery was comparatively certain. On that day Dr. Jesse Lazear was at work in the yellow fever ward of Las Animas Hospital in the suburbs of Havana. A mosquito settled on his hand. Lazear noticed the uninvited guest but believed it "a common ordinary brown mosquito." He allowed it to bite. Five days later, while James Carroll was leaving the hospital, Dr. Lazear was seized with a violent chill. Carroll examined his blood for malaria parasites; finding none, he termed the illness yellow fever.

The young man from Baltimore delivered his notes to Dr. Carroll and moved to the yellow fever isolation ward of the hospital. For three days he held his own. Then the dread black vomit made its appearance. His diaphragm contracted spasmodically. His eyes showed tense alarm. On the sixth day he died.

In a sense, Lazear's death was accidental. But it was also gallant and valuable to the Americas and to medicine.

Walter Reed, still in Washington, considered the evidence invincible. A month after Lazear's death he told the Indianapolis convention of the American Public Health Association that "the mosquito acts as the intermediate host for the parasite of yellow fever." [10]

But further proof was needed. The next step was the founding of Camp Lazear, in a sunny open pasture about one mile from the town of Los Quemados, Cuba, also a focus of yellow fever. Walter Reed took command. The original camp consisted of seven army tents and a flagstaff from which waved the Stars and Stripes. Reed, Carroll, and Agramonte moved to the location, taking with them Dr. Roger P. Ames, an immune, and Dr. Robert P. Cooke, a nonimmune, both of the Army Medical Corps; nine privates of the Hospital Corps, one of whom was immune, and an immune ambulance driver.

They established the camp in November of 1900 under strict quarantine—only the three immune men were allowed to leave or to re-enter. Temperature and pulse of all nonimmune residents were recorded three times daily so that any infected person entering the camp could be detected and removed.

Walter Reed and his associates proposed to try to produce the infection of nonimmunes in three ways—by the bites of mosquitoes which had previously bitten yellow fever patients; by the injection of blood taken during the early stages from those suffering from the disease; by exposure to fomites. To supplement the seven tents which quartered the camp's personnel, Reed directed the construction of two frame buildings, each fourteen by twenty feet and alike except that one, the "Infected Mosquito Building," was divided near the middle by a permanent wire screen partition and had good ventilation while the other, the "Infected Clothing Building," was purposely built to exclude ventilation. The houses were placed about eighty yards apart on opposite sides of a small valley, and both were provided with wire-screen windows and double-screen doors so that mosquitoes could be kept inside or outside as the experimenters desired.

The first need was for human subjects. Walter Reed called for volunteers among the troops. The first to answer were two boy privates from Ohio: John R. Kissinger, of the Hospital Corps, and John J. Moran, a headquarters clerk. Walter Reed explained to them the proposed experiment, pointing out the danger and suffering likely to be involved. When the youths expressed their willingness to go ahead, Walter Reed offered an official money reward.

Both young men refused to accept the money. Private Kissinger explained that he had volunteered "solely in the interest of humanity and the cause of science."

Walter Reed knew a hero when he saw one. He drew himself up before Kissinger and Moran and saluted his subordinates. "Gentlemen, I salute you!" he said.[11]

Private Kissinger was the first volunteer. On December 5th he permitted himself to be bitten by five *Aëdes aegypti* mosquitoes which had bitten yellow fever patients from fifteen to twenty-two days previously. Three days later Private Kissinger, who had been under strict quarantine for fifteen days, was seized with a chill which proved to be the beginning of yellow fever.

Walter Reed and his men, even Private Kissinger, were delighted. The commanding officer of Camp Lazear wrote to his wife:

Rejoice with me, sweetheart, as aside from the antitoxin of diphtheria and Koch's discovery of the tubercle bacillus, this will be regarded as the most important piece of work scientifically during the 19th century. . . . I do not exaggerate and I could shout for very joy. . . . It was Finlay's theory and he deserves great credit for having suggested it, but as he did nothing to prove it, it was rejected by all, including General Sternberg. Now we have put it beyond cavil. . . . Major Kean says that the discovery is worth more than the cost of the Spanish War, including lives lost and money expended. . . . I suppose that old Dr. Finlay will be delighted beyond bounds, as he will see his theory at last fully vindicated. 9:30 P.M. Since writing the above our patient has been doing well. . . . Everything points, so far as it can at this stage, to a favorable termination for which I feel so very happy.[12]

Two days later Reed again wrote to his wife:

Our patient . . . is doing very well. We had Dr. John Guiteras, Dr. Finlay and Dr. Albertini over here to see him yesterday afternoon. . . . Dr. Albertini did not hesitate to say "yellow fever." The others too regarded the case as one of probable yellow fever, but desired to see how his temperature and pulse would run during the next few days. Dr. Amadon, an expert in yellow fever, says the disease is undoubtedly that. . . . The case is as plain as the nose on a man's face. . . . Ah! wonderful is nature, and I thank God that he has allowed poor unworthy me to look a little way into this secret. Six months ago, when we landed on this island, absolutely nothing was known concerning the propagation and spread of yellow fever—it was all an unfathomable mystery—but today the curtain has been drawn—its mode of propagation. is established, and we know that a case minus mosquitoes is no more dangerous than one of chills and fever! Hurrah! [13]

At Camp Lazear, during the week that followed, four more cases of yellow fever were produced with the help of mosquitoes. Spanish immigrants, who had breezed into the camp and described mosquitoes as "little flies that buzz harmlessly about our tables," began to lose their courage. Spurning their agreements and specified rewards of $250 in gringo gold the Andalusians began to run. But United States troops continued to volunteer.

Meanwhile the fomite experiment was in progress. Three soldiers —Private Levi E. Folk, of South Carolina; Private Warren G. Jernegan, of Florida; Dr. Robert P. Cooke, of Virginia and the Army Medical Corps—all Southerners and nonimmunes, moved into the "Fomite House," sleeping in the filthy bedding of yellow fever patients, wearing castoff soiled clothes of yellow fever patients, and adorning their cells with all manner of contaminated articles reckoned to spread the contagion by direct exposure. In his paper, *The Etiology of Yellow Fever*, Walter Reed described the experiment:

On November 30 . . . three large boxes filled with sheets, pillow-slips, blankets, etc., contaminated by contact with cases of yellow fever and their discharges were received and placed there. The majority of the articles had been taken from the beds of patients sick with yellow fever at Las Animas Hospital, Havana, or at Columbia Barracks. Many of them had been purposely soiled with a liberal quantity of black vomit, urine and fecal matter. A dirty "comfortable" and much soiled pair of blankets, removed from a bed of a patient sick with yellow fever in the town of Quemados, were contained in these boxes. The same day at 6 P.M. Dr. Robert P. Cooke, Acting Assistant Surgeon, U.S.A., and two privates of the hospital corps, Folk and Jernegan, all nonimmune young Americans, entered this building and deliberately unpacked these boxes, which had been tightly closed and locked for a period of two weeks. These soiled sheets, pillow cases and blankets were used in preparing the beds in which the members of the hospital corps slept. Various soiled articles were hung around the room and placed about the bed occupied by Dr. Cooke.[14]

For twenty days the three *norteamericanos* followed through the repulsive experiment. After twelve days a fourth box of contaminated clothing and linen from Las Animas Hospital was distributed about the room, while heat and humidity were kept high. On December 19th the three experimenters were placed in quarantine for five days, then given the liberty of the camp. All had remained in perfect health.

After fifteen days in the pesthouse, the three volunteers heard of the successes with mosquito infection. . . . The observing Walter Reed noted:

With the occurrence of these cases of mosquito infection the countenances of these men, which had before borne the serious aspect of those who were bravely facing an unseen foe, suddenly took on the glad expression of school boys let out for a holiday, and from this time their contempt for "fomites" could not find sufficient expression. Thus illustrating once more the old adage that familiarity, even with fomites, may breed contempt! [15]

The fomite experiment was repeated three times. Volunteers slept in nightshirts that had been worn by yellow fever patients. Still they did not contract the disease.

With the fomite theory blasted, the next challenge was to show just how a house becomes infected with yellow fever. Accordingly, on December 21st, fifteen stegomyia mosquitoes, contaminated with yellow fever at intervals of five to twenty-four days previously, were released in one screened-in compartment of the Infected Mosquito

Building. Five minutes after the mosquitoes were released, Field Clerk John J. Moran, who had been in quarantine for thirty-two days, freshly bathed and clad only in his nightshirt, entered the mosquito room and lay down on the bed. On the other side of the partition, where no mosquitoes were allowed to enter, three more volunteers took up residence.

On Christmas morning, four days later, Army Clerk Moran was stricken with yellow fever. Luckily the gallant Ohioan recovered. The nonimmunes on the other side of the screen partition remained in perfect health during fifteen days of confinement.

On New Year's night, 1900, Walter Reed wrote his wife:

It has been permitted me and my assistants to lift the impenetrable veil that has surrounded the causation of this most wonderful, dreadful pest of humanity and put it on a rational and scientific basis. . . . The prayer that has been mine for twenty years, that I might be permitted in some way or at some time to do something to alleviate human suffering has been granted.[15]

The work at Camp Lazear was ended. The last successful case of mosquito infection was made February 7, 1901. Three days earlier Walter Reed had delivered a report of the Camp Lazear findings to the convention of the Pan-American Congress which met at Havana. The report was graciously received. Reed reported to his wife: "I received dozens of the warmest kind of handshakes from Cuban, Spanish, Mexican, South American physicians, men whom I had never met. . . . The hall was crowded and even the doors packed with listeners. It was a signal triumph for our work."[17]

Its work done, the Yellow Fever Board disbanded. Agramonte remained at Havana, a full-fledged member of the faculty of medicine. James Carroll returned to New York and Washington in company with Walter Reed. Yellow fever was being beaten from Cuba. Lives were being saved. For the American tropics a new era was dawning.

Reed appeared weary on his return to Washington. After Cuba he found the atrocious Potomac climate more than customarily distressing. Work waited and, rather eagerly, Walter Reed returned to it. His fame had spread far. But at fifty he was still harassed by lack of means.

A century earlier the British government had rewarded Edward Jenner, the country doctor of Gloucestershire who discovered small-pox vaccination, with a grant of £30,000. In France the great Pasteur, besides numerous honors, received a government pension of 12,000 gold francs a year. Joseph Lister, England's originator of antiseptic surgery, was made physician, knight, peer, and wealthy man in return for his achievements. In terms of human needs, the great findings and proofs of yellow fever were perhaps as beneficial to mankind as the work of Lister or Jenner. Together with the discovery of anesthesia, the yellow fever findings were the leading contribution to medicine of the United States. But the nation which spends millions for prize fights and fireworks displays, which now appropriates billions and tens of billions on war and devastation, granted Walter Reed no reward in money. Even his promised military promotion never actually came. Only after his death did Congress grant his widow a pension.

In spite of the harassment of his comparative poverty, Walter Reed's greatest work was done after he returned from Cuba, although he did not know, any more than most of the world knew, what it was that he had done. Little more than a year of life was left him, as it turned out.

During that year he became a teacher, one of the best in all the great roster of medical pedagogy. At the Army Medical School he was professor of pathology and clinical microscopy; at Columbian University, Washington, of pathology and bacteriology—hard subjects all, bristling with unsolved problems and clumsy nomenclature. But Reed studied while he taught. He led and encouraged. He gesticulated and accented. He remained patient and kind and he was inspiring. But he was tired. His posture was less erect. His step grew heavier.

Near Monterey, Pennsylvania, Walter Reed built a summer cottage, changed a barren rocky field into a modestly pleasant homestead. During June, 1902, he went with his wife to Cambridge, where he received Harvard's honorary degree of Master of Arts. A few weeks later the University of Michigan, not to be outdone, awarded him an LL.D. He spent more and more time with his family, regretting that his son had grown away from him. He cherished the company of his daughter and his wife. Frequently he rode horseback among the Virginia and Pennsylvania hills. He talked much of earlier days on the dying frontiers.

Throughout the autumn of 1902 he had been in poor health. On Wednesday, November 12th, he left his office early and remarked to his wife that his lunch had evidently not agreed with him. That night he was too sick to deliver his lecture at the medical school.

Next day he got out of bed, but complained of stomach pains which caused him to limp. On Friday, Major Reed approached his old friend, Major W. C. Borden, also of the Army Medical Corps, and diagnosed his own sickness as appendicitis. Dr. Borden made an examination and confirmed the diagnosis.

Saturday found Reed still ailing. On Sunday he sat up in bed, called for solid food, read letters, and talked of improvements to be made at his country home the following spring. But Sunday night he was worse. On Monday morning, Major Borden took his Virginia friend to the Army Hospital Barracks and made ready to operate. Major J. R. Kean, another devoted military friend, arrived just before the trip to the operating room.

Walter Reed said, "Kean, I am not afraid of the knife, but if anything should happen to me I am leaving my wife and daughter so little. My son is twenty-four now. He's in the Army with a commission. But my wife and daughter have so little." As he went under the ether Walter Reed continued to whisper, "So little, so little."

It was difficult surgery. The appendix was hard to find. When the surgeon did locate it, he discovered that it was filled with pus and at one point perforated. Dr. Borden did his best. He litigated the appendix stump, inserted a gauze drainage, and packed it carefully. Reed reacted badly. For eighteen hours he suffered intense nausea. When the worst pain was abated he remained unusually nervous and depressed.

Major Kean called every day. Reed talked fretfully of his poverty; of the bleak future facing his wife and daughter. Major Kean said he had heard a report that Reed was being promoted to the rank of colonel. But the Virginian frowned and said, "I don't care about that now."

On the fifth day symptoms of peritonitis appeared. Thereafter the patient sank rapidly, and on November 22nd, he died.

With his death the real esteem in which the world held him became apparent. The Medical Society of the District of Columbia held a memorial service. The New York Academy of Medicine, the University of Virginia, the International Congress of Medicine, and many other scientific societies passed resolutions of condolence and appreciation. Major General Leonard Wood said:

I know of no other man on this side of the world who has done so much for humanity as Dr. Reed. His discovery results in the saving of more lives annually than were lost in the Cuban War, and saves the commercial interests of the world a greater financial cost each year than the cost of the Cuban War. He came to Cuba at a time when one-third of the officers of my staff died of yellow fever and we were discouraged at the failure of our effort to control the disease. . . . To Major Reed belongs the honor of having led in the greatest medical work of modern times, and the results he accomplished will live for all time.[18]

In 1906, Dr. Howard A. Kelley published the only life of Walter Reed which has appeared in this country. It is no longer in print. There is no substantial account of him or his work available in all Latin America.

His greatest tangible memorial is the hospital in Washington that bears his name. Opened in 1919, seventeen years after the great Virginian's death, it is the kind of memorial he would have preferred. As for fame, Walter Reed would not have minded missing that. The esteem of his colleagues, of the men of medicine who knew what he really had accomplished, would have been enough for him.

That much he did have.

In 1903 the Walter Reed Memorial Association was founded and incorporated at Washington. Promptly the association undertook to raise by public subscription a fund of $25,000, interest of which was to be usable for support of the great Virginian's widow and daughter during their lifetime, the principal to be applied later to building an appropriate monument to the memory of Walter Reed.

The sum was never raised. That is probably not important, either. The single sentence on the shaft in Arlington says all that could be said, anyhow. Remembered, half remembered, or forgotten, Walter Reed belongs to the Americas, North and South. In the tropics and semitropics of both hemispheres uncounted thousands, perhaps even millions, of people are alive because of him. That is the intangible memorial that every doctor would wish to have. . . .

Chapter Six

GORGAS OF ALABAMA

ON October 3, 1854, Josiah C. Nott, an elderly country doctor of Mobile, was called to the Gayle plantation at Toulminville. Amelia Gayle Gorgas, the wife of Captain Josiah Gorgas, United States Army commander of the arsenal at Mount Vernon, Alabama, was in labor. She was twenty-six and fashionably frail.

One year earlier a ruinous epidemic of yellow fever had caused Amelia Gayle to hurry to Mount Vernon for refuge. Mount Vernon is in high country and the arsenal site was famed as a place "safe" from yellowjack. If the virus of yellow fever had been a sentient being and known what it was doing, it would never have permitted Amelia to escape from New Orleans. Had she never escaped she would not have met Josiah Gorgas, thirty-five, handsome and one of the most promising young officers. And had she not met Josiah, the daughter of the former governor of Alabama would not have given birth eleven months later to a son named William Crawford.

Six years earlier the little-noticed Dr. Josiah Nott, who attended William Gorgas's birth, had mildly but determinedly suggested that yellow fever is not a malady caused by miasms arising from hot lands and swamps. He had stated to a Southern Medical Convention

125

that the disease must have a "specific agent."[1] Dr. Nott thereby marked himself as the first pioneer along a tortuous trail which half a century later led to discovery of the etiology of the nineteenth century's most destructive disease.

Josiah Gorgas, whose boy Willie was later to win the title of conqueror of yellowjack, was born in 1818 at Running Pump, a village on the Lancaster Pike near Harrisburg, Pennsylvania. At six he was a newsboy; at eighteen an apprentice printer; at nineteen he gained admission to West Point and at twenty-three he graduated from the United States Military Academy sixth in his class and took up the study and use of heavy weapons as his military profession. In 1845 he was sent to Europe as an official observer of the armament policies of war-thirsty Prussia and war-weary France. At the outbreak of the Mexican War in 1846 Josiah Gorgas was twenty-eight and a first lieutenant of artillery. Like many other gringo soldiers he came to fear yellowjack far more than he feared Mexicans. His fears were justified, for he was soon stricken with the black vomit. Fortunately he recovered, but he saw hundreds of his fellow soldiers die of the fierce and agonizing plague. In a letter written to his mother during the siege of Veracruz, Lieutenant Gorgas noted: "Nearly all have been sick, and they have died by the hundreds."[2]

In 1853 Josiah Gorgas was assigned the command of the Army Arsenal at Mount Vernon, a short distance north of Mobile. There, as we have noted, he married Amelia Gayle. The first of their six children, William, was born in the luxurious parlor bedroom of the great Gayle mansion built in a grove of live oaks and approached by long tree-lined driveways. John Gayle, who had been governor of Alabama, and a member of Congress and a district judge besides, was definitely aristocratic.

Young William Crawford Gorgas, however, grew up as an army brat. When he was three, his father was assigned to command the arsenal at Augusta, Maine. According to his private journal, Captain Gorgas loathed New England and despised the damned Yankees.

He wearied of the transient life of an army officer and with his wife planned for a day when they could return to Alabama and own a cotton plantation.

Captain Josiah Gorgas further noted in his journal that "Willie is very bright, quite grave, and tolerably mischievous and trouble-some." [3]

When Willie was seven his father was given command of the armory at Charleston, South Carolina, and there the child beheld the actual beginning of the Civil War. Jessie, one of Willie's four sisters, recounts how her mother told her: "Willie and I were sitting in the open window at the armory at Charleston, South Carolina, about nine o'clock, his little hand in mine, listening to the guns at Fort Sumter, the beginning of the Civil War. He seemed much impressed and turning to me, said, 'Mother, isn't it solemn?' " [4]

For the Gorgases it was particularly solemn. Captain Josiah was torn between his love for the South and his oath as an officer of the United States Army. Deliberately he resigned his commission and joined the Confederacy. Jefferson Davis promptly commissioned him brigadier general and made him chief of ordnance for the Confederacy. General Josiah proceeded to Richmond, where Willie and the rest of the Gorgases spent four eventful years in the very heart of the Confederacy. They became socially acquainted with the austere, blue-blooded Jefferson Davis and his war cabinet; with the pious Robert E. Lee, the brilliant Stonewall Jackson, Albert Sidney Johnston, and other great personalities of the South. Willie Gorgas was eleven when Richmond fell. His father assigned him responsibility for the safety and protection of his mother, his four younger sisters, his baby brother Richard, and the family cow. Willie led the procession through burning streets, and watched the entry of the victorious Federal troops. A shell fragment grazed the cow and she bolted. Willie swung to the halter, was slammed to the pavement and left there unconscious. The cow was lost, but the Gorgas family survived and made its way to Baltimore.

Exactly fifty years later, William Crawford Gorgas, world famous as a sanitarian, and a major general of the United States Army, delivered a public address in Baltimore:

"I first came to Baltimore a ragged barefooted little Rebel, with empty pockets and an empty stomach. My father had gone south with the army. At the fall and destruction of Richmond my mother's house, with all that she had, was burned, leaving her stranded with six small children. . . ." [5]

After the war, penniless but undefeated, Josiah Gorgas led his family back to Alabama. There he became manager of a blast furnace at Brierfield. The mill failed and the Gorgases were again penniless. But the South was exceptionally loyal to its soldiers. In 1870, under the auspices of the Episcopal Church, South, the University of the South opened at Sewanee, Tennessee, as a sort of camp, with a handful of students and a few wooden buildings. Josiah Gorgas, ex-ordnance chief of the Confederacy, was invited to become its president. He accepted and held office for ten years.

William Gorgas grew up at Sewanee. He was a slender, handsome youth, energetic, hot-tempered, and generally popular. On first entering the college he was an extremely bad student. But during his final year he suddenly turned scholarly and won the Alabama medal for class leadership. Furthermore, he proved himself a distinguished performer on the baseball field, joined the Episcopal Church, and somewhat in anticlimax began pining for a military career, which his father energetically discouraged. Instead of heading for the Army, Willie went to New Orleans and spent a year studying law. He detested everything about the profession. Meanwhile he applied repeatedly and unsuccessfully for admission to the United States Military Academy. Finally he conceded that the only possible way he could ever own an army commission was to win a degree in medicine and thus enter the Army Medical Corps.

At that time Willie Gorgas had no interest in medicine. Joining the Army had been his one thought. Now he set out to learn medicine. His father, believing an army doctor to be approximately the lowest form of animal life—navy doctors, of course, excepted—discouraged the move. Nevertheless, in the fall of 1876, William Crawford Gorgas, twenty-two years old, enrolled in Bellevue Medical College of New York City and there spent four laborious years completing the same course which Walter Reed had so easily finished in one.

But at Bellevue the somewhat frustrated devotee of shell and cannon became interested in what he was doing. Casual interest soon changed to passionate enthusiasm. He worked overtime in the dissecting room. He studied while other medical students drank, gambled, and caroused. After his first two years, the elder Gorgas was no longer able to send his son money, but Willie stayed on, desperately poor, frequently hungry, struggling hard on borrowed funds. Nevertheless, he maintained his gaiety and was game. Also he was young, and New York was then, as it is now, a veritable Baghdad for the young. Willie Gorgas roomed with John Bowen, from Paris, Kentucky. The two Southerners kept house in a deplorable hovel and in a highly original way did their own mending, cooking, sweeping and cleaning.

Their one extravagance was the theater. In those days the Union Square Theatre, now a motion-picture house, was a Saturday-night paradise for the followers of the gaslights. The biography of *William Crawford Gorgas* by Marie D. Gorgas, his wife, and Burton J. Hendrick, offers the following bit of exposition, along with many others:

Medical students in those days did not engage the front row in the balcony; they simply took it, even defying the two policemen who stood guard. . . . If the curtain did not rise promptly enough, whistling and rumblings issued from the top gallery, and applause was more frequently manifested with the feet than with the hands. "The Two Orphans," with Kate Claxton, was now the rage of the town. The poignant scene when the little girls, one blind, were huddled under the gaslight, with the paper snow of Old Union Square falling upon their devoted heads, especially stirred the emotion of the young medicos. When the villain seized the blind girl,

Bowen, Gorgas's Kentucky roommate, leaped to his feet and yelled over the balcony rail, "Take your hand off that girl, you scoundrel, or I'll blow a hole through you!" putting his hand on his hip pocket. The house was in an uproar. Gorgas grabbed his friend and finally succeeded in forcing him to his seat.[6]

In June, 1879, at twenty-four, William Gorgas received his degree as Doctor of Medicine. Commencement was held in the old Academy of Music, then one of the handsomest of all New York's theaters. A ward nurse from Bellevue, who earned fifteen dollars a month, favored the handsome young Dr. Gorgas with a magnificent fifteen-dollar bouquet of roses.

The doctor's career began with a brief term on the staff of the Blackwells Island Insane Asylum, followed by a few months as intern at Bellevue. In June, 1880, he entered the medical corps of the United States Army. His father, by then president of the University of Alabama, continued to oppose his son's entry into the Army as a doctor, but he was unable to keep the young man from becoming a first lieutenant in the Medical Corps, with a salary of $1,500 per year and limited extra allowances. Young Gorgas's first five years in the Army were spent at Forts Clark, Duncan, and Brown in Texas. After that he had three years at Fort Randall, North Dakota, and thirteen years at Fort Barrancas in Florida.

These were typical frontier posts. Gorgas's life was filled with medical administration, sanitation of military quarters, inspection of kitchens, privies and muster rolls, dispensary and hospital registries, record-keeping, and red tape. In addition he found opportunity for independent practice; in those days this was permitted in the Army, even expected. Sick Indians and frontiersmen had to be treated; pioneer farm wives to be delivered of babies; all "fee work," though few patients had money with which to pay. There were blizzards, dust storms and hurricanes, floods and plagues. Most dramatic and tragic of all, there was yellow fever.

Even by the standards of his day, though, William Gorgas was more than a typical army doctor. In addition to pulling teeth, delivering infants, dressing gun wounds, treating sick soldiers, and the rest of his multifarious professional activities, he played poker conservatively, danced persistently, though badly, joined in the close-bound community life of army posts, juggled babies and played whist. Most important, he continued to study medicine, into the science of which new life had been recently injected by men like Lister, Pasteur, and Koch. Medicine was plunging forward. Yellow fever, as Gorgas soon learned, was unaware of, and apparently not subject to, the laws of medicine. It was increasing.

In the early eighties William Gorgas had been assigned to duty with the Nineteenth Infantry at Fort Brown, Texas, near the great battlefield of Palo Alto. The outpost town of Brownsville on the north bank of the Rio Grande had been quarantined. Matamoras, notorious Saturday-night town across the river in Mexico, was rotting with yellow fever which had been at first reported at the post as dengue, or breakbone fever. But Colonel Joseph Smith, medical director of the Southern Department of the United States Army, had investigated the Fort Brown epidemic and recognized it for what it was.

Down on the Mexican border, as almost everywhere else, mosquitoes were abundant and torturesome, but nobody associated yellowjack with mosquitoes. Some said the disease was being blown in by a "yellow fever breeze" from across the dirty Rio Grande. Many believed that oranges and bananas were the cause of the plague. Consequently, oranges and bananas were forbidden entry to the army camp. Whisky and mustardseed were the most commonly used preventives. Most of the establishment of Fort Brown partook generously of these stimulating specifics. When a person died of the yellow plague he was buried with the greatest possible haste, preferably within an hour or two.

William Gorgas was dispatched to Fort Brown, advance agent for several other military doctors. He arrived to find not merely the camp but all the surrounding countryside being devastated.

There were more than 2,300 cases of yellow fever. Towns were under rigid quarantine. Even mail was not allowed passage. The young Dr. Gorgas was halted by quarantine at San Antonio and again at Laredo. About sixty miles beyond Laredo he changed from train to stagecoach and spent a toilsome week in traveling the final two hundred miles to his station. At Fort Brown he was assigned to bachelor quarters and drew as roommate a lieutenant named Enoch Crowder about whom, like Gorgas, the world was to hear considerably more.

Gorgas was assigned as doctor to an infantry company and a cavalry troop and directed to avoid all contacts with yellow fever patients. He promptly defied the injunction, walked into the yellow fever ward of the post hospital and began attending the patients. The post adjutant, one of those inevitably literal United States Army disciplinarians, caught Gorgas redhanded, ordered his arrest and directed that he be confined to quarters in the infested area of the garrison. The division commander fortunately heard what had happened and promptly ordered Gorgas released. The drawling soft-voiced young gentleman from Alabama continued to attend the sick.

While fighting yellowjack, Dr. Gorgas met a girl named Marie Doughty, who was the colonel's sister-in-law. A few days after they met, Marie suffered a severe chill followed by high fever. The colonel sent for Dr. Gorgas. The colonel was sitting beside the girl's bed fanning her with a newspaper. When Dr. Gorgas entered, the patient roused and, somewhat deliriously tearing the newspaper from her brother-in-law's hand, said to the doctor, "*You* fan me!"

The trouble was yellow fever. Marie grew rapidly worse. On the fourth day a grave was made ready for her. Gorgas and a civilian physician from Brownsville, Dr. Melou, were not only tending the sick but conducting funeral services for the dead. Dr. Melou pointed to a newly dug grave. "This is Miss Doughty's grave. Will you read the burial service for her this afternoon?"

The young man from Alabama said that he would. But he didn't. She recovered. A few days later Gorgas himself was stricken, a severe case from which he also recovered. The Alabamian's quarters were next door to the colonel's. So Gorgas and Marie Doughty began courtship while convalescing. The wife of the overworked superintendent of the cemetery, a Mrs. Smith, undertook the task of feeding and nursing Dr. Gorgas. She promptly named him "that Gorgeous Doctor."

The Gorgeous Doctor, however, was brusquely ordered to Fort Randall, South Dakota—once more a solitary bachelor except for his speckled bird dog, Duro. In writing to Marie Doughty, he wrote of his dog:

Duro has improved immensely in personal appearance lately. He is a handsome and intelligent looking animal and a first-rate retriever, and has a good nose besides. He caught an uninjured quail on the parade grounds the other day. I think of him because he has his paws on the arm of my chair looking on as I write, as he sympathizes thoroughly with his master in everything. I know he wishes to send you his best love.[7]

Dr. Gorgas married Marie Doughty and took her to the desolate frontier post. During September, 1889, their daughter Aileen was born. During his bachelorhood Gorgas had favored army-post parents with a great deal of mellow advice on the proper care and training of babies, but when Aileen Gorgas made her appearance all his rules for the scientific upbringing of children were promptly discarded. The Gorgeous Doctor proved himself superlatively capable as a child spoiler, perhaps because little Aileen looked so much like her father that the post began to call her "little Doc."

As the years passed, Gorgas's interest in yellow fever, aroused by his experiences at Fort Brown, made him something of a specialist. His fame grew as a "yellow fever doctor" and wherever the yellow plague appeared the surgeon general was likely to send him. When the disease began its devastation of Fort Barrancas, Florida, Gorgas was ordered to that post.

The yellow fever doctor in those days had more than merely medical duties to perform; not infrequently he was undertaker, grave digger, even clergyman; so great was the fear of contagions that funerals were held at midnight, and even the family kept at a distance. One night at Barrancas, Dr. McCulloch, one of the Army physicians, and Mr. Richard Gorgas, the Doctor's brother, were awakened by Gorgas who asked for a prayer book.

Soon afterward, from the direction of the hospital, they could hear the measured tread of pall-bearers—hospital attendants—as they passed on their way to the cemetery in the woods. . . . In the light of the swinging lanterns that aided a cloud-obscured moon, the cheap, black-covered coffin on the attendants' shoulders was dimly visible. Gorgas afterward described the horrible details in which he took part—laboriously digging the grave in the wet, heavy soil, wrapping the corpse in its simple white shroud; filling the unoccupied spaces of the improvised coffin with quicklime; the difficult internment and the filling up of the grave, and the reading of the burial service by lantern-light.[8]

With the outbreak of the Spanish-American War, William Gorgas proceeded with troops from Barrancas to Siboney, Cuba. As United States troops arrived in Cuba and offered their fresh blood to the virus, yellow fever increased alarmingly. It attacked the clean and luxurious as well as the filthy and destitute and it began to demolish an otherwise victorious United States Army.

In Havana Dr. Gorgas made the enduring friendship of the stately and determined Carlos J. Finlay. Offhand the American did not believe in the great Cuban's theory of the transmission of yellow fever by mosquitoes. He was not particularly impressed by the surgeon general's appointment of another Army Yellow Fever Commission. Many other commissions had sought to learn of yellow fever, published reports, and promptly faded from the picture. But military eyebrows went up a bit, Gorgas's among them, when Walter Reed appeared at Havana. Reed's gaiety and wit and unquenchable enthusiasms were widely known in army circles even though he himself was a mere name to United States medicine at large.

William Gorgas worked and waited. On September 16, 1900, he

was called to visit another Medical Corps friend, Dr. James Carroll, who said he suffered from a "slight indisposition." Gorgas promptly diagnosed it as yellow fever. As Carroll reached the crisis period of the malady, Gorgas was called to attend still another member of the Army Yellow Fever Board, the youthful and lovable Dr. Jesse W. Lazear. Yellow fever again! Lazear became delirious, spouted black vomit, and died on the following day.

Dr. Gorgas pondered and worked. He took no active part in the dramatic experiments at Camp Lazear. When the experiments were far enough progressed to indicate that the *Aëdes aegypti,* or *Stegomyia,* mosquito is the carrier of yellow fever, he announced that he proposed to rid Havana of mosquitoes. Even Walter Reed termed that impossible. Then Bill Gorgas said, "It wouldn't hurt to try."

Generally speaking, the public of Havana failed to share that sentiment. The city was black and gray with mosquitoes, uncounted millions and even billions of mosquitoes. Havana had always been a mosquito mecca and the common opinion persisted that it always would be. To the man in the street it appeared that Finlay, Reed, Carter, and the rest were presenting a theory of despair. If mosquitoes carry yellow fever, there would always be yellow fever, for there will always be mosquitoes. North American medicine had never believed Carlos Finlay. North American medicine waited smugly to contradict the findings of Walter Reed and the gallant men of medicine who made possible his eventual fame.

In studying the diverse testimonies which weave together the story of victory over yellow fever in Havana occasional bits of comedy shine through the overlaid pattern of tragedy. For example, late in 1900, after the dramatic experiments at Camp Lazear had been glorified by the United States newspapers and received with dead calm by the American Medical Association, various medical men began making pilgrimages of observation to Havana. Most of them went as unbelievers and left still unbelieving. At Las Animas

Hospital, Walter Reed, receiving a delegation of fifteen doctors, all non-Cubans, undertook to explain the proofs of mosquito transmission of yellow fever.

The visiting doctors listened solemnly and with proper professional decorum, but obviously believing not one word of what they heard. At Gorgas's suggestion, and with the help of Drs. Finlay and Carter, Reed was illustrating his lecture with a glass jar which contained a collection of *Aëdes aegypti*. The jar cover was accidentally brushed off by a gesturing hand. The prisoner mosquitoes began to rise in the air. As one man the doctors sprang up and lunged for the door. Decorum vanished. The doorway became blocked with excited men of science. In the stampede they tore the screen door completely off its hinges.

When William Gorgas was appointed sanitary officer of Havana, he found himself in one of the dirtiest cities known to man. Yellow fever was frequent; typhus, typhoid, dysentery, and other filth diseases were rampant. Havana air was habitually crowded with flies and mosquitoes; and floors, grounds, and streets were alive with roaches and lice. Filth lay in the streets. Dead animals and sick people sprawled on sidewalks. Garbage was scattered in front of homes. Havana stank to heaven, earth and sea. Until the coming of Gorgas and his soon-to-be-renowned cleanup force, buzzards were the sanitation department of the city.

It is not surprising that General Leonard Wood and other military men anticipated a renewed outbreak of yellowjack with the arrival of United States troops.

William Gorgas's first strategy in the cleanup of Havana was to eliminate filth, to segregate the sick, and to enforce rigid quarantine. The great effort proceeded with plenty of publicity. Magazines and newspapers of the United States began publishing "before" and "after" pictures of Havana; camera-eye testimony of streets, avenues, and alleys changed from filth traps and buzzard roosts to immaculate thoroughfares. The Gorgas cleanup was amazingly efficient. It reached into homes, offices, back yards, roofs, and cellars. Citizens of Havana were astonished and sometimes infuriated, but Gorgas was masterly in diplomacy; and masterly, too, in the use of United States money. Where plumbing, new floors or new roofs were necessary he ordered his workmen to install them. Within six months Havana had become the cleanest of all tropical cities.

To the discouragement of the sanitary forces, however, yellow fever began sweeping into the immaculate city: yellow fever and new immigrants. During 1900 tens of thousands of immigrant Spaniards arrived in Havana. Poverty was rife in Spain. Now that Cuba was "salvaged" and governed by the United States, the grand island was again attractive to Old World immigration. This was just what yellow fever was waiting for, the coming of fresh blood. Newsmen began to describe the 1900 yellowjack epidemic as the worst in Cuban history. The Associated Press distributed incredible but authentic horror stories. The Spanish-American War was won. But the war against yellowjack had apparently been lost.

Leonard Wood, general and physician and newly appointed military governor of all Cuba, promptly ordered that the scrubbing and cleanup be continued. He designated Las Animas Hospital as a segregation center for the sufferers. Three officers attached to the staff of General William Ludlow, military governor of Havana, died of yellow fever. So did the newly appointed superintendent of San José Asylum. William Gorgas noted somewhat wistfully, "They press Wood and Wood punches me." [9]

As Gorgas was well aware, still another important North American doctor was in Cuba—an affable, stocky gentleman, with a square face, drooping walrus-style mustache, and a slow Virginia drawl. He was Dr. Henry Rose Carter of the United States Public Health Service, temporarily attached to the United States Marine Corps.

Dr. Carter was also attached to the all-important war on yellow fever. He had just completed an elaborate statistical study of the spread of yellow fever among houses, a paper which the foremost medical journal of the United States had declined to print because it was "too long."

Carter of Virginia was backed by five years of experience as a port quarantine officer. During those years he had noted many times that aboard ship one seaman would contract yellow fever, and though he slept and lived in a forecastle crowded with other seamen during the first week or two no other man aboard the ship would contract the disease. This suggested that yellow fever is not immediately or directly contagious. During 1898 Dr. Carter was chosen to combat yellow fever epidemics in the villages of Taylor and Orwood, Mississippi. In these rural settlements yellowjack was principally confined to farmhouses. Carter kept careful records of all homes where yellow fever was present. He noted that neighbors who visited a given patient within one to two weeks of the latter's contracting the disease did not, as a rule, take yellowjack. But those who visited the home later than two weeks after the disease had appeared frequently or usually came down with it.

Here was added evidence that the sick man is not the immediate source of contamination. Carter further noted that new infection sometimes took place after the original patient had been buried. This indicated an interval when the disease could not be transmitted from a patient to a visitor; and a later interval when the disease could be transmitted from the place of infection, even though the sufferer was no longer present. Here was material for the theory of "extrinsic incubation" of disease, at the time a most radical theory.

The North American doctors considered the possibility of inoculation against yellow fever. William Gorgas had little confidence in it. Instead he began a diligent study of the *Aëdes aegypti* mosquito, then known as the *Stegomyia*. He noted that this mosquito is an aristocrat of its kind, expert in the way of man; that it usually stings on the underside of the wrist where the skin is tender; that it usually avoids the head and face or other parts of the human body where it can easily be killed; that the female *Aëdes* must be nourished with blood before she can produce eggs; that she deposits those preferably in clean water, in man-made receptacles if available. She usually avoids mud puddles or filth.

In Havana the slow-spoken Gorgas continued his total war against mosquitoes. It was a task burdened with embarrassment and disappointment, with the unavoidable need for meddling in private homes. In the face of this problem Gorgas actually proved himself one of the very few United States officials ever to win the Cuban heart. The great doctor was to become more than a superior army doctor. He was also a crusader, an educator, and a masterly tactician in human relations. And he was an incessant worker. Quite regardless of latitude or social or economic position most Americans, whether in Cuba, Sioux Falls, Buenos Aires, or Quito, are prone to respect a man who does his job well and thoroughly. In Havana, and later in Panama, Gorgas's office was never locked. He worked ten hours a day and usually longer. His Sundays and holidays were also working days.

He prepared charts to illustrate the parallel declines of yellow fever and of the mosquito population. He rejoiced in the fact that the *Stegomyia* is primarily a house-breeding mosquito. This fact proved of particular help to his effort. The second and final stage of the great antiyellow-fever war in Havana began with the mosquito campaign of March, 1901. During July and August the city suffered only five deaths from yellow fever. During the remainder of the year, and for four more years, Havana had no deaths at all from that disease. At forty-seven, Gorgas had probably done as much as all men in all history to make tropical lands healthful.

Walter Reed was dead, but Gorgas stayed at work in Havana. His rank was raised from major to colonel. Late in 1902 he was recalled to Washington and promptly left on an official journey to Egypt, Suez, and Paris. Next he paid a preliminary visit to the Isthmus of Panama, which James Froude had so effectively described: "In all the world there is not . . . concentrated in any single spot so much swindling and villainy, so much foul disease, such a hideous dung heap of physical and moral abomination. The Isthmus is a damp tropical jungle intensely hot, swarming with mosquitoes, snakes, alligators, scorpions and centipedes, the home, even as Nature made it, of yellow fever, typhus and dysentery." [10]

On June 5, 1905, the S.S. *Allianca* docked at Colon. William Gorgas led a party of eight down the gangplank. The group included Joseph L. Le Prince, chief sanitary engineer; Mary Hibbard, head nurse; Dr. Henry R. Carter, grown plumper and more self-assertive; the fiercely energetic Dr. John Ross, of the United States Navy; Dr. Louis A. La Garde, Dr. Louis Balch, and Major James Turtle of the United States Army. These eight medical missionaries landed without benefit of any impressive authority and with a minimum of equipment.

When Gorgas appealed to the Canal Commission for workmen to put his program into effect, his appeals were promptly denied. He cabled Washington for help and in reply received a reminder that cablegrams are expensive; that it would be advisable to use the mails.

Gorgas's missionaries occupied the forlorn Ancon Hospital, where they were presently joined by Drs. Deeks, Perry, Herrick, and others. Gorgas himself returned to Washington to appeal for help. Although the medical world had at last accepted the findings of Walter Reed and was faced with the fact that Oswaldo Cruz, inspired by the great Havana experiment, had rid Rio de Janeiro of the yellow fever which had harassed Brazil's great capital for centuries, Congress was not impressed. Neither was the Canal Commission, whose chairman, Admiral John G. Walker, was an able pennypincher. The admiral knew nothing of the tropics. Washington was his world. He had heard of Walter Reed and come to believe him an absolute lunatic. Admiral Walker knew all he wanted to know. Habitually fierce, he could and did laugh heartily at the idea that a puny mosquito could possibly transmit a man-killing disease. He said if Gorgas would only clean up the Canal Zone, remove filth, dead rats, dogs and cats, and whitewash the buildings diseases would vanish.

The first governor of the Canal Zone was General George W. Davis. Davis was an engineer who had supervised the building of the Washington Monument. It was his stated opinion that "a dollar spent on sanitation is like throwing it into the Bay." He also said that the whole theory of disease transmission by mosquitoes was insanity; that all who believed it were mad. It is noteworthy that the membership of the first Canal Commission rarely went closer to Panama than Washington, D. C.; and that, while squelching efforts to bring about sanitation of the Isthmus, they never hesitated to provide generous appropriations for the purchase of coffins. As well they might. When the steam-shovel men took over, when engineers and office staffs took their places, yellow fever was waiting. An architect who flippantly refused to authorize an appropriation for wire screening was one of the first to die of yellow fever.

By November, 1904, the disease was no longer dormant. An Italian opera company appearing at Panama City was struck down by yellow fever to the last member of the chorus. As thousands of new workers swarmed into the Isthmus, the disease began its attack all along the fifty square miles of Canal Strip. As the yellow plague gained strength, so did the panic of the people. To get out of Panama became the foremost ambition of the company of adventurers from the north. Twenty-two workers in the Canal Administration Building were stricken by the fever. Bosses and workers alike were dying. Ships brought cargoes of would-be workers who, as soon as they had set foot ashore, frantically applied for return passage aboard the very vessels that had brought them.

A bad situation grew rapidly worse. Senators roared denunciations of the Panama route and declaimed that the Big Ditch could never be finished. Through all the shouting William Gorgas remained at work, gambling his reputation on what he called a flank attack against the army of mosquitoes. Panama towns lacked modern water systems. Open rain barrels and troughs were standard equipment everywhere and they were ideal breeding grounds for *Aëdes aegypti*. Gorgas's cleanup gangs and oiling crews took over.

According to a story told by Gorgas, a weary sanitary inspector came back to his hotel one hot day and, as a gesture of final exhaustion, dumped his remaining supply of crude oil into the cistern on the hotel roof. Shortly thereafter a fat and blowing naval captain arrived at the hotel, went to his room and happily made ready for a shower bath. He stripped off his clothes, smeared his body with liquid soap, stepped under the shower and pulled the chain. Instead of fresh cool water the shower produced sticky oil which mingled with the soap to make a sort of stubborn coating that could not be washed off. There was no fresh water on the premises. The captain couldn't put on his clothes. So, having slithered and sworn for an entire night, he wrapped himself in a sheet and set out to track down and kill the sanitary inspector. In due course the outraged gold-braid was informed that the sanitary inspector had caught yellow fever and was dying. Thereupon the man bellowed, "I'm damned glad of it!"

After what seemed an interminable delay, the help which Gorgas prayed for arrived, more doctors and a group of registered nurses from the United States. Some of the nurses, Dr. Henry Carter observed, had been with the Army in the Philippines, others with Gorgas in Cuba, and some apparently with Washington at Valley Forge, but whatever their age or condition, yellow fever or matrimony, sometimes both, awaited them in Panama. Dr. Carter told in particular of one nurse who had slipped away from her quarters and joined a young doctor in a jaunt to Panama City, then a particularly dangerous focus of yellow fever.

I was rushed . . . to the nurses' quarters at Anconcita. I found her with yellow fever, tossing from one side of the bed to the other. . . . Neither morphine nor cocaine quieted her. Finally I said, "Child, you have a fine constitution and you ought to get well. But if you don't lie still in that bed you are going to die." She insisted that she couldn't keep still, but suggested if Major —— (calling the name of one of the younger doctors on duty) would hold her hand she would try. I gave Major —— a call and stationed him at his post. She quieted down immediately and the major sat by her all night. The girl got well, and it wasn't long after when I got cards to their wedding.[12]

The flank attack began to gain ground. One day in September, 1906, Dr. Gorgas stopped at Ancon Hospital and noted a band of white-clad doctors viewing the corpse of the latest yellow fever victim. Gorgas said, "Take a good look, boys! That's the last case of yellow fever you'll ever see!" [13]

Though the sanitation of Panama was continually handicapped by stuffed-shirt politicians from the United States, yellow fever was being beaten and the building of the canal was beginning to look like a possibility, even though the Isthmian Commission continued to brand the chief of its sanitary department a failure. Early in 1906 Dr. Charles A. L. Reed of Cincinnati, formerly president of the American Medical Association and chairman of the association's Committee on Medical Legislation, went to Panama and investigated the efforts of Gorgas and his helpers, approved the work, then returned to the United States and promptly launched a scathing, hide-removing attack on Admiral Walker and all his bungling commissioners.

Dr. Reed's most forceful bombshell was his story of a nursing bottle and nipples:

A woman in the insane department [at Ancon Hospital] was delivered of a child; her condition was such that she could not nurse her offspring; the nurse applied to Major La Garde [of the hospital staff] for a nursing nipple and a nursing bottle; he had none—the requisition of last September had not yet been filled; he made out a requisition, took it to Colonel Gorgas for endorsement, then to Mr. Tobie, chief of the Bureau of Materials and Supplies, for another endorsement, then to a clerk to have it copied and engrossed; then a messenger was permitted to go to a drug store and buy a nursing bottle and nipple, which finally reached the infant two days after the necessity for their use had arisen. The articles ought to have cost not more than thirty cents, but . . . the cost to the Government of the United States was in the neighborhood of $6.76—all due to the penny-wise-pound-foolish policy of the Commission.[14]

Dr. Charles Reed's story of the nursing bottle found its way into print throughout the United States. Certainly it reached the White House and the desk of the President. Whether or not Theodore Roosevelt saw it, he promptly discharged all seven members of the Isthmian Commission. Unfortunately his replacements were no more helpful to William Gorgas than the originals had been. Theodore P. Shonts, succeeding chairman of the commission, proposed to discharge Gorgas and replace him with an osteopath, who presumably had voted the right way.

Accordingly, Mr. Shonts, railroad promoter, and his new commission recommended to William Howard Taft, Secretary of War, that Gorgas, Carter, La Garde, and indeed all who believed in the silly nonsense about transmission of disease by mosquitoes be discharged and replaced by "practical men." William Howard Taft, who had personally viewed the sorely bogged canal effort and who should have been more intelligent, approved the recommendation and referred it to the President.

Theodore Roosevelt refused and ordered Shonts to support Gorgas. A few months later the President visited William Gorgas and the Ancon Hospital in person—the first time in United States history that a president had gone beyond domestic boundaries. At last William Gorgas found himself in command of an independent department. After two more years he was made a member of the Isthmian Commission—in company with Gaillard, builder of Culebra Cut; Sibert, who directed the building of Gatun Lake; and Lieutenant Colonel George W. Goethals, of the Army engineers, who became chairman of the commission and chief engineer of the canal. In 1908 William Gorgas was also elected president of the

American Medical Association, which apparently did not impress the cold, power-loving Colonel Goethals whom Gorgas called Mister X.Y.Z. Goethals ridiculed Gorgas, protested at his extravagance (sanitation appropriations for the canal averaged $350,000 per year); declared that every mosquito killed in Panama was costing the United States ten dollars. The great Gorgas answered, "But just think, one of those ten-dollar mosquitoes might bite you and what a loss that would be to the country!"

Despite political corruption, despite jealousies and bickerings, Gorgas carried on his war against disease. When yellow fever was beaten he threw his huge energies into the struggle against malaria, curse of tropical natives and newcomers alike, in ultimate effect as serious as yellowjack, if not as deadly, and much harder to control.

Through a sweaty and tumultuous decade of canal building, William Gorgas carried on. The Canal Zone begot its own brand of social life; a scrambled American frontier dropped into an alien jungle; a society of starched linens and mud-caked overalls; of Panamanians learning to speak English; of *norteamericanos* disdaining Spanish; of *polleras*, señoras, and wives from Sioux City; of bimonthly dances at the Hotel Tivoli. Gorgas was able to fit his private life into that bizarre pattern. He made many friends. He attended and promoted frontier church services. He laughed, danced, and worked. Perhaps he was no longer gorgeous, but hospital patients frequently called him the cheerful doctor.

The world soon learned that he was also the successful doctor. In 1914, when the Panama Canal was opened, the annual death rate of the Canal Zone was 6 per thousand inhabitants. The general death rate of all the United States was 14.1 per thousand. Nebraska was the healthiest of the states, yet its death rate was 9.2 per thousand. Minnesota was second with 9.4; Washington State third with 9.5 per thousand. In terms of vital statistics the Isthmus of Panama, pesthole and death trap of the centuries, was changed into the healthiest land area in the world.

Gorgas closed his Panama service in triumph. He was the first to cross the Isthmus—in a canoe. Far more important, he was first among all sanitarians. His election to the presidency of the American Medical Association preceded many other honors—honorary degrees from Harvard, Brown, the University of Pennsylvania, and his own alma mater the University of the South. His aging but still illustrious teacher at Bellevue, Dr. William H. Welch, "dean of American physicians," now conferred upon his renowned student Johns Hopkins degree of Doctor of Letters. During 1911, while his mother was still alive and he was in Panama, William Crawford Gorgas had been offered the presidency of the University of Alabama, at Tuscaloosa where his mother lived. Gorgas confessed his eagerness to follow in his father's footsteps as president of the university. He wrote his mother: "But it seemed to me that this was my life work upon which my scientific reputation rested. That if I separated from the work before the Canal was opened, I would lose a good share of this reputation. So very reluctantly I declined. After the Canal is finished . . . I would jump at it." [15]

Two years later he was offered the presidency of the University of the South at Sewanee, but the canal was still unfinished and Gorgas remembered his place as a man of medicine. He knew that the Big Ditch would soon be carrying ships from all ports of the world and that, with them, it would carry all the world's diseases. At fifty-nine he could not help thinking what the things he had learned in Panama, applied to human health problems elsewhere in the world, might accomplish. He knew, for example, that in the Rand regions of South Africa thousands of Negroes were dying of pneumonia. In general the black race seems to have more resistance than the white to mosquito-borne diseases, but with pulmonary diseases the opposite is the case. The resistance of the black race to pneumonia is particularly low.

When the world-renowned gold and diamond mines of the Rand were opened, British mining companies began to recruit tens of thousands of Negroes for mine labor; Britain's pocketbook aristocracy, which had brought misery and degradation to so many colonial territories, began the decimation of the South African native. Unintentionally, of course, but certainly and surely.

The expropriation of Dutch African mines, followed by the ruthless exploitation of African mineworkers, was one more major blot upon an already besmirched white man's civilization. In 1913 the prevalent death rate of Negro mineworkers in Rhodesia was approximately 30 per cent each year. The evil had been long-standing. Hundreds of thousands of Negroes, duly shanghaied by contract recruiters, were working the richest mines in the world for wages averaging considerably less than one shilling a day, frequently three or four pennies. "Contract" Negroes went underground, were fed in the manner of starving dogs, quartered much like corralled sheep. Death took no holidays. Cecil Rhodes was the king of diamonds. Newly titled colonial society was beginning to bring prosperity to tropical watering places, but at heart Africa was dying and even his Majesty's government, much against its apparent inclinations, threatened to halt labor recruiting unless "miners' pneumonia" was checked.

Samuel Evans of the Transvaal Chamber of Mines had heard of William Gorgas. The astute Mr. Evans pondered the proposition that this fabulous Dr. Gorgas might be the one man most needed in South Africa. Dying Negroes were a threat to British income; alive they were wealth. The future of the Transvaal rested upon the continued abundance of coolie-waged native labor. Mr. Evans boarded a ship, proceeded to Panama, met William Gorgas, studied his work, and became his friend.

In Panama, five years earlier, Gorgas had met and solved on a smaller scale a problem of Negro deaths from pneumonia. The beginning of canal construction had seen the employment of thousands of Jamaican and other West Indian Negroes. By 1906 pneumonia was taking an alarming toll among them. Gorgas investigated and promptly realized that living conditions were at fault. When North American operations in the Canal Zone began, Negro laborers were quartered in the very huts and palm shacks which the ill-fated De

Lesseps Company had abandoned. Wages had been low in the early days. Negro employees could rarely afford more than one outfit of clothing. Much of the time they worked in the rain. They slept at night in their wet clothes in crowded tiers of bunks. Small wonder that pneumonia appeared among them and spread like wildfire.

William Gorgas proposed to eliminate the crowding. He called for new and better barracks and careful segregation of the sick. The government provided plots of land and encouraged Negro employees to build their own houses, well separated from adjoining houses. Wages were raised. With his habitual diplomacy Gorgas urged the Negroes to provide themselves with more clothes and to live with their families. Promptly and with a minimum of effort the pneumonia epidemic in the Zone was beaten.

Late in 1931 Gorgas accepted the Transvaal invitation and again sailed for Africa. There must have been considerable twitching of eyebrows in British medical circles. His Majesty's pacificators had deliberately gone out of the Empire to take on an American sanitarian. The American sanitarian stopped in London on his way to Africa. He dined with Sir Ronald Ross in London and with Sir William Osler at Oxford. Then on November 15th, accompanied by his wife, Marie, and Dr. Sam Darling, a Canal Zone veteran, William Gorgas sailed for Capetown.

There the S.S. *Briton* landed on December 2nd. The medical ambassadors from North America proceeded by train to Johannesburg—about a thousand miles to the north. Mr. Samuel Evans and the Chamber of Mines had established offices for the newcomers in the Carlton Hotel. Gorgas lunched with Viscount Gladstone, the governor general, interviewed diamond kings, and made a tour of the hospitals of the Rand. Next he studied the miners' barracks, the provisions for space, the varieties, quality, and quantity of food provided for the Negroes. Evidently Gorgas was not pleased. It did not take him long to recommend immediate abandonment of the existing barracks and the establishment of open villages for laborers.

The plight of the Rand was basically the same as that of Panama during the early period of canal building.

Gorgas next set out to investigate British methods of recruiting mine labor. He found that the required labor force was about 200,000. The standard contract period was six months, which meant the recruiting of at least 400,000 Africans each year. Without successful recruiting the economic background of the Union of South Africa faced collapse. Wholesale deaths from pneumonia were proving a serious threat to its prosperity.

Gorgas dispatched Dr. Darling to Portuguese East Africa to make a further study of Negro recruiting. On Christmas Day Gorgas recorded: "Darling and Noble are studying my commercial code, trying to send Christmas greetings to their wives. Unfortunately this kind of code does not lend itself to love letters. Darling has triumphed. He has found two code words that mean 'Love in carload lots!' He thinks this will satisfy Mrs. Darling." [16]

Dr. Gorgas proceeded to Kimberley and the De Beer mines, where he noted that working conditions within the mines were not wholly unbearable. Dr. Darling, however, returned with distressing reports. Laborers were being lifted from the jungle, transported by crowded ships and on crowded freight cars, and without being given additional clothing, moved from humid sea levels to altitudes of five thousand feet and higher. Thus laborers reached the recruiting camps already afflicted with pneumonia. Before transfer to the mines many more were sick. Transfer from the deep and hot working shafts to cool surface levels added to the havoc of the disease among those well enough to work. Furthermore, barracks were pitifully overcrowded. Bedding consisted of one shoddy blanket to a man. Ventilation was almost nonexistent. Hot-country Negroes had no understanding of the type of clothing required for high altitude. They would not have known what to wear even if they had the means of obtaining it.

Sick at heart and depressed, Gorgas went on to Salisbury, capital of Southern Rhodesia, where among newcomers malaria was prevalent. Gorgas began his visit by calling on Sir William Milton, the governor. The governor addressed him as "General Gorgas." Colonel Gorgas proffered a polite correction, but the governor repeated the "general" and handed his guest a cablegram from Washington announcing that President Woodrow Wilson had appointed William Crawford Gorgas surgeon general of the United States Army.

General Gorgas and his party toured Rhodesia, speaking to farm audiences on sanitation and malaria control. They toured the mining lands of lower Rhodesia, the probable Biblical Ophir where Solomon and the King of Tyre secured their stores of gold. They saw a troop of baboons playing in the ruins of Khama. Gorgas noted, "They did not seem particularly shy or unfriendly. We did not do anything to provoke them." [17]

Within three months Gorgas had covered much of South Africa, completing a detailed report and recommendation which he presented to the Transvaal Chamber of Mines. It was not by accident that Dr. Lewis Ornstein, a Gorgas assistant in the Canal Zone, was made sanitation director of the Central Mining Company of the Transvaal. By 1919, or within four years, the mortality from pneumonia among Negro mineworkers had fallen from more than 300 per thousand to approximately 3 per thousand. Gorgas had quite candidly informed the Chamber of Mines: "The success of any system of sanitation . . . will depend a great deal upon the choice of the man who has charge of carrying it into execution." [18]

Returning by way of London, Gorgas addressed the Royal Society of Medicine and received a tremendous ovation. Oxford University promptly honored him with the degree of Doctor of Science. Back in Washington Congress recognized his Panama services by promoting him to the rank of major general. John D. Rockefeller, the elder, had established the International Health Board, which now was grown from an incorporated crusade against hookworm to a disease-fighting agency not limited in scope to any part of the world or any one disease. The International Health Board proposed a final knockout war against yellow fever. During 1915 it was common knowledge that yellow fever, whatever might have been done to it in Cuba and the Canal Zone, remained alive in Africa, particularly along the west coast. Still more menacing to the United States, it waited in Mexico, in Central America, and in the Isthmus.

The spread of yellowjack to regions whose inhabitants are not immune was (and is) a continuing nightmare. Completion of the Panama Canal, as has been suggested, added vividness to the nightmare. Dr. Wickcliffe Rose, president of the International Health Board, worried about the possible dissemination of the disease and sought the advice of William Gorgas. He had no difficulty in getting the advice. It was definite and convincing. Destroy all remaining foci of yellow fever, said Gorgas. That would be the best and easiest insurance against epidemics.

During 1915 Gorgas and two other stanch warriors in white, Dr. Henry R. Carter and Dr. Joseph A. White (the latter at eighty-five has read and discussed the text of this book), called on the Executive Committee of the International Health Board in New York to make fighting plans. The First World War was making more noise than Latin-American mosquitoes. Public attention was riveted more upon high explosives than upon health. The war against mosquitoes was, however, declared.

The International Health Board needed exact information as to the localities where yellowjack persisted. The board invited General Gorgas to spend several months traveling through the American tropics in search of the required information. During June, 1916, Gorgas, with Dr. Juan Guiteras, of Havana, and other medical men, set out to tour Brazil, Ecuador, Venezuela, Peru, Colombia, Central America, and Mexico. It was a delicate mission. Without masterly tact it might have proved irksome, even insulting, to the admirable and duly sensitive medical talent of Latin America. Once more William Gorgas demonstrated his superlative qualities as an ambassador. He was a world-renowned authority upon yellow fever, a proved conqueror of the plague, and a completely engaging and disarming medical leader. Latin America welcomed him with open arms. Presidents, governments, mayors, and bishops waited to greet him. The International Health Board benefited enormously. Doors to the south were opened.

William Crawford Gorgas was sixty-two, but he planned his new crusade with the enthusiasm of an adolescent. The International Health Board made him director of its world-spanning campaign against yellow fever. At this point the United States declared war on Germany. William Gorgas was a general and his country was at war.

The importance of the Army Medical Corps grew. In 1916 the United States Army had only 435 medical officers plus a medical reserve corps which included slightly more than 2,000 civilian physicians. When the Armistice was signed the Army had about 32,000 medical officers in active service, about 35,000 civilian doctors and dentists in the reserve corps, a medical corps enlisted personnel of about a quarter of a million men, and about 22,000 nurses. Under Gorgas the Medical Corps was substantially larger than the entire peacetime Army of the United States. In numbers it was the largest command assigned directly to any one major general.

Although Gorgas was old in years when the war began, his administration is commonly regarded as the most aggressive and capable in medical history. It included building and equipping thirty-two base hospitals at principal training centers throughout the United States, providing domestic hospital accommodations for more than a hundred thousand men, and in France a hospital network to accommodate approximately one-fourth of all the United States soldiers reaching the front line.

During the First World War the Medical Corps examined more than six million men, attended about four millions, cared for sick and wounded at home and overseas. Gorgas accented preventive medicine; directed that the Army be provided with wholesale vaccination, antitoxin, and serum against infectious diseases. The Medical Corps approved all military buildings and directed the inspection of barracks, kitchens, and field encampments as well as hospitals, clinics, sick camps, and dispensaries. Gorgas commanded the Medical Corps, served as a member of Council of National Defense, chose as assistants many of the ranking surgeons, physicians, and laboratory technicians of the United States, ensconced Drs. Will and Charles Mayo in his office, and otherwise proved himself a pre-eminent leader of American medicine.

At sixty-four he continued to dream of leading troops into actual combat. Burton J. Hendrick describes the general's official pilgrimage to Macon, Georgia, one of the first centers of epidemic influenza in 1918. Officers of the Alabama brigade gave a dinner honoring the renowned son of their state. Gorgas addressed his hosts:

I have had every honor my profession could give me. My government has given me every honor it could bestow on any physician in its medical service. Yet I am not satisfied. I still have one ambition to realize before I can count my life happy and rounded out. I wish it were possible for the President to reduce my rank as Major-General to that of Brigadier-General and put me in command, in active service in France, of that brigade of splendid Alabamians whom I have seen here.[19]

Perhaps that was merely a daydreaming mood. Dr. Franklin H. Martin, of Chicago, a World War aide under Gorgas, tells how his commander remarked, "I wish this horrible war were over." Dr. Martin asked what the general would prefer to do if the war should end tomorrow. Gorgas answered, "I would ring off, call New York City, and order a passage for South America. I would go to Guayaquil, Ecuador, the only place in which yellow fever is prevalent, exterminate the pestilence and then return to Panama, the garden spot of the world, and end my days writing an elegy on yellow fever."

In a measure the wish was fulfilled. After the Armistice was signed, General Gorgas was retired. He said that he was still young and still ready for work. Since the Army would have him no longer, he returned to the International Health Board. At Guayaquil,

Ecuador, the late Dr. M. E. Connor was effecting a magnificent cleanup of yellowjack. Reports of new outbreaks, however, came from West Africa. A British medical commission confirmed the reports. William Gorgas conferred with the Rockefeller men and then, accompanied by his wife and a few friends, he sailed from Quebec en route to England and Africa. Belgium had awarded him the Harbin medal for services to mankind. The medal was to be presented by King Albert at the International Hygiene Conference at Brussels in 1920.

On the day following his arrival in London, Gorgas was taken ill. The next night he summoned Marie, his wife, and told her that he had suffered a paralytic stroke. Sir John Goodwin, surgeon general of the British Army, took his American colleague to a military hospital at Willbank. English physicians predicted an early recovery. Gorgas stated quietly that he would fight to the last, though he believed that he was dying. From his hospital bed he watched the Thames and its busy traffic of ships. He smiled and said he was fortunate to be among friends. Otherwise he might have died alone at sea or in the jungle.

One day the King himself called at the hospital at Willbank. His Majesty entered without fanfare and spoke to the brown-skinned, white-haired man who was now known as the greatest sanitarian in all the world. The King talked of Panama and Cuba and of the services which Dr. Gorgas had rendered the Empire. He motioned his equerry, took the insignia of the Knight Commander of the Most Distinguished Order of St. Michael and St. George, and presented it to William Crawford Gorgas. "I very sincerely appreciate," he said, "the great work which you have done for humanity—work in which I take the greatest interest."

Next day General Sir William Gorgas received the King's greetings and his expression of hope that no harmful effects had resulted from His Majesty's visit. Gorgas answered, "The King's gracious visit has done me a world of good. I feel decidedly better for my decoration, and I am ready for another!"

Four weeks later, still in the bare hospital room which overlooked the Thames, William Crawford Gorgas died. At St. Paul's Cathedral he was accorded the funeral of a British major general. His body was brought back to Washington and buried at Arlington among the graves of other great warriors. His spirit, his work of administration and the practical application of common sense and uncommon ingenuity, his rare diplomacy and human sympathy live on. Wherever he went he won friends. In Latin-American eyes he remains the most illustrious of North American medical men. His career was both a primer and a gospel for succeeding generations of ambassadors in white.

Chapter Seven

DEEKS OF CANADA

WHILE Gorgas, the greatest sanitarian among our ambassadors in white, was winning world renown by bringing tropical sanitation into existence, one of his less publicized colleagues, Canadian-born Dr. William Edgar Deeks, was blazing a pioneer trail into the almost virgin field of tropical nutrition.

The careers of both Gorgas and Deeks began outside of the tropics. Gorgas was in his late forties when he first saw Cuba. Deeks was in his late thirties when he first reported at the Panama Canal Zone. Both were entering the tropics in pursuit of interests aroused by the impact of their particular personalities upon the medical problems of their time.

During May, 1906, a trim white banana ship was plowing her way through the Caribbean. Taking their leisure in deck chairs were two youngish men who were engaged in earnest conversation. One was Dr. William Deeks, whom Gorgas had hired as chief of clinic for the rapidly expanding Ancon Hospital, medical base for the Panama Canal. Dr. Deeks, who preferred to be called Bill, was broad-shouldered, round-faced, and rather good-looking, somewhat

British in bearing, extremely good-natured, and intensely curious. Already this curiosity had led him to study medicine in order to learn more of human nutrition; to serve as doctor to obsolete Indian tribes of the remote Canadian Rockies; to win a faculty post at Mc-Gill University and Bishop's College; to produce an imposing list of scientific papers and to study clinical medicine in Vienna.

It was at Vienna that Bill Deeks had first given serious attention to tropical medicine. At Vienna where, at the time, the theory and practice of medicine was finding the most fertile soil for its development, he rather suddenly became convinced that the tropics are actually the greatest of all laboratories in which to study human nutrition and health. His presence on the banana ship bound for Colon was the immediate result of this conviction.

Dr. Deeks's companion on the starboard deck was Dr. William James, who was returning for a second "term" in the green hell of Panama. Dr. James's personal conception of an ideal day at sea was one match and fourteen mellow, oversized cigars.

"Science," said Dr. James, "is for the smoothies. Malaria and yellowjack are the jobs for tropical tramps. In these mosquito hells all a medical man can do is work till he falls in his tracks. The only way you ever get to rest is to die."

"What about malaria?"

Dr. James sighed with infinite boredom. "Everything south of Mobile is rotten with it. They shake with chills and fevers. They curl up with brain clog. They rot with blackwater fever. Amoeba bugs play leapfrog down their guts. . . . Talk about cultured Europe! It's those so-called cultured Europeans from those ancient art centers that have set Panama to rotting."

"Why?"

Dr. James lighted another cigar. "You like that word, don't you, doctor? 'Why this?' and 'Why that?' " The younger medical man sighed again. "Well, there're bound to be answers. I don't know what they are. Been too damned busy to find out. I've only been with the Big Ditch one year. Haven't had time to blow my nose but once since Gorgas signed me on. Let's talk over the whys, say, a year from now. By then you may not be such a whyer."

But Dr. Deeks was not so sure. He recalled that he had been asking why all his life, or at least most of it. He recalled one of his first school days. That was back in Canada, near Williamsburg, Ontario, a farming village in the valley of the great St. Lawrence.

At recess time one day, a little girl was describing to a group of children an extremely funny book she had read, a book about a Mr. Pickwick who was bowlegged, so bowlegged in fact that a pig could run between Mr. Pickwick's knees without anyone but the pig being the wiser. Little Bill Deeks listened intently. It happened to be the closing day of school, and there was no chance of his reading the book. Because he had seen many bowlegged people, he could appreciate Mr. Pickwick's lamentable defect as a pig drover.

One of the girls turned to little Bill and pointed at his legs. "Billy Deeks's legs is already curvin'. If he's not careful, he'll be just like Mr. Pickwick."

That prophecy was immensely funny to the other children, but not to Bill Deeks. He trudged home in grave meditation. He knew he was getting bowlegged, and he wondered why. There had to be a reason. Here it was springtime, and here a long hard-working summer waited for all the Deekses. There would be pigs to herd. Little Bill Deeks again considered his legs. Yessir, he *was* getting bowlegged. And he had to find out the reason for it.

A few nights later the country doctor came by for supper with the family. Little Bill Deeks rarely spoke at the family board, but on this particular night he screwed up his courage and asked the doctor, "What makes people bowlegged?"

The doctor was flustered and the entire Deeks family was properly embarrassed.

The doctor said, "Well, sometimes mothers let their children walk too soon. That makes them bowlegged. Then sometimes when boys and girls are growing up, they carry burdens that are too heavy.

Maybe that causes it. Then again bowed legs may be due to what people put into their stomach. Who knows?"

Little Bill sensed an honest but unsatisfactory answer. Bill's father changed the subject by announcing that he had bought the neighbor's farm. That meant more work for all the Deekses. It suggested that young Bill could stop puttering around with school and silly questions and take up real man's work on the new farm. There's no time for school pranks when a boy's father has a square mile of field land that has to be plowed, planted, and harvested all within a hundred working days.

But young Bill Deeks continued to ask questions. He couldn't find many answers in books. For one reason books were extremely scarce in the Williamsburg countryside. For another, some of the most urgent questions which popped up in late-Victorian Canada had never been answered in books or by wise country schoolteachers or even by honest, hard-working farmers like the elder Bill Deeks.

Good citizens were simply too busy to answer questions. They had to change little farms to big farms—small barns to giant barns. To do this they had to beget big families and work in the fields from dawn until dark. Why? Well, because down in the States, Yankee factory hands were beginning to buy Canadian farm products. So was Europe, particularly a silk-stockinged, fiercely industrial England. In Canada agriculture was life, seasons were short, and man power was precious—all of which called for bigger families and bigger farms.

When Bill Deeks, Senior, married Martha Merkley, they set out to conquer the deep rich earth and replenish it without asking questions. During the first eleven years of their marriage they produced seven children and doubled their original half-section. After a ten-year work interval, four more children were born to the hard-working couple. Bill Deeks gave the second son of the final four his own name and considered the naming entirely appropriate. For the child was sturdy and "sensible." At five little Bill worked in the gardens. At eight he joined his brothers in the fields.

But the boy was a habituated question-asker, and his round, black-thatched head was crowded with peculiar ideas. About bowlegged-ness, for example. Throughout his ninth summer little Bill was absolutely certain that the whole Deeks family would be bowlegged before the crops were made. And he continuously bombarded the family with unanswerable questions about what makes bones hard or soft; why people sweat, and what makes bodies grow tired.

Five years of hard work followed, years without school and without satisfying answers to questions. One August day, young Bill Deeks, who was now fourteen, walked home to supper, faced his father and announced that he planned to leave home. The Deeks family listened, their mouths open. Old Bill gazed sternly at his son and asked for a reason. Young Bill could think of only one answer.

"Because I've got to know things."

Old Bill Deeks made a somewhat unexpected answer. He said, "If you want to go, then go ahead."

It was dark by the time supper was finished. Young Bill walked out into the night and down the darkening road to the village. First he found work at a country store; hours, six in the morning till nine at night; pay, three dollars a week. In spite of all that, Bill Deeks liked the store and the people who came to its counters. He liked the school children who came to buy books and tablets. He read some of the books and found them good company. After a year in the store, he went to the storekeeper, thanked him, and resigned.

"Why?"

"I've got to learn things. I've got to find answers."

Bill Deeks went home. The family welcomed him to a prodigal breakfast of buckwheat cakes, fat sausages, fried eggs, and black coffee. It was Sunday and the homecomer rode to church with all the family. After church the two Bills talked. Young Bill declared his intention of going to school—to McGill University down in Montreal. As he talked, he sensed paternal admiration. Old Bill had no money. His wealth and his poverty were his land. Neither father nor son mentioned money. Old Bill said that in order to go to college a man had to be a scholar. The only man in those parts who could make a scholar out of anybody was the parson. If the parson would consent, young Bill could hire himself as a student, and pay for his tutoring with chores.

The parson agreed, and young Bill Deeks spent two years getting in shape. When he was ready, with fifty dollars sewed into his clothes, dressed in a ragged woolen suit at least two years too short, with an apple box packed with food contributed by his mother, and a giant, black, crook-handled umbrella donated by his father, Bill Deeks proceeded to Montreal and McGill University. A great, scientific curiosity was on its way toward the medical problems of the tropics. As Deeks gaped at the great buildings, he noticed another shabby youth standing beside him.

"I came here from the West," said the youth, "a year ago. I was homesick then—same as you are. I stood and hoped for somebody to show me around, like I'm ready to show you around. My name's John Goff."

John Goff and Bill Deeks became roommates and friends. They took an unheated cell-like room out in a slum section of the city. They began the assiduous cultivation of first mustaches, which in wintertime acquired icicles after morning face-washings. They learned that men can live month in and month out on rice, milk, and apples—raw apples and rice cooked in water over a lamp chimney.

Shortly after his arrival Bill Deeks appeared before the dean, Sir William Dawson, applying for admission to the university. Sir William considered the candidate. Abashed by the consideration, the candidate sought vainly to hide his shabby clothes. It was soon apparent that the dean was not interested in appearance. He was interested in questions and answers. He asked questions for two grueling hours. At the end of the two hours Bill was accepted as a "preliminary" student.

After two years, during which he came very close to starvation,

Bill Deeks finished the academic course as class valedictorian. His father quit farming long enough to journey to Montreal for the occasion—as proud a father as ever strolled across a college green.

The following year Bill joined John Goff in the long grind of medical school. Like grass blades working through hard-crusted soil, they pushed to the lead of their respective classes. After Deeks's first year, he found himself again penniless and in rags, but stubbornly determined to remain a scientist. Apparently Dean Dawson held the same belief, for he again summoned Bill Deeks.

"You need to travel; to see new country; to study outside of college."

Sir William then explained that he proposed to send Bill to Saskatchewan for a summer to perform certain services for the university and to observe the life and health of Canadian Indians—all expenses paid.

Heretofore Bill Deeks had seen only a few of the St. Lawrence villages and Montreal. He now went out into a new, breath-taking world. From the railway terminal at Whitehorse he rode horseback into the far mountains, stopped at a solitary hut and saw a woman in childbirth—without a doctor, a neighbor, or any other human attendant. Deeks served as obstetrician, helped by his home experience in watching the foaling of mares and cows. The fact that the woman and her baby lived had its effects. Bill was doubly resolved to practice medicine. These Indians seemed to him the most capable of physicians. They practiced prevention before cures. They used food instead of pills and powders. They were meat eaters, but along with lean meat they also ate the fat and entrails, the hearts and lungs, of freshly slaughtered cattle and deer. Bill Deeks noted that most of the Indians were good physical specimens. Certainly they were not bowlegged. Unlike most other rural people, their teeth were sound and clean. Bill pondered upon these realities.

Sir William welcomed his returning scholar. "You'll not stop at being an ordinary doctor. You are much too inquisitive for that."

Deeks won an instructorship in the medical school and, accordingly, he did his dissecting work and most of his laboratory exercises after school hours and on Sundays. When final graduation came, he was tired and, like most of his classmates, aged far beyond his actual years.

For a second time he was chosen valedictorian, but this time he was sick. Graduation finished, he walked painfully to the college hospital and went to bed. Once more Sir William Dawson gave him counsel.

"When you are rested, I'll find you a place as ship's doctor. Salt air and open ocean will bring back your health."

So young Dr. Deeks went to sea as surgeon on a lumber ship. After some six months he returned to Montreal to hang out his shingle and search for patients. He found one whom other physicians of the neighborhood had assiduously avoided. A certain nosy widow of the block was notorious as the most effective scandalmonger in all Montreal. The old lady had an invalid daughter who had been more or less bedridden for nine years. Each physician who attended the girl had left with a very much enfeebled reputation. In spite of the record, Bill Deeks attended the girl. Since he had no other patient, he resolved to turn heaven and earth to help this one. He succeeded. The girl recovered after he had successfully removed an unsuspectedly troublesome appendix. The gossipy mother went through the neighborhood telling the miraculous news. She told it from rooftops, street corners, shop counters, and church aisles. Bill Deeks was made. Within a week he had other patients, and his practice began to multiply.

Dr. Deeks was happy in his practice, but he was poor. Most of his patients could not afford sufficient food, much less pay doctor bills. Much of the time he gave his medical services free. Frequently he gave groceries instead of pills or tonics. As his practice grew, he began to think again of Mr. Pickwick with the bowed legs. He was distinctly aware that hunger and malnutrition were among the foremost allies of disease; that substantial areas of Montreal were islands of starvation in a figurative ocean of plenty.

Deeks continued to study nutrition. He pondered on the challenging immensity of his unfocused subject. He resolved to save until he could go to Vienna. Saving was slow and tedious. Though his practice flourished, his fees continued to be skimpy. Moreover, his father's farms were beginning to fail. Bill Deeks undertook to restock the lands with pure-bred cattle, much to the delight of his father, who was no longer the strong man of Williamsburg.[1]

Meanwhile Bill continued to study and to publish scientific papers. By 1902 he was chosen lecturer on medicine at the University of Bishop's College of Montreal. With the issue of July, 1902, he began publishing in the *Montreal Medical Journal* studies of old age, of cardiac maladies, of suprarenal extract treatment for Addison's disease. The succinct, fact-crammed papers demonstrated great curiosity; also an ever-present interest in human nutrition and the conviction that food is the staff of life and improper food the main barrier to health.

The doctor was getting along in his profession, but he did not forget his resolve to study at Vienna. To this end he not only saved money, he studied German. In the comparatively good year of 1904, Vienna was gay. To it came doctors from five continents, some to study, and perhaps more to make merry and study later—after waltzes, love, and drinks were finished, after horse-chestnut blossoms no longer festooned the Prater.

But William Deeks came to Vienna to study, and his arrival marked the second stage of his trip to the tropics. Wagner, Strauss, beer, and love-making were purely incidental. Bill was especially anxious to study human nutrition—not in a classroom or in lecture halls but in hospital wards, clinics, farm homes, and city tenements. So he came to Vienna as an "auditor," seeking to learn, not to annex additional degrees. By noteworthy coincidence the Vienna of 1904 was beginning to think about tropical medicine. Malaria, dysentery, typhus, pellagra, and other cosmopolitan diseases with important tropical significance were being treated and studied in its clinics and hospitals.

Due attention was being paid to the memorable proofs offered by Walter Reed and his associates of the United States Army Yellow Fever Board; to the noteworthy findings in malaria reported by Sir Ronald Ross and French and British researchers in Algeria and India. The fame of Sir Patrick Manson, called the father of tropical medicine, was spreading throughout the medical world. Colleges of tropical medicine were being founded in various capitals—Hong Kong, London, Hamburg, and Brussels. It was an era of imperialism and Sir Patrick Manson had taken the lead in proclaiming that tropical medicine was as profitable as it was interesting. Deeks had no particular interest in money for its own sake. But he remembered vividly the brief, busy growing seasons of Canada and the long sterile intervals of winter. He could not help thinking of the tropical earth which raises crops and foods every day and month of the year. Though he had never traveled toward the equator, he began to visualize the tropics as a potential refuge for the harassed peoples of an overcrowded world. He pictured the immense possibilities of the lush hot countries as laboratories and study centers for work in nutrition.

Late in 1905 Dr. Deeks decided to set up practice in New York, which people said was on its way to becoming a New World Vienna. He rented an office in a then typical white-collar apartment block. Fate, or perhaps a particularly well-satisfied patient, brought to his waiting room Colonel and Mrs. William Crawford Gorgas, who were in New York on vacation from Panama and were looking for a good family-style doctor.

Dr. Deeks had heard a great deal about Dr. Gorgas. The gigantic adventure called the Panama Canal was the talk of the day. Medical journals were already describing Gorgas's work in the "pesthole of the Western World." New York newspapers, which had previously recorded "pre-Gorgas" and "post-Gorgas" accounts of Havana, now published lurid stories of sudden death in the Panama jungles, of disease-carrying mosquitoes, of ruthless maladies which blew in like tropical hurricanes.

Gorgas said he had long wanted to meet Dr. Deeks, whose published papers had come to the favorable attention of the great Alabamian. Reciprocity was complete. Gorgas, like Deeks, was a delightful individual to meet—soft-voiced, handsome, and reassuring. After his first visit Gorgas returned to discuss symptoms. But he forgot to mention symptoms because he was too preoccupied with offering Dr. Deeks the post of clinic director at the refurbished Ancon Hospital.

Dr. Deeks promptly accepted, closed his office and sailed for Panama, the jungle hellhole which awaited transformation into a land where healthy men might work. Gorgas had said that Panama was a proving ground for medical techniques. All the world now knew that Gorgas had good reason to know what he was talking about. So, in the spring of 1906, Dr. William Edgar Deeks, near forty, unmarried, renowned, and still asking why, was sitting in a deck chair on a banana ship, anticipating his first sight of the American tropics.

When the banana ship pulled into Colon its passengers plunged into a thick, fetid atmosphere of heat, filth, and disease. Colon's disease and attendant crime were notorious. Gorgas field crews, assisted by United States soldiers, were beginning the long-projected "clean-up offensive." Parts of the Big Ditch were beginning to show the work that had been done on them. Piers were piled high with machinery and steel. Ships were arriving, their decks black with West Indian Negroes. Work camps and railheads were appearing by the hour throughout the jungle.

Swarms of flies and mosquitoes came scouting from the lowland villages. Sick camps were becoming crowded even before their tin roofs could be set in place. Gorgas was on the scene. Gorgas doctors and nurses were arriving from various corners of creation. The marines had landed. But only the mosquitoes had the situation well in hand.

Dr. Bill Deeks proceeded by two-coach railway train across the Isthmus to Panama City and thence by mule-drawn army ambulance to Ancon Hill and the already aging, flat-roofed, much-annexed institution serving as base hospital and medical center for the entire Canal Zone. Its considerably scattered clinic, which awaited the new director, had already become one of the busiest in the Western Hemisphere. Patients were clamoring for admission at a rate which the rapidly increasing staff could not handle.

Bill Deeks went to work. Before the first day was finished he learned that Dr. William James's assertion that a Canal Zone medical man is too busy to ask questions was highly factual. A Jamaican orderly showed the new doctor to a cot in a cluttered lobby near the clinic and admonished him not to fret about the many bad qualities of the bed, since in any case he wouldn't have much time or opportunity to use it.

Within a few days the medical newcomer was assigned to bachelor quarters—a one-story screened bungalow on the green hillside beyond the hospital. The veranda faced the Pacific. There was a flower garden, planted many years before by French nuns, and a convenient scattering of orange trees and tall poplarlike Castilloas. The veranda was an ideal spot upon which to sit and sip a highball and ponder the eternal verities—when and if time allowed.

Deeks began to learn about Panama. Though work frequently kept him from going far into the country, the same work quite literally brought Panama, and indeed all the American tropics, to him. The ever-questioning doctor began to note his findings:

Since the American occupation of the Canal Zone its inhabitants may be divided into two groups: the one composed of those who work for the Isthmian Canal Commission; the other made up of natives of the country, with such immigrants as have been attracted by the increase of business.

The first group comprises three distinct races: the American, which is Anglo-Saxon in origin; the European, made up mostly of Spanish and Italian laborers, with considerable preponderance of Spaniards; and the West Indian Negro, coming in greater part from the islands of Jamaica and Barbados. . . .

These three races are natives of localities where, broadly speaking, malaria does not prevail to any great degree. The Italians are mostly from the north of Italy; the Spaniards from the north of Spain; and Jamaica is not badly infected with malaria, while Barbados is said to be free from endemic cases. Such immunity against malaria as is present during the earlier stages of a residence here, is therefore racial and not acquired. . . . Americans and Europeans are alike susceptible to the disease, while the Negro possesses a partial racial immunity.

The same general conditions of sanitation, such as drainage, water supply, sites from which grass and underbrush are removed, and inspection of quarters by the Department of Sanitation, obtain equally among the three races. . . . The American employees of the Commission . . . almost without exception live in houses provided by the Commission. . . . Among these employees the use of quinine at the first onset of fever is universal, and prompt consultation with the nearest Commission physician is the rule. Each employee is granted six weeks' vacation, with pay, for twelve months' service, and the vacation must be taken in the States or a malaria free country. . . .

At night the Americans do not frequent the native quarters in the Zone towns, do not expose themselves unnecessarily to malarial infections, and of their own initiative aid greatly in preserving their health and in keeping sanitary regulations. . . .

Those of the European laborers who so desire, live in well-kept and carefully screened barracks, and for their families screened quarters are provided. But no amount of advice seems to be effective in securing among them individual prophylaxis against the disease. Every sanitary regulation needs to be rigidly enforced. They often prefer to sleep in hammocks or even on the ground under their quarters. . . . They mingle freely at night with the natives, and cannot be kept indoors. They are indifferent to personal hygiene and equally indifferent to their state of health, until illness compels them to seek aid.

As elsewhere in the world, the enforcement of sanitation among the Negroes is a gigantic task. A small percentage only of this race lives in the free quarters provided by the Commission. The rest prefer cheap lodging houses where they huddle together like so many sheep, or else they live in straw-thatched huts after the manner of the natives. . . .[2]

In a region which was a center of malarial infection, employed in a hospital where staff members (including Dr. William Gorgas himself) were working from twelve to twenty-four hours a day, Sundays included, Bill Deeks learned about malaria. During 1906 Ancon Hospital treated and discharged 7,561 cases of malaria. During 1907 this total passed the 8,000 mark, and during 1908 it reached almost to 9,000. There was every reason for Dr. Deeks to continue his study of malaria which was causing between a half and three-quarters of all hospital admissions. The questioning Canadian, still questioning, was almost instantly elevated to an important lieutenancy in the most aggressive warfare man has ever waged against one of the world's worst scourges.

Malaria stubbornly kept its place as the "universal disease" of the Canal Zone. During 1906, Bill Deeks's first year there, 821 canal employees out of every thousand were admitted to commission hospitals for malaria treatment. During that year Dr. Deeks and the much-overworked Ancon Hospital staff, received about 12,500 of the total of 30,400 admissions to all hospitals and sick camps of the Canal Zone. During the following year, hospital admissions along the Big Ditch had reached an all-time high of 58,521. Of these Ancon Hospital admitted more than 14,000. Virtually every employee on the canal went to a hospital at least once during that year. The daily hospital train had become a routine institution. Wet seasons brought still more malaria. And wet seasons were as wet as they were regular. November of 1906 saw 19 inches of rainfall. November, 1909, touched a record high of 28 inches.

Dr. William Deeks was impressed with the vagaries of malaria recurrence. "In our opinion . . . variations in malaria occurrence is due more to relapses than to primary infections or reinfections. . . . In untreated syphilis, patients will return repeatedly with malaria relapses. . . . Influenza is also an important factor in the production of malarial relapse. . . . It is not unusual to observe a patient develop a chill while under treatment for influenza. . . .

Injury, an operation, administration of an anesthetic, childbirth, any severe shock . . . may interrupt the temporary immunity established in latent malaria. . . . Muscular fatigue has long been known as an important means of participating a malarial chill. . . .[3]

In front-porch conversation with Drs. William James, Herbert Clark, Alfred Herrick, and other bright young men of Canal Zone medicine, Dr. Deeks had proclaimed that malaria is more than a disease. Like marriage, politics and war, it is also a social-economic institution. During man-breaking days and nights spent attending a perennially overcrowded hospital clinic Deeks became convinced that malnutrition, another social-economic institution, is a fundamental factor in most important tropical diseases, malaria not excepted.

"Malaria remains a gigantic problem, difficult to solve. . . . Hookworm and other intestinal infestations play minor roles in their attendant economic loss, but of outstanding importance in raising the efficiency of labor in all tropical countries is the influence of nutrition. The effectiveness of the natural defensive agents of the body, through which diseases of all kinds are prevented and cured, rests in its final analysis on nutrition, and this necessitates a satisfactory, well-balanced diet."[4]

From one of the world's best vantage points, Dr. Deeks was learning that even in the tropics, where vegetation has the benefit of an eternal spring, where jungles are so inordinately crowded with life that there appears to be neither time nor space for death, tropical peoples are nevertheless pitiably undernourished and most frequently sick because they are badly fed.

The Canadian's thought went back to his childhood and recalled the schoolhouse episode of Mr. Pickwick, the pig, and the bowed legs. Bill Deeks was still thinking about the reasons for mortal bowleggedness. Here in the canal-side jungles, testimonies of human malnutrition were not limited to everyday Temperate Zone deformities such as bowleggedness, rotted teeth, rickets, and potbellies.

Day and night the great Ancon Clinic served as clearing center for those more virulent and spectacular tragedies of malnutrition which are common in the tropics. Through the humid and seemingly interminable office hours Dr. Deeks, drenched in sweat, served as recorder and physician to hundreds of human beings sick for no other reason than that their stomachs were improperly filled or, worse yet, left pitiably empty.

Deeks saw pellagra in all its confusing multiplicity of symptoms. One day the hospital train brought three sick children. One, a boy of thirteen, who was approximately the size of a normal five-year-old, was tormented by a severe skin rash. The back of the child's hands, forearms and neck, as well as his forehead and cheeks, appeared to be severely sunburned. "Sunburn" was written on the entry card. Bill Deeks threw aside the diagnosis. Though still new to the tropics he had learned in Vienna the symptoms of third-stage pellagra.

The next child was suffering from bloody diarrhea; the third from skin irritation similar to that of the first, except that the inflamed patches were dull brown, as if burned by acid. The doctor began to question the children about their usual diet. The three answered, almost in chorus:

"We eat tortillas and beans except when we don't have any beans and then we eat tortillas."

The questioning doctor had already learned that field corn, ground into coarse meal and fried as thin, flapjack-style tortillas, is the principal food of most Panama Indians. He knew, also, that pellagra, a disease of general food deficiency aggravated by an infectious factor, is frequently associated with a diet consisting of little but corn. He recognized the varying symptoms of the three Indian children as standard symptoms of pellagra. So he put them in the hospital and prescribed diets of fresh meat, green vegetables, and fresh milk. All three recovered.

He treated pellagra in a dozen other disguises, particularly in native women, many of whom suffered extreme depression of spirit, or severe headache, or relentless insomnia, or tremors of the tongue or hands, or sudden attacks of giddiness which caused them to fall to the ground (and frequently to be inaccurately listed as cases of heat prostration), or confusional insanity, or various combinations of these unhappy afflictions. All of these, Dr. Deeks discovered, may be symptoms of pellagra, and are frequently curable by diet correction.

Pellagra, he found, was bad enough, but it was not the only nutritional ailment. A gruesome procession of beriberi cripples trooped through Ancon. That was more than a third of a century ago and knowledge of dietary diseases, still much too feeble, was then almost nonexistent.

Beriberi had been called the rice disease, or more exactly the polished rice disease. Its most conspicuous endemic centers were, and are, such rice-eating nations as Japan, Thailand, the Netherlands Indies. Dr. Deeks promptly renamed it the excessive-starch disease. There was no sizable rice-eating public in the Canal Zone at that time, but natives and many imported laborers were starch-eating peoples. And there certainly was beriberi.

Many years later other distinguished researchers, such as Wellman and Bass, confirmed Deeks's contention by pointing out that one of the world's three largest endemic centers of beriberi includes Brazilian areas where rice is not an important food, though corn grits, boiled white potatoes, macaroni, and sago are predominant. Certainly beriberi is a poor man's disease, most prevalent in warm, damp climates and bad hygienic surroundings.

Deeks's first care was to relieve the tragic symptoms—the numb legs and feet, which incapacitate the sufferer for work, the skin blotches, which develop into running sores, and other chronic and lingering deformities. He watched tortured fellow beings die of heart failure—a frequent accompaniment of beriberi. He became grimly acquainted with the "hobbles," a manifestation in which the leg muscles begin to fail and the sufferer, his feet far apart, staggers and lurches as if groping with an imaginary cane.

At least once the questioning doctor saw a case of "beriberi corset" —one of the most terrible causes of death known to man. An old Negro came to the clinic complaining of a hellishly painful chest. "Mistah doctah," he wailed, "I'se bein' squshed to death!" The old man's diaphragm was paralyzed. Quite helplessly, Dr. Deeks watched the sufferer fall to the floor, wail, writhe, and die.

One night when Deeks was resting on the cool veranda of his bachelor quarters, relaxing in the sleepy tropic night, he indulged his taste for questioning upon a rough, tough field doctor newly arrived from the wilds of Texas.

Deeks proposed question after question about jungle fare. Presently the Texan finished his drink and answered, "What the hell do you care? You don't have to eat with 'em, do you?"

"Yes," said Dr. Deeks, "from now on that is part of my job. And if you only knew it, it's part of yours too."

He began to learn at first hand what tropical diet was really like. He joined the ragamuffin sons and daughters of misery who strolled streets and jungle trails chewing strips of sugar cane. He concluded that if Canadian food was inadequate, tropical food was positively lethal. For Canadians had meat—good beef and pork, including active metabolic tissues, such as liver, kidneys, and heart. In the lowland tropics, production of cattle and swine was, and still is, rare and discouraging. Cattle are grown in the grassy tropical highlands, but even in the highlands there is little grain feeding and therefore no adequate production of milk. In the lowlands few of the native inhabitants keep cattle. The beef which they occasionally have an opportunity to buy is usually of deplorable quality: scrawny, fly-stung, and too often, filthy.

Moreover, no system of preservation and distribution of fresh meat and milk has been devised except in a few localities where foreign influence is in operation. In the Island of Puerto Rico, Ashford states that the consumption of fresh milk per capita averages less than one ounce a day. Imported canned and powdered milk have a limited consumption . . . the same may be said of fresh fish, which are available as food stuffs only in the localities where they are caught. . . .

Very little poultry is raised in the country districts, as they are prone to disease and preyed on by many wild animals. Consequently the protein supply from this source, or from eggs, is exceedingly small. The chief protein sources are those from cereal grains and beans, which are not as suitable for human growth as proteins from animal sources because of the disproportional relationships of their amino-acids, as compared with those from animal proteins. This may account for the small stature of many of the native inhabitants, particularly in the coastal plains.

The fat supplies are mainly vegetable oils and imported lard substitutes, none of which contain adequate supplies of vitamins. Their carbohydrates are derived mainly from starchy roots, such as yucca yams, sweet potatoes, etc., and in some localities rice and maize cereals. . . .

Green vegetables are difficult to grow in the coastal plains because of insect pests and the necessity of labor and skilled attention; and although some excellent spinach-like plants grow wild, they are not utilized to any extent. Several varieties of cultivated fruits are obtained at certain seasons of the year, but only bananas and plantains the whole year round. The average native gives little thought or care to fruit culture, and depends more or less upon an inadequate supply of native wild fruits. . . .

We are accustomed to consider only a few syndromes as directly resulting from deficiency in diets, such as beriberi, scurvy, rickets, pellagra, and sprue. This is far from the fact, as an extensive clinical experience demonstrates.[5]

As Bill Deeks learned more about the commonplace tropical diet, and more about its insidious wreckage of tropical health, he also learned more of the insurmountable difficulties of improving the common man's eating habits.

The nature of a daily ration is rarely the result of accident. There are sound, tough climatic and environmental reasons for tropical fondness for over-starchy foods. There are also financial, traditional, and horticultural reasons. Work, planning, and objective skills are required for changing luxuriant vegetation into an adequate food supply. Deeks had learned from earlier and personal experience that a hungry man is not inclined to consider complicated theories of balanced diet or to reflect that it is possible to starve even with a full stomach. He observed, too, that culinary prejudices can be as forceful in the tropics as anywhere else, and still more discouraging, that the provision of canned foods and other commercial processed products can prove even more ruinous to consumers in the tropics than to their more habituated victims in the United States and Canada. For dietetic needs are even more exacting in hot countries than in cold countries.

Impossible as it seemed, something had to be done. No doctor worthy of the name could deliberately and indefinitely avoid the issue. The busy wards, corridors, and clinic rooms of Ancon Hospital produced superb testimony that good life arises from good earth and that the basically good tropical soil was poorly tended and tragically misused.

The discerning and fact-hungry Deeks studied obstetrical cases and saw plainly the serious situation of women in the tropics, who, because of faulty nutrition, are unable to produce sufficient milk to feed their babies. The doctor began to compile ingenious tables of infant nutrition and to ponder the comparative effectiveness of the milk of various animal mothers:

Animal	Time Required for Doubling Weight at Birth	Protein	Ash	Lime	Phosphoric Acid
			Per Cent		
Man	180 days	1.0	.2	0.032	.047
Horse	60	2.0	.4	0.124	0.131
Calf	4.7	3.5	.7	0.160	0.197
Goat	19	4.3	.08	0.210	0.322
Hog	18	5.9	...	....	....
Sheep	10	6.5	0.9	0.272	0.412
Cat	9.5	7.0	1.0	....	....
Dog	8	7.3	1.3	0.453	0.493
Rabbit	7	10.4	2.4	0.891	0.996 [6]

The questioning doctor concluded that the place to begin a campaign to defeat tropical malnutrition was the nipple. Better formulas for babies would result in better adults. In spite of incessant interruptions and overlong working hours he developed several of the earliest successful feeding formulas for infants. News of this work, then unprecedented, reached food manufacturers of the United States. One of his first baby food formulas he contributed to the Nestle Company. One after another he gave his feeding formulas without charge to manufacturers who promptly exploited the formulas to their own advantage.

It is not strange that, in Ancon Hospital, Dr. Deeks won the enduring title of "Daddy." Though a bachelor and a moderately gay one, from the time of his infant-feeding study, he was Daddy Deeks and his increasing force of physician assistants were Daddy Deeks's boys.

In the tropics that was what passes for fun, and Daddy Deeks was a man to cherish fun. Nature had provided him with twinkling eyes and a genius for easy laughter, and he was among the gayer of the gay-blade medicos of Ancon, which is not saying little. "The Three Bills"—Deeks, James, and Herrick—presently occupied the same bachelor's bungalow, and inaugurated a regime of more or less open house, enthusiastically attended by dozens of Canal Zone medical men, including the great Gorgas.

The Three Bills called their tranquil veranda the Highball Deck. Some of the material for merriment was purely liquid, some indigenous, and some incidental to the work at hand. For example, one day two of the Three Bills noticed the Ancon maternity ward in the act of receiving an inert, potbellied priest. The fat padre, touched by heat, had collapsed at the foot of Ancon hill. Hospital orderlies, Jamaica Negroes (and Protestants), had sighted a human being in distress; noting the long skirts, the rolled-brim hat, and the impressive bulge of the mid-section—also the pallid face and the black raiment—then standard for Central American womankind—had assumed that the maternity ward was the place for the patient. They promptly placed the padre next to the delivery room, and with much bowing and babble reported an imminent blessed event.

In this atmosphere of evil enemies and good friends Bill Deeks continued to work and learn. In collaboration with Dr. William James, he prepared and published an elaborate report on hemoglobinuric (blackwater) fever in the Canal Zone. The work, a highly scholarly report to Colonel Gorgas, was published in 1911 by the Isthmian Canal Commission. It remains one of the most respected studies of malaria and malarial complications ever published in American medical literature.

When Bill Deeks found time to stop and take stock he noted, with considerable amazement, that he had spent nine years in the infinitely fertile laboratory of the tropics. The Big Ditch was nearing completion. Great ships were waiting to ride its miraculous locks. Within the Canal Zone disease was materially reduced. Hospital admissions had at last begun to show a noticeable decline.

Europe was beginning to rumble with the then greatest of wars. Deeks realized that he was forty-nine and beginning to grow bald. His eyebrows and cropped mustache were turning gray, and he was tired. Gorgas was studying pneumonia in Africa. Daddy Deeks's boys had learned the hospital ropes. So Deeks himself announced that he was going to take a long leave for a world cruise. The "boys" listened in understanding silence. They weren't misled by a chronically busy man's professed desire to rest. Britain was at war. The Empire was calling its man power. Bill Deeks's "world tour" would most probably end at an army camp somewhere in England.

So it did. At Hull, the Medical Corps of the British Army put him to work as a civilian volunteer.

"I was set to examining recruits. In all the hundreds I examined, I didn't find one set of perfect teeth. The more I traveled, the more people I saw, the more completely convinced I became that diet is the all-important factor in life." [7]

Britain's army of 1915 had plenty of doctors—in fact, more than it could use. Dr. Deeks felt justified in deciding to return to Canada for a visit to his boyhood home. Although ships were scarce and the Kaiser's submarines voracious, he finally succeeded in booking passage on a rusty old tub called the *King Edward*.

It was a stormy voyage. The *King Edward's* engines broke down among the icebergs off Greenland. There were cold, slow days of waiting. With few exceptions, the passengers were desperately seasick. One exception was a table of five bachelors, including Dr. William Edgar Deeks. The other was a young lady, who had been in Paris studying voice. The young lady was charming, and her gowns were as interesting as she. The bachelor's table collected a pool of a hundred dollars as a regard for the one who could make the most headway with the lady. Bill Deeks won the hundred dollars and the girl; she was Clara Cramer Strunk, of Pennsylvania. They landed at Quebec with the wedding planned. But at that point Dr. Deeks received a letter with a Boston postmark.

The United Fruit Company, with plantations, towns, fleets, and railways scattered throughout much of the American tropics, desired the services of a superintendent for its already renowned medical department. The United Fruit Company, "after long and studious consideration," had chosen Dr. William Deeks for the position.

It is more or less axiomatic that men so "chosen" by the United Fruit Company become members of that company's staff. Dr. Deeks was no exception. He was already acquainted with the company's brilliant progress in tropical medicine and sanitation. At Ancon Hospital he had repeatedly rubbed elbows and swapped conversation with members of the company's medical department. The story of the United Fruit Company's place and work in tropical health administration is told in better detail in the chapter on "Banana Medicine."

While Gorgas was directing the epic cleanup of Havana, and while Walter Reed and his fellow workers were making medical history at Camp Lazear, the United Fruit Company was building and equipping in Panana a base hospital and clinic for the benefit of tropical plantation workers. During the ten years of canal building, the United Fruit Company's investments in tropical medicine had multiplied until by 1916 the company was using a dozen field hospitals and a medical personnel of more than five hundred to pioneer field sanitation and social medicine throughout a trade sphere which include Cuba, Jamaica, and much of the Caribbean frontage of Mexico, Central America, and Colombia.

Now that the canal was nearing completion the medical loads of the Isthmian Commission were abating. But the great banana company was only beginning to fall into its stride. It needed Dr. Deeks and it would have places for a number of his Ancon Hospital "boys." Accordingly, the questioning doctor got married, went to Boston, and once more sailed south on a trim white banana ship for an inspection tour. Unlike his earlier trip, this one was also a honeymoon.

Deeks now found himself a family head and a ranking medical executive. Like mallards and managers of baseball teams, banana company executives are usually highly migratory and much given to flying south in cold weather. In spite of these frequent intervals of migration, the doctor's married life was happy and serene, with much music and increasing ranks of friends. On Lincoln's Birthday, 1917, his wife gave birth to a daughter, Kathleen. Enormously pleased, the doctor assured his friends that at last he had a home consumer of some of those baby rations on the data for which he had spent so many thousands of off-hours.

Family life could not, however, interrupt Bill Deeks's study of tropical nutrition. He saw that the need for such study increased by the day. Then, as now, precise statistics about the extent of tropical malnutrition were not to be had. In tropical medicine it has for too long been tacitly assumed that there is no need to compile statistics about the effects of improper diet on a population which has been so consistently underfed that malnutrition is practically normal.

Furthermore, much depends upon the point of view. Even in our own country the relation of diet to disease is still in dispute in many, many cases. When poor food results in a case of rickets, everyone agrees that it is dietary. If an undernourished person contracts tuberculosis, the role of malnutrition is much more speculative.

So far as Latin America is concerned, tables of figures and columns of percentages are not needed to prove the wide incidence of malnutrition. Anyone who has had opportunity to learn the incredibly limited lists of foods available for rural populations knows that the problem exists on an enormous scale. The basis of rural diet in Latin America is the crop or crops easiest to grow or to gather. Corn, plantain ("cooking banana"), and wild fruits, where there are any, or freshly slaughtered beef and pork, when and if available, are the week-in week-out fare of millions. Even if there are a few pesos to spend on food in the local *tienda*, or crossroads store, José Mozo tends to buy heavy starchy food because it provides the most filling for his very limited money. The idea that children require special body-building foods and vitamins is still little known in a great many areas outside of the larger and more progressive cities.

Tropical people working for the United Fruit Company and other established employers have an earning power capable of noticeably improving their diet. Dr. Deeks promptly observed that regular wages were not instantly or completely converted into better food. But he also noticed that, as a matter of hospital and clinical record, improved earning power lowers the frequency of nutritional diseases —despite the fact that so many commercial food products were and are very bad foods.

These busy years would not let Deeks forget that combating malnutrition is a slow and complex warfare, never clearly limited as to place or time. He was persistently aware of the medical side of the problem: that there were huge gaps in the science of dietetics; that the definition and classification of vitamins—in which achievement he himself was winning a distinguished place—was full of grave dangers. Even if you were right about vitamins your rightness could be wronged by dishonest commercial exploitation. Deeks kept clearly in mind the necessity of objective research and stubborn scientific toil.

During January, 1923, he was invited to lecture at the Harvard Medical School on food requirements for the maintenance of health —with particular reference to the American tropics. His address summarized the accrued convictions of seventeen years as an ambassador in white:

We develop certain habits, and on entering new conditions in the tropics, we carry our food habits with us. A great many of the vegetables so common in our northern latitudes, do not grow in the tropics, and consequently we are inclined to use canned goods (which are largely devitamined in their manufacture) instead of adjusting ourselves to the new conditions and using the vegetables and fruits which grow abundantly at hand. . . .

From an extensive clinical experience in the tropics I am fully cognizant of the ill effects of an excessive starch and sugar diet deficient in meats, green vegetables and fruits. I was aware of the tendency to fermentation and systemic autointoxication in a diet in which carbohydrates predominate, and traced a great many morbid conditions to their excessive use. . . . The newer studies of nutrition not only verify the clinical experience then obtained, but explain the fundamental reason for the morbid processes. [He added sternly:] If you want to live long and remain healthy, select a mixed diet properly balanced . . . and avoid as much as possible the refined foods of commerce. . . .[8]

Through busy years Dr. William Deeks continued to study that childhood problem—what makes people bowlegged. He encouraged others to ponder the question. He improved and continued the superb annual reports of the United Fruit Company's medical department, and encouraged his staff of physicians, more than fifty, to contribute reports and deductions from their individual studies and experience to the annual volumes which soon gained international recognition as boons to the study and understanding of tropical medicine. He made extensive studies of hookworm and its relation to diet and living standards.[9] He prepared and published noteworthy reports on the influence of nutrition upon dental symptoms and tooth decay.[10] He made extensive study of the prevention and treatment of tropical pneumonia [11] and other respiratory diseases.[12] He continued research in pellagra.[13]

Through fifteen years with the United Fruit Company this questioning doctor continued to study nutrition and malnutrition while directing an incessantly busy and fast-growing federation of hospitals and medical centers. His scientific publications followed in rapid and impressive succession. The ranks of the Deeks boys doubled and tripled. Most important, he watched the persistent reduction of the death tolls and sick lists of banana lands. He saw initial malaria indices fall to a half, a fourth, a tenth, or a twentieth. He watched hookworm disappear from place after place. He watched memorable improvement in the surgical records of banana-lands hospitals. He saw a gradual but widespread reduction in the toll of acute dietary diseases.

At Kingston, Jamaica, during June and July of 1924, supported by his company, Deeks assembled an international conference on health problems in the American tropics. To this conference came leaders of tropical medicine throughout the world—great medical names from South America, Central America, the West Indies, the United States and Canada, the British Isles, Europe, Africa, India, China, and the rest of the Far East; among others, Drs. Hideyo Noguchi, of the Rockefeller Institute, John G. Thompson and Aldo Castellani, of the London School of Tropical Medicine; Milton R. Rosenau, of Harvard; Albert R. Patterson, of East African Kenya; Sir Thomas Oliver, of Durham University; Joseph A. Le Prince, senior sanitary engineer of the Panama Canal; Dr. Henry Rose Carter; Sir James Fowler, of Britain's Colonial Medical Advisory Committee; Aristides Agramonte, of Cuba; Miguel Arango, of Colombia; Dean Charles C. Bass, of Tulane; Frederick G. Banting, of the University of Toronto, and dozens more of the great medical names of this century.

Dr. Deeks considered the conference the greatest ever held and the high point of his long, busy medical career.

The doctor bore his years gracefully. At sixty-four, he was still directing an extremely busy medical office in New York, making frequent study and inspection trips to the tropics, attending many medical clubs and study groups, and finding life good. As the years hurried on, he found more and more laughter in them.

Dr. Deeks came to feel at home in New York, even though his oversized handbag was usually packed ready for quick departure to the tropics. His life continued happy. During 1924 he had become a citizen of the United States, explaining that he "liked Canada none the less, but he had come to like the United States more."

He began writing a book on nutrition, hoping to make it a guide book to inter-American health. The book was never published, for during his sixties he began to suffer from a failing heart. On the morning of July 25, 1931, he finished breakfast, donned his hat and started for his office. But he collapsed before he reached his apartment door. His wife hurried to help him and to call the family doctor. But before night he was dead.

Bill Deeks had earned a place as one of the great clinicians and medical administrators of the American tropics. There is good reason to believe that his studies of nutrition and malnutrition within the American tropics have helped pave the way for better agriculture and better life throughout much of the Western Hemisphere.

Chapter Eight

NOGUCHI OF JAPAN

WHEN and if the last fertile but now dangerous acre of tropical America is thrown open to the uses of the hungry, materials-starved population of the Western Hemisphere, the names of a great variety of men of many races will be remembered as pioneers. Among them will be men who have given what they had to give for many reasons, men of many origins and many types of character. None of them will prove more fascinating, more inscrutable, none will, by their careers, give rise to greater controversy than Hideyo Noguchi, the great Japanese-American scientist of New York—Rockefeller Institute for Medical Research—whose name is inseparably associated with the disease, supposedly conquered by the Army Yellow Fever Board in 1900, from which Noguchi himself needlessly died.

How this son of Japan reached his eminence among students of tropical medicine is a story worthy of Horatio Alger. How he died is a tragedy worthy of Shakespeare. Between his birth and his death lies one of those mysterious applications of human intellectual force which change the face of the world.

Noguchi was a queer and, by ordinary standards, a careless fellow. When the great 1924 international conference on tropical medicine was being held at Kingston, Jamaica, under the auspices of the United Fruit Company, Noguchi was supposed to read two scientific papers and was duly registered at conference headquarters in the luxurious Myrtle Bank Hotel. He could not be found. He did not appear in the dining room, his room was unoccupied. He was not seen in the patios and lobbies nor found talking to his medical confreres.

At first the hotel manager was somewhat concerned, perhaps because he discovered that two Negro bellboys also were missing. Sober thought suggested that the bellboys would probably reappear to collect their pay. If and when they did they could be called upon to locate Noguchi.

After nightfall the first day of the conference, Noguchi and two boys emerged from the twilight. Noguchi was carrying a stuffed and wriggling pillow case. With the help of the Negroes he had spent most of the day chasing lizards through pasture lands and hillsides beyond the hot city of Kingston. They had picked up a handsome collection of big and little saurians. Noguchi proceeded to his room and unpacked his microscope and slides. With the aid of a sharp penknife he began to dissect the lizards, squeezing their "juice" out on the glass slides, and recording his findings. As the conference downstairs talked of human parasites, Noguchi spent his days and nights observing the parasites of lizards. He confided to a curious associate director of the American College of Surgeons: "Inside these leetle leezards, ah, you find wanderfall microorganism. Wander-fall!" A titled British man of medicine stared at him in casual astonishment. "Odd about those Rockefeller Foundation chaps!" he said.

Odd or not, it is certain that Noguchi lived and died a mystery man in the changing world of tropical medicine. At Kingston he read two papers, listened patiently to protest and agreement, and once more vanished in quest of the material, discoverable only in Central America, which he felt he must have. He carried away from the conference a mangled collection of Jamaica lizards and the text of a controversy that has not yet been settled.

Hideyo Noguchi was born near the Japanese farm village of Okinajima of poor, sickly farm people, devout Buddhists, devoutly destitute. He was raised by the toil and care of a peasant mother who was strong, clean, and honorable, proud of her son and sure of his greatness.

In infancy Noguchi suffered a decisive accident. He crawled into an open fire. The finger tips of his left hand were burned away. His left arm and right hand also were badly burned. No one could doubt that he would always be a cripple.

At his country school Noguchi proved an exceptionally good scholar. He could not study at home, because his family could not afford lamplight. So the crippled boy tended the fires at a local bath-house and, in lieu of pay, was allowed to read books by the firelight.

Noguchi could never be a farmer. So for a time he became a teacher, earning a few sen by teaching country louts to read and write—rebellious students, most of them, older and bigger than their teacher.

One day a civil examiner noticed Noguchi, the cripple, and invited him to study at a preparatory school not far away. The one-handed boy, poor and farm born, soon stood at the head of his class. Then he met a great Japanese doctor, home from studying at the University of California. Inspired by the achievements and renown of this Dr. Watanabe-san, Noguchi resolved that he, too, would be a doctor. The great physician began work on Noguchi's hands. Within a few months the right one was almost normal. Meanwhile Noguchi became the doctor's drug-boy. Drug-boys were expected to supply their own beds. Noguchi was too poor, so he slept for three or four hours each night under the desk of Watanabe-san.

When the doctor was called away to the China wars, Noguchi, though the youngest and newest of five drug-boys, was made leader of the group. His service was so outstanding that Dr. Watanabe-san, on returning from the war, suggested that his chief drug-boy appeared ready to stand the first examination in medicine.

Noguchi, who had managed to save a few yen, tramped to Tokyo to study. His entry into the capital was his first sight of a great city. When his tiny savings had vanished, he found work at two yen monthly and lodging, as janitor in a dental school. Finally, the very day when his drudgery-driven mother was appointed to a country school of midwifery, back in the home village, Noguchi was admitted to a medical school in Tokyo.

That was in 1896. The Saiseigakkusha in Tokyo was a private medical school with a thousand students. Lectures began before dawn and lasted through a fourteen-hour college day. At twenty-one Noguchi finished the course, passed his examinations, paid his six-yen license fee, and became a practitioner.

Being crippled and moneyless, he despaired of making a success of medical practice. He wanted to study bacteriology, but for a long time his nearest approach to that was a job writing for a hospital journal at starvation rates. Finally he was able to manage a few months of actual study of microscopic work, which gave him the determination to study more of medicine in America and Germany.

He could have done so after a preliminary two months' course, but he continued preparatory laboratory work for five years during which time he studied English. He gave up this work to become a port quarantine officer. Then he joined a Japanese government mission of fifteen doctors dispatched to China to study contagious diseases. There were no definitely outstanding contagions at the time, but there was sickness on every side and hordes of patients eager to benefit from the wisdom of foreign doctors. For the first time Noguchi began to earn well from the practice of medicine, sometimes as much as 300 yen, or $150, a month.

With the advent of the Boxer uprising, his source of income was cut off and he returned to Tokyo jobless and moneyless. For a time he became lecturer at a dental school, but he hated the work and presently managed to borrow enough for a journey to America. On the long sea voyage he read Shakespeare, saying that it was better to begin a new language at the beginning. He landed at San Francisco and proceeded to Philadelphia; there he applied for an assistantship in pathology at the University of Pennsylvania, only to learn that the university had no provision for the sort of laboratory job he expected. Quite evidently there had been a misunderstanding. Noguchi was miserable in a strange land. But, as the stars of Nippon directed, he carried a letter of introduction to Dr. Silas Weir Mitchell. Fortunately Mitchell saw something in the eager, lonely little Japanese and staked him to a job, salary payable from his own pocketbook.

Dr. Mitchell was, at the time, much interested in the study of snake venom. That was a reason, or at least an excuse, for his interest in Noguchi. Far deeper was the beloved Pennsylvanian's interest in the phenomena of human immunity to disease. Vaccines, as we all know, are merely dead bacteria used to destroy their living brethren within the human body. Bacteria give off poisons, or toxin. So medicine also employs antitoxins as immunizing agents.

The story of snake venom belongs in this vast and exciting field of medical endeavor. Injection of certain snake venoms destroys the ability of human blood to clot and in other ways changes corpuscular status, as Dr. Mitchell's own researches had clearly shown. So Noguchi began work with snake venom, extracting the inexplicably deadly fang fluids, feeding snakes, "milking" snakes, studying snakes through long busy days and nights. He learned to hold tubes and instruments in his stub of a left hand—about which he remained extremely sensitive. He learned to correct his own blunders and to develop a high degree of technical skill. Within a year he was invited to appear before the National Academy of Science to discuss venoms in blood.

At the recommendation of the same benevolent Dr. Mitchell he was made a Bach Fund Fellow. Busy years followed. Noguchi proved again his amazing genius for concentrated research. He loved

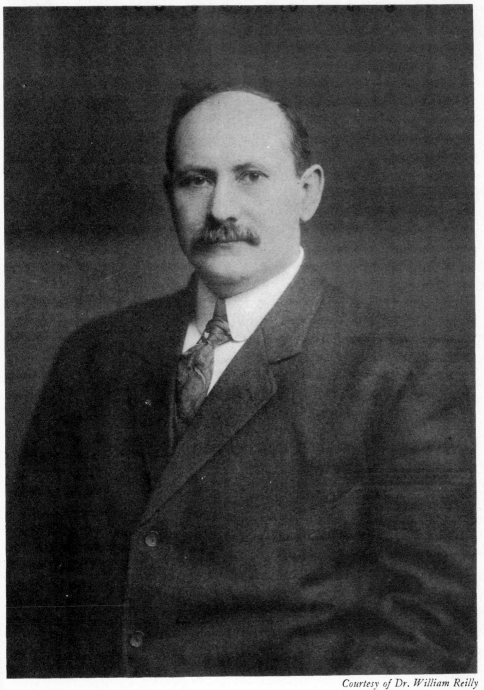

Dr. William Edgar Deeks.

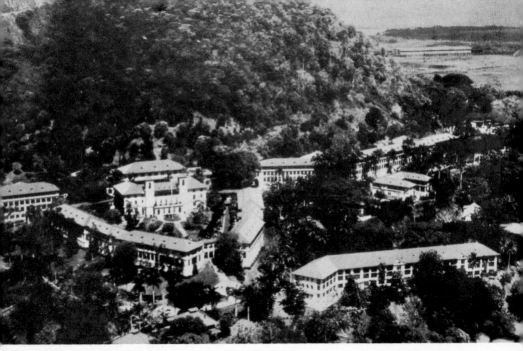

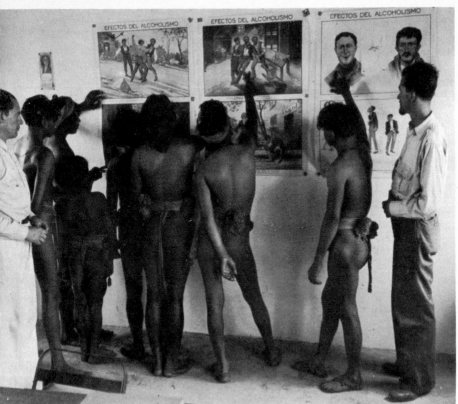

(Upper) Gorgas Hospital (Ancon), Panama Canal Zone.

(Lower) Backcountry Indians of Colombia view Colombian Government health posters.

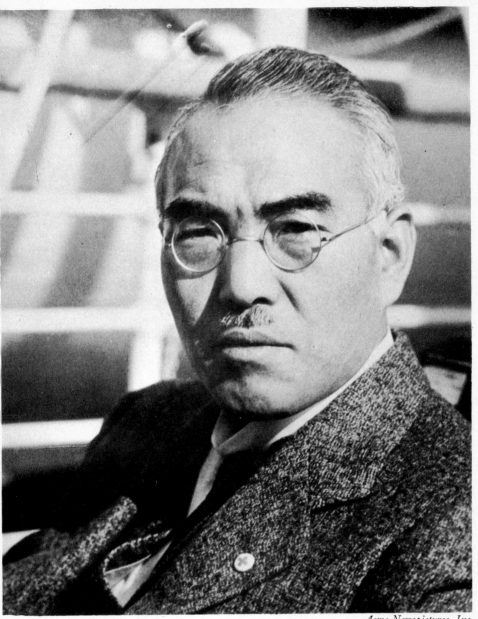

Acme Newspictures, Inc.

Noguchi

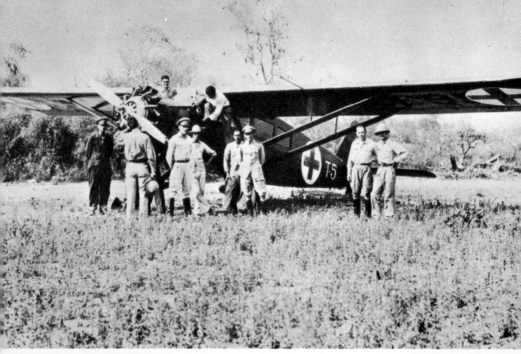

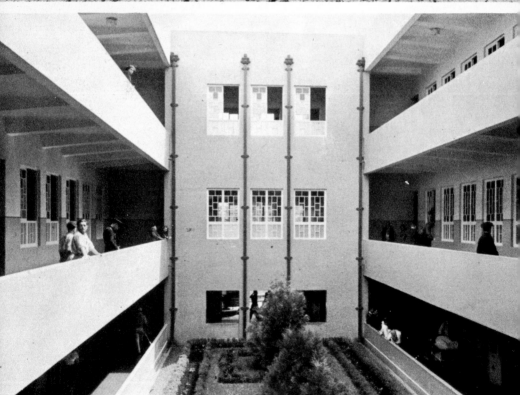

(Upper) In the Chaco War Paraguayan wounded were carried by plane to Ascunsion Hospitals.

By Iris Woolcock

(Lower) Streamlining Latin American hospitals.

the white rats with which he worked, and carried them about in the capacious pockets of his white smocks. He learned to laugh, drink, and be one with Americans, but he maintained the ritualistic courtesy of the Japanese. He continued to bow low, and to shake hands stiffly, like a child just learning. His laboratory was pointed out as a frightful example of slovenliness and he himself was known to his professional seniors as the "messy lab boy."

In Pennsylvania there were fortunately professors who realized that material neatness and orderliness can sometimes be evidence of profound inner laziness and disorder: that, like gentility or veracity, neatness can sometimes be a front for chronic mediocrity. Noguchi, at any rate, was not lazy. He worked until midnight, until two or even five in the morning. He was not mediocre, for after three years he was granted a Carnegie Fellowship for study abroad. Within another year the elder John D. Rockefeller had appropriated a million dollars for founding an institute for medical research. Noguchi was promised a place on its staff. But first he returned to Europe, to Paris, then to Copenhagen where he studied at Staateus Serum Institute with Dr. Thorvald Madsen. The Carnegie Institution informed him that it had appropriated $5,000 to publish his researches on venom and another $800 for illustrating the book. But Noguchi resolved to study longer before offering his work for publication. He was enormously impressed by Copenhagen, and by Madsen, a reflective young bacteriologist who was barely thirty-two and looked even younger.

With Madsen, Noguchi continued his work on toxins and antitoxins. Noguchi had brought several hundred grams of dried rattlesnake venom from Philadelphia. With Madsen helping, he produced a first serum for protection from that venom, a serum obtained by injecting repeated doses of the venom into a goat, bleeding the goat, and separating the serum from its blood. The work progressed rapidly. When an animal was bitten by a rattlesnake and promptly treated with the serum, the wound healed without swelling or festering. Noguchi's results were distinctly impressive. The King of Denmark visited him at his laboratory.

From Copenhagen, Noguchi watched the conflict of ideas which attended the Russo-Japanese War; the French press rabidly pro-Russian, Germany pretending to be neutral but actually conspiring in every possible way to help Russia; the English both openly and backhandedly acting to help Japan. The lack of ethics in Europe's power politics of the day made him resolve to return to America.

Back in New York, Noguchi began work for the Rockefeller Institute at $1,800 a year. His laboratory was at Fiftieth Street and Lexington Avenue. He rented a single room near by, continued to work hard and to make friends, both Japanese and American. He began to study the bacterial properties of wounds: how one species of bacterium follows another in incessant parade across a given patch of mangled flesh; how other microbe invaders soon overcome the ranks of the pioneers, and how men frequently die of infections which presumably were unknown to the fresh wound.

He carried on his work with syphilis. The Rockefeller Institute built a new research building. Noguchi had a laboratory on the third floor, overlooking the East River and Blackwells Island (now called Welfare Island). He began to write articles for scientific magazines. He was now third man among a staff of six. He noted with interest the appointment of Dr. Alexis Carrel as a fellow in experimental surgery. It should have been a happy situation for a scientist, but Noguchi worried sometimes because his earnings vanished without his knowing where they had gone. He worried because of piles and insomnia and overwork. He worried because he seemed unable to save and help other students.

In Germany, Schaudinn had found the cause of syphilis—isolated (some said discovered) the tiny spiral organism called *Spirocheta pallida*, and ended a quest which had continued through centuries. Noguchi remembered that years before, as a drug-boy, he had seen such a spiral organism through his first master's microscope. Schaudinn announced his findings in April. By the middle of June, Noguchi and Flexner, his superior at Rockefeller, announced that they had verified the spirochete, as had other researchers in Europe.

The fact that the now celebrated Schaudinn was only thirty-three goaded the young Japanese to greater activity—activity of more than one sort. When in Rome do as the Romans do. He learned to smoke cigars—as many as fifteen every day, to drink whisky straight from the bottle, to amuse himself by gazing pensively at the ceiling. He had resolved either to make his life a great success or to kill himself. In the first decade of the twentieth century he found less and less reason for killing himself.

The University of Pennsylvania awarded him an honorary Master of Arts degree. The list of his published scientific papers was growing. He was becoming one of the most renowned of America's young research workers.

The Wassermann test for syphilis was devised in 1906. It made use of the principles of serology upon which Noguchi had already been working for seven years. It involves the dissolving of blood corpuscles. Noguchi saw the opportunity for improving the technique of Wassermann preparation and of further increasing the value of an enormously valuable test. He also realized the importance of syphilis as a social disease. He knew that the world, certainly the American world, would listen to anyone who knew something about syphilis. He began a frantic study of the vast and complex background of the disease. As he worked he published what he learned. Medical men better known than he began to look for and attend his lectures on serology. American medicine was becoming serum conscious. The practitioner began to be interested in syphilis. Since Noguchi had something to say, he became world famous as a student of the bacteriology of syphilis.

At first his knowledge produced no tangible results, only a greater interest in the disease. Before 1915, however, he had two real advances to his credit. He was able to substitute human blood corpuscles for those of sheep in the Wassermann test and he developed an independent test for detecting syphilis of the brain and spinal cord. This test (the Noguchi butyric acid test) is a matter of extracting fluid from the spinal canal and testing it for protein content. A high protein content proves the existence of syphilis.

As his work expanded, Noguchi realized that to accomplish what he wanted to accomplish he must produce a pure culture of syphilis. He saw that it was necessary to develop a standard feeding for such cultures. This he succeeded in doing and became the first to cultivate the syphilis-producing spirochete organism. That was an advance which brought Noguchi to the attention of the entire medical world, a lifesaving medical revolution. Honors came to him from all over the world. He bore the honors well. He simply worked harder. He married an American wife and settled, American style, in a five-room apartment.

In his laboratory he began consolidating his achievements, preparing for a new advance. He developed a successful standard culture medium—a food upon which the organism of syphilis would thrive and multiply. For this he chose a mixture of one part serum to three of water plus the fresh kidney and testicle tissues of rabbits. He prepared and filled hundreds of oversized test tubes, which he checked and rechecked for sterility. He then inoculated his feeding media with syphilitic materials, sealed the tubes in airproof jars and placed them in incubators.

Every day he examined every test tube. He improved techniques for filtering viruses from bacteria. From the successful development of a pure culture of the spirochete of syphilis he proceeded to the successful cultivation of other spirochetes: those which infest the teeth of pyorrhea-infected mouths; those which produce mucus; still others which produce odors; and the spirochete of European and African relapsing fevers. He began a laboratory study of trachoma, that terrible disease of the eyes. He propagated the microorganisms discovered in the brains of rabid dogs. He studied infantile paralysis, which was then epidemic in the eastern United States.

He began to collect sections of the brains of people who had died of paresis, to preserve them and make slides. He developed incontrovertible proof of the true cause of syphilis, shed new light upon syphilis of the brain, and developed culture techniques invaluable to the understanding of numerous diseases.

He lectured in Vienna, dined with German royalty, spoke before the medical societies of Munich and Frankfort, Berlin and Copenhagen. At Copenhagen he received the Royal Medal of Denmark. He found himself recommended for a decoration by the Swedish crown. He made triumphant visits to Heidelberg and London. When he returned to New York he was asked to take up the study of the etiology of hog cholera. He was offered also the research directorship of Mount Sinai Hospital in New York and declined it when the Rockefeller Institute raised his salary to $5,000 (the hospital had offered $6,000). The institute gave him a bigger laboratory and several capable assistants.

During May, 1915, Noguchi received the Imperial Prize of the Japanese Academy. He asked that the great medal be first shown to his old teacher, then to his mother. As soon as he could he returned to Japan for a final visit with his mother and presented her with part of the thousand-yen ($500) award from the Imperial Academy. His mother promptly redistributed the gift—to the temple, the priest, and the village master for gifts to the aged and the school principal.

Though he had never visited the tropics, Noguchi's research on syphilis, one of the more destructive enemies of tropical peoples, made him well known in tropical medicine. On returning from Japan he visited the Harvard Medical School and, through Wolbach, became interested in the search for the organism responsible for Rocky Mountain spotted fever and, as a matter of course, for the wood ticks which carry that infection. Rocky Mountain fever is identical with, or closely similar to, a Japanese malady called *tsutsu-gamushi*. Jaundice fever, another disease common in Japan and in many parts of the Western world, also attracted his attention. It, too, is a spirochete disease. Noguchi proved that it is transferable by rats.

In New York he suffered a severe attack of typhoid, probably acquired from a self-imposed build-up diet of oysters. He left the hospital weighing 97 pounds, though his ordinary weight was 130. This was his forty-second year, and every Japanese knows that the forty-second is the bad year of a man's life.

Noguchi recovered. His next great undertaking was a study of yellow fever. It was June, 1918. The United States and most of the world was at war. Yellow fever was active in many regions, as it is today and as it probably will be tomorrow. Nott, Finlay, Walter Reed and the Army Yellow Fever Board and many others had studied and fought the malady sincerely and at times dramatically. Defense against malaria had been a distinctive American attainment. So had been the foundation work in yellow fever research. Much had been done in sanitation, but the problems of yellow fever as a disease remained serious. In areas where yellow fever is endemic most inhabitants are subjected to the disease during infancy or early childhood, when resistance is fairly high, and in surviving become immune. Migrations of people, however, to a great degree cancel such immunity. Nonimmune people from the high Andes, for example, where mosquito vectors are relatively scarce, die like flies upon descending to the lowlands.

In 1918, as mentioned in an earlier chapter on the achievements of General William C. Gorgas, yellow fever was rampant in Ecuador, particularly at Guayaquil, principal seaport of that beautiful and unfortunate republic. Human material was available at Guayaquil—and plenty of *Aëdes aegypti* mosquitoes. Gorgas, then studying the Ecuadorean problem, had heard of Noguchi. He knew that he needed the man; he made him a proposition.

On July 7, 1918, Hideyo Noguchi arrived at the Canal Zone en route to Guayaquil. He was very much preoccupied with the chaperoning of several cases of laboratory guinea pigs. When his ship called at the Ecuador seaport some of the passengers refused to disembark. Noguchi and three American nurses landed. The Japanese doctor from the Rockefeller Institute addressed a delegation of Ecuadorean doctors—in Spanish. The Ecuadoreans noted with smiles that Noguchi had brought guinea pigs from New York and the guinea pig is native to Ecuador. Their smiles broke into laughter. Noguchi noted that Guayaquil, a city of 80,000 people, had hospitals devoted exclusively to bubonic plague and yellow fever. He noted that they were crowded and he did not laugh.

In a wing of the yellow fever hospital he set up a laboratory. There he located what he believed to be the spirochete of yellow fever, which, as Gorgas had predicted, closely resembled that of infectious jaundice. He began an ambitious and what might seem to the layman a pointless study of the animal and bird life of Ecuador. Children brought Noguchi turtles and newts and lizards and he thanked the children and patted their heads. He continued to study animals because he was always interested in animals and, not at all incidentally, because he had scientific reasons to suspect that certain of these animals were carriers of serious diseases. Within six weeks local newspapers announced that Noguchi had probably isolated the organism of yellow fever and that this organism, directed into the body of a guinea pig, had produced all the clinical symptoms of yellow fever.

Guayaquil was hospitable. There were many gay parties for Noguchi. But the work was heavy. The little doctor had succeeded in finding the spirochete in six out of twenty-seven alleged cases of yellow fever under observation. He developed a vaccine and used it to inoculate a battalion of highland troops coming down to the lowlands for the first time. Ecuador was grateful and paid him glowing tribute.

Noguchi left Ecuador without having completely solved the

riddle of yellow fever, but he left with real accomplishment behind him, having given the world sound, durable scientific information. Though far from final, his work proved the stupidity and the peril of assuming that yellow fever had been conquered by Walter Reed or anybody else in 1900, or any other year.

Back in New York, Noguchi declined to offer any particular claims for his Guayaquil research. He admitted that yellow fever and infectious jaundice are very much alike. He knew that his work was not finished and went on learning more about the symptoms of yellow fever and their terrifying consequences.

Usually in yellow fever the patient comes down suddenly. His head and loins ache. His flesh is sensitive. He is drowsy, yet complains of acute belly pains. Then vomiting begins. Gums and mouth bleed. The patient grows thirsty. The whites of his eyes turn yellow. The skin becomes discolored, an orange yellow which changes to pallid green. The first nausea leads to "black vomit." The blood in the stomach congeals and becomes like tar. Sometimes the nose bleeds. The face becomes smeared with clotted blood. As a rule death comes on the fifth or sixth day. If the patient survives the fourth or fifth day after the climax, a jaundice appears, spreads, and finally vanishes.

Noguchi continued to study and record. He treated infected animals with his serum and the animals recovered. He began to transmit the disease to mosquitoes. Favorable results from the vaccination of the highland soldiers of Ecuador's army were reported.

At the Rockefeller Institute and in Cuba and Mexico his work went on. He proved that the spirochete of the disease diagnosed as yellow fever in Cuba was identical with that of diagnosed yellow fever in Mexico. He became enormously fond of Mexicans and Cubans, even as he had of Ecuadoreans. He returned to New York and, hearing of a new outbreak of yellow fever on the west coast of South America, turned about and sailed for Peru, proceeding to

Paita, the northernmost port, where Dr. Kligler was using a wooden shack on the beach as a laboratory.

There *was* yellow fever in Peru. The great Dr. Henry Rose Carter had made the diagnoses. Kligler appeared at Paita with blood cultures taken from people in all walks of life, from the dwellers in thatched huts to those living in high-class residential districts. The cultures showed positive reactions and the same spirochetes found in Ecuador, Mexico, and Cuba. A Peruvian doctor took the disease, was treated with Noguchi's serum, and promptly recovered.

Noguchi journeyed to Lima, the capital. The President offered him the directorship of the Peru Research Institute. Meanwhile the British Government had offered him the directorship of a commission to study the hoof and mouth disease of cattle. Noguchi stayed with the Rockefeller Institute, writing reports on yellow fever, resuming his study of syphilis, of Rocky Mountain spotted fever, and following up his lines of research. He developed a serum for Rocky Mountain spotted fever, carried the serum to Missoula, Montana, and described it to the membership of a medical study conference there in convention. Much of this extraordinary man's research was extremely dangerous—to Noguchi. Accidental self-infection was a perpetual hazard. One of his laboratory assistants died of the spotted fever and Noguchi, momentarily heartbroken, swore a renewed warfare against the disease.

Nothing, however, could hold him down when a serious yellow fever outbreak was reported. This time it was in Brazil. The year was 1923, the place Bahia. Noguchi began work in the Institute Oswaldo Cruz. Drs. White and Scannell had been supervising mosquito eradication in the locality. They had done too good a job of it—according to Noguchi. Only three cases of yellow fever could be found in Bahia. Plenty more waited in the interior, but men would have to travel through the jungle and seek them out. Blood cultures might become contaminated en route and patients might die. The tropics are not the ideal place for a man who likes to work twenty hours a day. And the laboratory, though handsomely housed, was poorly equipped. At every turn Noguchi met with languor and procrastination. His instrument cases were lost in transit. He was unable to find the sort of microscope or sterilizing equipment which is considered necessary for investigating the yellow-fever organism.

While waiting for equipment he began to study other tropical disease, particularly the flagellates found in ulcers. An outbreak of measles occurred and he began to look into that. Noguchi observed that, while men frequently move slowly in the tropics, microorganisms usually work, move, and propagate with uncomfortable speed, making deadly and disastrous scourges of diseases which in temperate climates are generally mild.

Yellow fever sufferers and recent convalescents came to the institute and offered their blood. Thus Noguchi was able to collect serum and to learn, with the collaboration of the medical faculty of Bahia University, that Brazilian yellow fever was serologically identical with that of Ecuador, Mexico, and Peru. With superb diplomacy, Noguchi enlisted Brazilian medical talent; explained the trying technicalities of his dark-field microscopes (which finally arrived), and otherwise proved himself a superb teacher and scientific leader. Brazilian medical men were appreciative. A Brazilian doctor was able to verify the microorganism which Noguchi had described.

Meanwhile Noguchi was keenly aware of what a stupendous natural laboratory the American tropics really are, and how infinitely complex their medical problems. He had only four months to spend in Brazil. That was not time enough to tell him what he wanted to know.

He returned to New York in February, 1924, and immediately received from Dr. William Deeks, superintendent of the medical department of the United Fruit Company, an invitation to attend the International Conference on Health Problems in Tropical America at Kingston during the following summer.

Noguchi, eager for more work in the tropics, accepted. When June 22nd, the date of the convention, arrived, he was at Kingston, as we have already noted, searching for lizards. In spite of his unconventional attendance he did favor the conference with the two addresses he had scheduled: one dealing with flagellates, the other describing his work with yellow fever in Brazil. He spoke briefly and his English, as usual, was not easily followed. Dr. Agramonte challenged him. Dr. Castellani accepted what he said. Dr. Henry R. Carter defended Dr. Noguchi's vaccination for yellow fever, but offered certain scientific doubts about the spirochete. Dr. Henry J. Nichols, director of laboratories of the United States Army Medical School, came out unreservedly in acceptance of all that Noguchi had said, written, and done about yellow fever. The gentleman from Japan calmly and modestly discussed his work with the flagellates— whiplike growths of cells and threadlike runners; a vast field of bacteriology which comparatively few scientists find time to know or to appreciate. In Brazil, Noguchi had learned that lumbermen or lumber bush choppers are frequently infected with these living and poisoning threads. At Brazilian hospitals he had seen the resulting ulcers and running sores. He had taken one strain of the Brazilian type back to New York, acquired other materials from Nichols, and by means of rabbit inoculation had developed and classified several pure cultures of the flagellates, thus taking still another step into the vast dark field of tropical medicine.

Dr. Gustav Eckstein summarizes:

He [Noguchi] began his career with venoms, the venoms took him to serology, serology to syphilis, syphilis to the spirochetes, the spirochetes to these strange and little studied diseases of tropical medicine; diseases where science has made least inroad, where treatment is still in the hands of miracle workers, horrible diseases, fatal like the diseases of the north a century ago; causes unknown, carriers unknown, the human being never certain from where the malevolence will strike, but romance in the study of them.[1]

In the midst of the Kingston Conference, Noguchi left it. He sailed for Tela, Honduras, and the Lancetilla Experiment Farm near by, where he found plants infected with flagellates. He boarded a ship for New York, and filled his bathtub with the prized vegetation. The arrival of a testing sample of blood from a patient in Lima, Peru, switched Noguchi abruptly back to the study of Oroya fever, that mysterious disease which reputedly has harassed Andean people since the time of the Incas.

Oroya fever and verruga warts are believed to be complementary —the fever, the acute form; the blood warts, the chronic. The martyrdom of the Peruvian medical student, Daniel Carrión, supports that belief. Carrión, as we saw earlier, inoculated both his arms with liquid pressed from an active verruga wart. He promptly developed Oroya fever and died. Carrión's was another heroic death and important. For the strange fever and the strange warts are common in parts of otherwise healthful highlands. They may infest one valley and be unknown on the other side of the mountain.

During 1913 the Harvard School of Tropical Medicine had sent an expedition into South America to study verruga and other tropical diseases. The expedition concluded that verruga and Oroya fever, although frequently occurring in the same individual at the same time, are entirely separate diseases; the boils caused by a parasite, the fever by an "indefinable virus."

There was rather impressive evidence that the disease was being carried by insects—perhaps nocturnal insects, since Andean folklore has it that the affliction is acquired at night. The fact that the disease is segregated in particular highland valleys was another significant hint. Charles H. T. Townshend, an American entomologist in Peru, began work on the insect theory, suggesting first the tick as carrier, then isolating approximately fifty blood-sucking insects common to the region where the disease is most frequent (9 to 15 degrees south latitude). One by one, Townshend eliminated the suspects until finally he had reduced the eligibles to the horse fly, buffalo gnat, and phlebotomus—the "vein opener." The first two he eliminated because they bite only during the daytime. The third he chose because it is nocturnal. Peruvian newspapers followed the reasoning quite easily. But not the gentlemen from Harvard. It wasn't "scientific." The nomenclature and deductive processes were entirely too obvious.

During September, 1925, Noguchi attacked the same problem. He propagated in pure culture the organism with which the Harvard medicos had struggled. He worked stubbornly from September through February inoculating large numbers of animals, monkeys, dogs, rabbits, guinea pigs, and mice. Steadily testimony grew in support of the belief that Oroya fever and verruga warts have one and the same cause. Noguchi said nothing. By successive animal passages he managed to increase the virulence of his culture until it produced remittent fever and an extreme anemia, which caused the blanching so graphically described by Inca historians.

Noguchi imported warts cut from a patient in Lima, macerated them in salt solution, and inoculated two monkeys. Both animals promptly developed remittent fever. From the blood of each monkey Noguchi cultivated an organism indistinguishable from that cultivated from the blood of sufferers from Oroya fever. Having produced warts from fever and fever from warts, Noguchi was figuratively hauling in his catch. In his own laboratory he had been able to control several phases of the vastly complex disease: the degree of the malady; remittent fever; anemia; fever from the warts, warts from the fever; the spontaneous wart, the irregular fever. Then coldly he reported:

The data obtained justifies the conclusion that verruga peruana is caused by *Bartonella bacilliformis*. They also definitely establish the fact that the inoculation of blood or *sanguineous exudate* from lesions of verruga peruana is capable of inducing in susceptible individuals a severe systemic infection, such as that to which Carrión succumbed. The designation "Carrion's disease" is therefore the appropriate one for both forms of the infection.[2]

Once more Noguchi had let fly the golden arrow of scientific proof and it had punctured the ponderous and inflated reports of the Harvard Medical School on the subject. The Harvard "expedition to study and collect pathological materials and study certain tropical diseases, particularly verruga and Oroya fever" had undertaken a hugely important mission and published an influential report.[3]

Noguchi graciously and completely blasted the report, which seems to have deserved just such a fate. For the Harvard report had gone far out of its course to discredit Latin-American testimony. The assertions about "definable parasite" and "indefinable virus" were slovenly. Barton, a Peruvian physician, had previously reported (1909) that in the red corpuscles of Oroya fever patients he had seen bodies that looked like bacteria. He suggested that the bodies were protozoa. The Harvard doctors asserted that these bodies "lay somewhere between bacteria and protozoa." They severely discredited the heroic experiment of young Dr. Carrión, who had given his life to prove that the two diseases are really the same. The Harvard report read:

Although it has been stated that Carrión during his illness kept notes and gave a minute description of his symptoms to his companions, unfortunately it appears that none of these were preserved and published. No accurate record of Carrión's case and of the necropsy is available. It has been suggested since that he died of typhoid fever or a more acute form of septicemia, and it is also quite possible that the patients from which he infected himself were suffering with Oroya fever as well as verruga at the time.[4]

It seems probable that Noguchi took great pleasure in doing justice to Carrión. Certainly Harvard did not choose to contradict.

Noguchi's next project was trachoma, that cruel malady which destroys eyesight and particularly persecutes the poor.

Throughout the Americas trachoma is an especial enemy of the Indian. For generations it has afflicted our great Indian reservations. During most of the past half century the results from surgery have been extremely bad. In 1924 and 1925 "the scourge of the Reservations" was receiving more than ordinary attention from the surgeon general and the United States Public Health Service at Washington. Doctors realized a paramount need for better research; for getting at the organism involved. Noguchi heard and agreed to go to the Indian lands—provided there were real cases to study. Presumably there were (and are) millions of cases in the world. Of our own third of a million Indians it is estimated that no fewer than 30,000 suffer from trachoma with symptoms ranging from granular lids to complete blindness.

In the government hospital for Indians at Albuquerque, New Mexico, Noguchi found plenty of material for the study of a disease that is scarcely known in New York. He noted the symptoms— watery eyes, small ulcers or granules on the eyelids, lids drawn from processes of scarring, lashes raking the eyeball surface as a result of lid shrinkage. Dr. Polks Richards, an authority on Indian diseases, was assigned to be Noguchi's assistant. The two men viewed a procession of blind Indians; they began examinations of eyelids, the granules, the late and the early symptoms. Noguchi began taking cultures, vetoed a project for experimental inoculation of human eyes. He believed that monkey or other animal eyes would do as well, at least for the preliminary stages of research. He announced that when the time came to use a human subject, he would inoculate his own eyes. Back in New York he tried the cultures on the eyes of monkeys, chimpanzees, and orangutans. He noted a bacterium that had never been described. Perhaps it was the organism of trachoma. He inoculated the animals and waited. Trachoma is a slowly developing disease. But within ninety days Noguchi's rhesus monkeys and chimpanzees began to show granular conjunctivitis of the eye. It looked like human trachoma. Painstakingly Noguchi proved that serum from trachoma cases in the Kentucky mountains reacted positively to the organism from New Mexico. That was good evidence and good detective work.

Before his trachoma work was complete, Noguchi decided to return to yellow fever research. There were criticisms of some of his earlier tenets; criticisms which could be answered only by further work. More immediately pertinent, there was yellow fever in Africa. And there was the researcher's burning desire to be right. He knew the elusive resemblance between yellow fever and Weil's disease, or infectious jaundice. He also knew the possibility of clinical error beyond his personal control. He had been dependent upon others for the securing of human blood samples; upon many doctors and laymen in many countries. Perhaps some of his past yellow fever blood samples had not been real yellow fever at all. Perhaps there are two or more kinds of yellow fever. Maybe he had worked with only one. Africa would be a better place than South America for studying the disease. Not that Africans could possibly be more charming people. Noguchi had learned to love South Americans. They inspired him to run his hand through his black mop of silky hair and smile, and sometimes to write poems.

But at this time he must have felt many reasons for going to Africa. For one, Dr. Nichols, of the United States Army Medical School, had died in Panama; Nichols had been the most loyal champion of Noguchi's work with yellow fever. Gratitude required that the work be finished. Moreover, this yellow fever of Africa was, according to reports and to Adrian Stokes, also of the Rockefeller Institute, capable of being transmitted to monkeys. Stokes had succeeded in making the transmission in East Africa. And Stokes could diagnose yellow fever as well as any man living. The best authorities agreed that jaundice virus cannot be transmitted through monkeys.

Noguchi applied to the Rockefeller Institute for permission and funds to undertake the African adventure. It would be a perilous mission, as he had every reason to know. Adrian Stokes was reported dead of yellow fever. At the institute in New York, Stokes had been a close friend of Noguchi's. Stokes had died as a true and brave scientist. His death was sufficient proof that the conquest of yellow fever had not been attained.

Stokes had gone to Africa with complete confidence in his ability to withstand the plague which he had elected to fight. He had over-stayed his African leave by two weeks. During those two weeks he had contracted the disease.

Noguchi was fifty-one. His health was not of the best. His heart condition was reported bad. He was developing diabetes and a nervous insomnia. He was not yet seasoned to the tropics. In terms of yellow fever he was very probably a nonimmune, and worse, a transient nonimmune.

In terms of bacteriology it was another story. If Noguchi stayed in New York he would merely be juggling test tubes and toying with blood which somebody else had collected weeks earlier. He could not be sure that it actually came from yellow fever patients. Most probably the material would be contaminated or improperly drawn. There would be the usual list of error factors inevitable at long range.

There was no doubt about it. Noguchi knew he had to go to Africa. He began preparation for the great journey. He worked with Dr. Alexis Carrel in developing methods of tissue culture for possible use in Africa. He made plans for continuing research on Oroya fever and trachoma, purchased huge quantities of laboratory equipment and other supplies for jungle work. Two days before he sailed he gave a preliminary report on trachoma to the institute staff. It has been called one of the finest discourses in medical litera-ture.

Aboard ship he dispatched radiograms to the European head-quarters at Hagenbeck's circus, ordering monkeys and chimpanzees to be forwarded to Dakar. At Freetown two doctors of the Rocke-feller Foundation boarded the S.S. *Scythia* to accompany Noguchi on the remainder of his journey. The immediate destination was Accra. At Dakar, French doctors were already using Noguchi's yellow fever vaccine with good results. But yellow fever was still the biggest news of west-coast Africa. Accra, the principal city of the British Gold Coast, appeared to be a focus for the yellow plague.

At Accra, Noguchi met Dr. William Alexander Young, director of a small but capable research station maintained by the British government. Dr. Young welcomed the distinguished visitor and provided him with livable quarters and a native cook.

Noguchi began work, making blood cultures from local yellow fever cases; using horses, monkeys, and chimpanzees as laboratory subjects. A virulent outbreak of yellow fever occurred in near-by French Togoland, within a day's ride of Accra. Noguchi worked in a happy frenzy in the murderous climate. Reports went about that the great man from the Rockefeller Institute had been bleeding himself and using his own blood to inoculate monkeys.

Presently Noguchi isolated a new organism. Deliberately he abandoned his theory of the spirochete. He was now convinced that African yellow fever and South American yellow fever are not the same disease. More samples of yellow fever blood came to him from the Belgian Congo.

He considered the newly discovered parasite, a simple spore-bearing organism. Perhaps this, at last, was the true causal agent of yellow fever. He would return to New York and finish his work there. As an afterthought, he decided to pay a visit farther down the coast before sailing from Accra for the New World. He chose the port of Lagos, overnight by ship from Accra.

During his first morning in Lagos, Noguchi suffered a severe chill. He insisted on returning to Accra. Accra is one of the many shallow-water ports of Africa. Passengers must embark and land by surfboats—for a twenty-minute ride from shipside to harbor. While on the surfboat Noguchi was soaked by a cold blowing rain. The boat crew had provided no shelter. As a rule exposure to rain is the worst possible treatment for a tropical chill.

Noguchi believed he had malaria. But blood tests did not confirm that diagnosis. The port physician suspected the worst, persuaded the distinguished physician to go to the hospital. Next morning Noguchi was certain that he had yellow fever. A week passed and symptoms grew steadily worse. The medical staff, including Young, was deeply concerned. They needed Noguchi. His greatest work was still unfinished. In their makeshift laboratory Dr. Young had worked with him on the new, unfinished research. The genius of the work, however, was the personal possession of this strange little Japanese. If he died, that which he could impart to no one would die with him.

There was good reason to believe that Noguchi would die. Both his heart and his kidneys were failing. Yellow fever is particularly hard on the kidney tract and on the heart. There were *Stegomyia* mosquitoes at Accra, perhaps all over West Africa. Chances of a research man's contracting the disease were great. In any case, Noguchi had contracted it.

On the eighth day of his illness Dr. Young called on his famous guest. Dr. Noguchi inquired about Dr. Young's health. Young answered that he felt fine. He did not know that he, too, was marked as a victim of the same disease.

After nine days of illness Noguchi lapsed into unconsciousness. He suffered a slight convulsion and clasped his nurse's hand like a fearful child. On the tenth day he died. And within a fortnight Young was dead. So passed three great ambassadors in white: Young and Stokes, two medical men of promise never to be realized, and Noguchi, perhaps the greatest bacteriologist the world has ever known. His life proved that the war on tropical disease is an international matter, limited to no one race and segregated in no one hemisphere. His death proved not only that such diseases as yellow fever are far from conquered, but also that man has the courage and the wisdom necessary for ultimate victory.

Chapter Nine

MICROBE TOURISTS

IT was New Year's Eve aboard a pitching banana boat out of Santa Marta, Colombia. The eight passengers, all more or less seasick, sat in the tilting saloon, drinking and talking. I was one of those passengers, bringing to a close my first session in the tropics. I had become an incurable tropical enthusiast.

Late in the evening, when the ship's bar had closed, the conversation turned, perhaps in recognition of our common quandary, to the subject of democracy. The bar steward and I were having difficulty agreeing on the fact that the decisive forces creating democracy are economic; that democracy is essentially an institution of frontiers and requires for its success abundant, cheap, or free lands in which free men may earn a livelihood and upon which they can escape the realities of tyranny and want which prevail in settled communities.

I contended that the American tropics are today the brightest hope for the continuation of American democracy. They include millions of miles of fertile, winterless lands still awaiting human settlement. Much of our tropical land is cheap, rich, and readily habitable. Its producing power is varied and immense. Reliable surveys indicate that barely two per cent of the tillable part of tropical America is actually under cultivation. In Continental United States the topsoil is rapidly vanishing. Agriculture in the north is making a gallant and perhaps final bid for survival. Latin America is literally the last great American frontier. Now that our original wilderness has been tamed and filled with men, American democracy can only look to the south for the soil and space in which to survive.

Among the listening passengers on that fruit steamer were three medical men. One, a handsome, fiercely energetic Colombian physician employed by his government's system of socialized hospitals; another, a drawling, towering Texan who had spent sixteen years as clinic director of the great Ancon Hospital of the Canal Zone; and the third, a chubby, gruffly amiable doctor from Carolina who had served a third of a century as tropical field man for the Rockefeller Foundation and earned his place as one of the greatest living authorities on parasitic disease.

The three men listened in tolerant skepticism until suddenly the Colombian made a gesture, as if he were disposing of a troublesome fly, and smiled with fierce intensity: "Señor, unless great changes come—in health, sanitation, quarantine, and preventive medicine here in the tropics—the first act of your seekers after new land and renewed democracy when they come to Latin America will be to die. Those thousands of immigrants to the tropics—from the long-ago followers of Columbus to the many who now come from northern lands—have learned this. For wherever there are many *turistas* there will be still more touring microbes."

The physician from Colombia knew what he was talking about. Like travelers from Brooklyn and from Iowa, tourist microbes go everywhere and see everything with or without the help of Thomas Cook & Son or the American Railway Express. The Colombian knew this all too well. So fresh in his mind was the death of an entire Mexican village from the effects of an alien's visit that he could hardly speak of it. Yet speak he did, in eloquent Spanish. The alien visitor was smallpox and the year was not 1600, it was 1935.

This particular village, which might have been any one of thousands scattered throughout rural Latin America, was in the state of

Campeche, on the mesa about forty miles southeast of the Yucatan frontier and about the same distance from the port of Campeche on the Gulf of Mexico shore of that huge, blunt boot, the Yucatan Peninsula.

Antonita, as the Indians call it, was an Indian community of some four hundred people. Imagine yourself to be, not surrounded by a barrier of immigration officials, forts, and naval bases, but open to all comers, vulnerable and unsafe. That is what, said the Colombian doctor, the little village of Antonita was like, but its enemies were not men and they did not come with planes and tanks and guns.

There are hundreds of Indian villages like Antonita, as much like it as peas from the same pod. There is an adobe church with a pretentious white spire topped with a golden cross; six or seven tiendas grouped about a plaza shaded with orange trees and otherwise ornamented with bright flowers and strolling belles; about twenty one- and two-room adobe dwellings, and a public watering trough fed by a big deep-set spring which bubbles out of heavily fissured limestone.

In 1935 Antonita's women, girls, and old men kept the shops and worked small outlying fields of corn, squashes, and melons. Some grew henequen plants and took out the fibers by hand. A few were able to grow patches of pineapple. But the principal livelihood of the community was provided by the young men, most of whom were tree-climbing, jungle-prowling *chicleros*, free-lance harvesters of chicle, the valuable sap of a rather rare jungle tree from which the cud-loving *yanquis* make chewing gum.

Actually Antonita was the best part of a hundred miles from any important stronghold of chicle trees. But anyhow the chicle is far-scattered among the denser bush of the Yucatan and North Guatemala country and it is virtually impossible for a chiclero to keep his family in the steamy jungles where the precious trees still hide. So chicle harvest remains a trade for hardy, pest-bitten wanderers.

During Holy Week of 1935 two chicleros from Antonita, the brothers José and Eduardo Calias, both stalwart, honorable young men, came home to die. They were desperately sick. Their bodies were disfigured by a repulsive red rash. They had been taken sick while in the jungle and they had traveled more than a hundred miles afoot. On the way they had been further tormented by pelting cold rains.

Having arrived at their home village, the Calias brothers proceeded immediately to the chapel to make confession. The padre heard their confessions and prayed for their return to health. But the padre could hardly disguise his alarm. He had seen smallpox before; in fact he had seen it carried home from the chicle jungles in exactly this manner. He knew the inevitable agony and tragedy. With as much diplomacy as possible he urged the brothers to leave the chapel, lest the holy place be contaminated, and to seek refuge at a monastery several villages beyond.

The brothers agreed but begged permission to visit their families and loved ones before leaving. When the padre hesitated they explained that many chicleros were suffering from the same fierce rash and that others would unquestionably be returning to the village bearing the same mark of God's punishment. The padre mumbled a prayer and gave his consent.

That is how smallpox came to the village of Antonita, once a stronghold of the great Mayas. Within a week nine more weather-beaten chicleros had returned from the jungles bearing the terrible disease. José Calias had collapsed on reaching his home. He never left it. Smallpox began to spread through the village like a storm. Within a fortnight many were sick, children and women as well as men. The younger ones did not recognize the affliction, for it had been more than a third of a century since the village had suffered such a pestilence.

The padre worked frenziedly administering to the sick. But their number was rapidly increasing and young and old, strong and weak, were dying. Unwilling to leave his flock the padre dispatched messengers to seek help from the government office at Campeche port, and to explain that the shops were closing and that supplies of food and patent medicines were almost gone. The sick were going hungry. The padre feared that the water supply had been contaminated. At any rate his parishioners were refusing to drink.

The padre's lay messenger explained also that neighboring villagers were deathly afraid to go near the stricken village and that those of Antonita who fled were being turned away from public inns and plazas. He said that the hardware shop had already sold its entire supply of coffins and that no others could be bought and that the padre himself had labored like a common peon to help dig graves for the dead. The messenger also reported that the village had never had a learned medico. But two countryside herb doctors, yerbateros, were helping as best they could. The two local midwives were working valiantly at nursing the sick, though one was already broken out with the disease she was trying to cure.

It was at this point that the young Colombian medical school graduate, then a junior employee of Mexico's public health department, journeyed to Antonita, riding a mule and leading a burro loaded with five hundred shots of typhoid vaccine and various other medical supplies and equipment.

It took him two hard days to reach the sequestered village. On arriving he found sixteen dead and a sick population of nearly two hundred. One of the midwives was dying of smallpox and one of the native yerbateros had collapsed. Promptly the young doctor began vaccinating the sick and well alike, for he quickly learned that at least nine-tenths of all the people were nonimmunes and that Antonita was one of the hundreds of remote communities which had not been reached by Mexico's campaign for public vaccination.

For eighty unbroken hours the student doctor attended the sick. He did not sleep. The second day brought nine deaths; the third, seven more. With the assistance of the surviving midwife, the doctor delivered a sick mother of a healthy baby. On the fourth day he made a brief expedition to outlying districts and began vaccinating citizens who had not yet been exposed to the pestilence.

He was appalled by the feebleness of individual resistance to the disease and the grim uniformity with which the pestilence struck down all age groups. Babies and very young children were the one exception. These showed considerable inherent immunity. The death toll was highest among men between twenty and fifty. A few of the older villagers had already survived smallpox and were therefore immune, but eleven of the chicleros, twelve other men of the village, nine children, and fourteen girls and women died. During three weeks there were also seven deaths from pneumonia and two from dysentery—all aggravated by smallpox.

The doctor began a series of incidental tests which disclosed about twenty cases of syphilis and more than a hundred of malaria. He estimated the malaria index as approximately forty per cent of the entire population and he found the zygotes of malaria in the blood of virtually every child examined.

Following departmental instructions he attempted to place the entire village under quarantine. But before police could arrive survivors and escapers of the pestilence were beginning to disappear. Within a month the village was almost deserted. The churchyard was crowded with new graves, and the good padre celebrated mass in a chapel that was almost empty. Within another month the village was completely abandoned, a total social and economic loss.

"That," said the Colombian doctor, "was how a village died even as a pestilence was beaten. It could happen again to any one of ten thousand villages between the Rio Grande and the Straits of Magellan. Yes, señores, it probably will happen again."

The story of Antonita is the skeleton in the closet of Latin America. It is the story of the world of today, a world in which the undefended community is at the mercy of the invader. In Latin America, although there are undoubtedly certain indigenous pathological states, disease is almost always an alien invader against whom there is no defense other than an often too costly immunity.

Addressing the Ninth Annual Meeting of the Population Association of America at Princeton during May, 1941, Dr. Aristides A.

Moll, secretary of the Pan American Sanitary Bureau, and one of the most capable students of Latin American disease and health problems, made a number of noteworthy comments on alien diseases south of the Rio Grande. He stated among other things that according to Mallo's researches pestilences, presumably of foreign origin, killed at least 2,000,000 natives of Bolivia, Argentina, and Chile between 1590 and 1610; that in five years between 1798 and 1803 European or African yellow fever killed seven-eighths of a French army of 25,000 in Haiti; and that during the Mexican War we lost 1,549 soldiers in battle while 10,951 died of disease. (See Appendix C.)

For five centuries past there have been Antonitas in Latin America. This is not to say that there are not indigenous diseases in the American tropics nor is it to claim that all diseases which have been imported could not have originated in the Western Hemisphere without foreign instigation.

Whatever the truth of the matter, it is fairly well agreed that before the white men came, the Western Hemisphere suffered from few contagious diseases. As already noted, there is indisputable evidence that most of the principal Old World diseases did travel to the Americas. For example, it seems probable that the first devastating epidemics of cholera began in India during the years between 1817 and 1823. They did not reach the New World at that time. But the second great epidemic of cholera which blackened India and the Near East during 1826 and for several years thereafter did find its way to our hemisphere. By 1837 a cholera plague was devastating Guatemala and many other areas of the American tropics deep within the South American continent.

Twenty years later cholera again burst out in the warmer Americas. Thereafter its history is comparatively well recorded. By 1855 it was widespread in Nicaragua. It decimated Mora's army and shattered the filibustering forces of William Walker. It spread with hurricane speed throughout Central America and for two years continued its ravages. It again appeared in Nicaragua in 1866. It was causing wholesale deaths in Honduras during 1871. By 1892 the disease had appeared as far north as New York City. Although there is no information of the exact number of deaths resulting from these epidemics,[1] it is a reasonable assumption that huge numbers of Latin-American Indians were victims.[2]

Perhaps because in the fortunate north it is regarded as an almost necessary minor evil of childhood, the medical history of measles is not very well known. We do know, however, that measles has been a deadly scourge to Indians throughout Latin America as well as in North America. According to Dr. Henry R. Carter, Mexico suffered a severe epidemic during 1531.[3] From Mexico, where it developed into a full-fledged pestilence, it swept south, wiping out cities, villages, and nations of Indians. In Guatemala, which included most of present-day Central America, Alvarado, Spain's royal governor ordered that Indians be freed from their labor bondage and that all holders of royal grants of lands should release their peons from field work so that they might attend the sick and dying. Territories vast and rich were being depopulated. Fuentes y Guzmán recorded that the disease spread "like fire in grass destroying entire cities of thousand of inhabitants." [4]

Typhus, a malady carried by rats and transmitted to men, has for centuries toured the New World leaving death in its path. For four hundred years or more typhus was the curse of European armies both in the New World and at home. It traveled with the troops but did not withdraw when they withdrew. Time and time again it has held up shipping and ravaged seaports. Two centuries ago the disease was so prevalent in Latin-American jails that a jail sentence became all but identical with a sentence of death. During the eras of New World conquest in fact, typhus became known as army fever, jail fever, famine fever, or ship fever. Juarros wrote of an outbreak of typhus which attacked Antigua in Guatemala during 1774, one year after a ruinous earthquake had all but demolished that great capital. "The fatal results of the last calamity still afflicted the wretched population; a fatal fever soon showed itself and raged until the month of May, 1774, before it could be subdued, making a horrible increase to the already lengthened list of mortality." [5]

Hans Zinsser, the distinguished physician who wrote *Rats, Lice and History*, points out that typhus depopulated great areas of Spain after 1577, and quotes the Spanish historian Villalba's suggestion that the fever was transported directly from Spain to Mexico. [6]

According to Zinsser, there are two distinct types of the virus that causes typhus: the murine type, still present in rats of Latin America, which is carried from rat to man by the rat flea and from man to man by the louse; and the European type, which has not been identified in rats and is therefore believed to be carried from man to man by lice. [7]

Smallpox is even more certainly a migrant from culture-loving Europe and perhaps incidentally from Africa. Bernal Diaz, the Mexican historian, wrote of a great smallpox epidemic in Mexico during 1520. "Navarez brought with him a Negro who was in the smallpox; an unfortunate importation for that country, for the disease spread with inconceivable rapidity and the Indians died by thousands; for, not knowing the nature of it, they brought it to a fatal issue by throwing themselves into cold water while in the heat of the disorder." [8]

Don Domingo Juarros described the Central American capital of Antigua, Guatemala, in 1601: "Pestilential distemper carried off great numbers. It raged with so much malignity that three days usually terminated the existence of such as were effected by it." [9] Eighty-five years later the inhabitants of the same infinitely lovely highlands were again ravaged by smallpox: "Some of them died suddenly; others expired under the most acute pains of the head, breast and bowels. No remedy was discovered that could check its destructive progress." [10] There were not enough priests to administer the sacraments and hundreds were buried in common graves. Smallpox spread from the capital to villages, then to open country. Adults died. Children starved. Fuentes y Guzman tells how Indian capitals such as Santo Tomas, San Mateo, and Santa Lucia were wiped out.[11]

A hundred years later smallpox was again sweeping the American tropics. Juarros recorded in Guatemala City: "This distemper was of so malignant a character that in a few days great numbers fell victims of it. . . . The defunct were not permitted to be interred in the churches, both on account of their numbers and because serious injury might be done to the survivors . . . three cemeteries without the city were therefore consecrated for their sepulchre." [12]

During the entire nineteenth century smallpox continued to spread death throughout Latin America. As late as 1905 ruinous epidemics were still in progress south of the Rio Grande. In 1890, according to Gaitan, Guatemala's death toll from smallpox was 20,000, while the toll for all Latin America was possibly a quarter million. Today vaccination for smallpox is practiced throughout most of this hemisphere. In the United States and Canada the disease is comparatively well in hand. But there is indisputable evidence that it continues to linger in hundreds of remote areas of present-day Latin America. However, the organisms of disease being the ready travelers that they are, no disease can be said to be extinct in one part of the world while it exists in another. Thus the eradication of smallpox in Latin America is the condition of its total eradication elsewhere.

Medical scholarship is generally agreed that whooping cough also was brought to the New World from Europe. Apparently the scourge was at its worst during the nineteenth century when it spread from Europe and the British Isles, after causing thousands of deaths, to Mexico and South America, where the mortality from it was even greater.[13]

Perhaps most tragic of all was the importation of tuberculosis, which, according to Hrdlicka, probably made its way into the New World through Mexico, spreading north and south through the Indian nations. There is extensive testimony to support the belief that [14] before the coming of white men consumption was entirely unknown among the Indians of North America. Hrdlicka points out that "as yet no bones of undoubtedly pre-Columbian origin have been found that show tuberculosis lesions." [15]

Other scholars, such as Shattuck and Hooten, however, report possible pre-Columbian indications of tuberculosis among the Mayas, Toltecs, and perhaps other ancient Indian nations of Central America. In his *Medical Survey of Guatemala*, Dr. George Cheever Shattuck summarizes: "It appears . . . that pulmonary tuberculosis and glandular tuberculosis were not indigenous in America, but that tuberculosis of the bones may have existed in pre-Columbian times. Certainly, tuberculosis has not been in the past a frequent cause of death among the Indians of Guatemala." [16]

There is considerable controversy as to whether or not pneumonia came as an immigrant from Europe. Dr. Shattuck again suggests: "It is probable that pathogenic pneumococci were brought to America by ancestors of the Indian tribes, and that more or less pneumonia resulted therefrom; but, whereas many different strains of pneumococci and certain other organisms as well can cause pneumonia in man, it is equally probable that some of these strains were brought in by the conquering races and that they have caused an increase of pneumonia mortality among (American) Indians." [17]

Unquestionably epidemic influenza came to America from the Old World, though the basis for diagnosing this particular public enemy remains far from satisfactory. Hirsh suggested that the first epidemic of influenza known to the New World occurred in New England during 1627.[18] Dr. Henry R. Carter declared that "influenza must be considered a probability in the great epidemic which occurred among the Indians on the New England coast about 1618, which was the salvation of the Plymouth colonists." [19]

Perhaps the Plymouth colonists survived merely because Indians of those parts were too much preoccupied with influenza and were not in the mood for taking scalps. Even so, Carter was convinced that the Indians got their infection from the Europeans.

He pointed out that by 1732 the disease had appeared in epidemic proportions in the West Indies, Central America, Mexico, Peru, and perhaps other areas of South America, and that, according to Antonio de Ulloa, during 1759 a widespread and highly fatal epidemic of influenza-pneumonia swept over the Andes highlands.[20]

Like a great many contemporary travelers, influenza behaves very badly once it reaches the tropics. There is good reason to believe that Latin-American death rates from the fast-moving "flu" are between two and three times that common to the United States.[21] Latin-American deficiencies in housing, clothing, and average family income may have a great deal to do with the mortality rate.

Still another unwelcome and highly destructive visitor is leprosy. Amoebic and bacillary dysentery are probably in the same class. Giglioli presents effective evidence that paratyphoid was imported into South America, particularly British Guiana, by the contract labor brought from India and China.[22]

Dengue, that mosquito-borne cousin of yellow fever, which rarely kills but frequently causes men to consider death a kind interposition, is the result of still another virus migrant to the New World. Dr. Henry R. Carter states that the first recognizable account of dengue tells of an epidemic which struck the West Indies in 1827, having been brought by slave ships.[23] Almost certainly chickenpox, diphtheria, mumps, scarlet fever, and cerebrospinal fever are infections imported from the Old World. Perhaps the same is true of the venereal diseases, trachoma, and the scores of diseases resulting from fungi. The importation of infectious or epidemic disease is a continuing nightmare throughout Latin America, and a menace to the United States as well. Microbe tourists are the most skillful hitchhikers and the most successful stowaways known. By land, sea, and air inter-American travel is increasing and will continue to increase. Where trains, motorcars, planes, ships, and armies go, there also go the hidden organisms of disease.

According to League of Nations reports, Latin America provides a large part of the fast-diminishing world totals of anthrax, tetanus, and rabies,[24] tourist diseases like the others. The same sources indicate that Latin-American and North American losses from venereal diseases are closely comparable; that the war against syphilis is another high-ranking challenge to Pan-American health activities.

As never before, the American health front is a community problem. As never before, the threat of migratory diseases must be studied. Microbes are still tourists and, tourist-like, success among them encourages new waves of migration. As Pan-American union becomes more close and boundaries come to mean less, the exploits of disease as well as the intercommunication of men will be facilitated. Americans must realize that if their efforts toward the eventual solidarity of the hemisphere are to meet with durable success the warfare against disease must be increased and its battle lines better solidified.

At this point, having presented an outline portrait of the expeditionary horde of European diseases, it might be interesting to shift the point of view and look at a section of the Latin-American scene as the invaders themselves might see it. The invading disease organism finds in much of Central and South America not only primitive conditions which are ideal for his undercover work, but also almost everywhere outside the cities a primitive state of mind. As a case in point, consider the native yerbatero, the herb doctor, of the Andes, inland Central America, and many parts of Mexico where he is often the only representative of the forces of men arrayed against sickness and premature death.

While directing a survey of the Yucatan peninsula, Dr. George C. Shattuck, already frequently quoted, described his introduction to the indigenous medicine men of the Mayas:

On the day of our arrival at Chichen-Itza it was a great surprise to us to see an Indian medicine man bringing two patients of his own for a consultation. He had semi-semitic features of a peculiar type which we came later to recognize as typical of the Maya. His expression was thoughtful and the eyes intelligent. He wore a large pair of horn-rimmed glasses and carried a silver-headed cane. His hair was done up in a white cloth, a loose white cotton tunic covered his body, and short white trousers and sandals completed his attire. . . . Our microscopes, specimens and laboratory equipment greatly interested this *curandero* (healer) and he interested us. . . .[25]

Mayan medicine is fundamentally the practice of herb doctoring, a native and ancient form of pharmacology, but it also includes religious and ritualistic functions. Dr. Shattuck visited the Mayan yerbatero, Balbino Ek, of Chankom, Yucatan.

The date and hour had been determined by consulting the crystal, and noon was the hour selected. From the interpreter we learned that the ceremony was intended to encourage some hived bees to produce much honey and that it would take place at the house of their owner. When we arrived a few men were already assembled there with Ek. They were digging up great loaves of coarse bread. The loaves were wrapped in leaves and had been cooked in a hole in the ground by covering them with hot ashes. Great quantities of cut-up fowl and of other meats were also being unwrapped. The viands were then stacked upon or placed close to an altar which had been erected at one end of the apiary.

Upon the altar were several *jicaras* (gourd bowls) containing food or liquid. When all was ready, Ek, standing before the altar and looking very solemn, made a long invocation interspersed with the names of Christian saints. Meanwhile, as he prayed, Ek frequently dipped out a little fluid from one of the bowls, using a rolled leaf for the purpose, and tossed the fluid to the four points of the compass. This over, other men carried the bowl to the hives and poured a few drops of fluid into the entrance of each. When all this was finished the guests fell upon the viands with enthusiasm. . . .[26]

Besides being an herb doctor, the Mayan medicine man claims, as a priest, the possession of supernatural wisdom. His name in the Mayan language is *h'men*, or star. He directs rites of fertility and rain-bringing; he administers steam baths, practices simple surgery, pulls teeth, usually by tying around the tooth a strong cord made of snakeskin, and makes and applies splints for the treatment of broken limbs. He is probably the most completely indigenous physician within our hemisphere and as such he deserves sympathetic notice. Through unrecorded centuries the yerbatero has remained the guardian of common health. In hundreds of remote regions of Latin America he is, as I have said, even today the only medical practitioner. But generally he is not, and never has been, an effective guardian against invading contagions.

In addition to the yerbatero, Mayan medicine places much emphasis upon the function and sagacity of the midwife. Miss Katheryn McKay, registered nurse for the Chichen-Itza Project of the Carnegie Institution, presents the following manual; its information takes from Georgia Canul of Piste, Yucatan, and Leandra Caamal of Chankom, both Maya Indians, and from other practicing midwives of the Mayas. I quote the document because I believe it illustrates particularly well the inherent competency of yerbatero medicine:

Pregnancy—During the entire period of pregnancy the patient is massaged monthly by the *partera* (midwife). The object is to keep the uterus in place and the child in correct position. The massage is given with a rotary motion in an upward direction, starting from the groins and passing along both sides of the abdomen. Great care is taken to prevent the uterus from becoming tilted or remaining too low as the child grows heavier. Spontaneous abortions are rare. They are usually attributed to lack of some much desired kind of food, such as acid fruit or salty meat. . . .

Labor—The period of labor usually lasts from 8 hours to 12 hours. After 4 hours have passed a hot infusion of herbs is given. This potion is made by boiling together mint, or *yerba buena*, cinnamon bark, or *canella*, and chips or bark from a native tree called *pixoy*. The latter is supposed to have dilating properties. During this state of labor the abdomen is well massaged with hot oil.

If labor lasts more than 12 hours, the body is douched for several minutes by pouring hot water over it from a gourd. Hot drinks also are administered. They are made of beaten eggs mixed with hot honey to which has been added a spoonful of powdered sulphur. This mixture is believed to have dilating properties.

Great importance is attached to breathing. It should be very slow and deep to give expulsive force. . . . Malposition of the child is very rare. Should one foot present, it is well oiled and pressed back. The child is then turned into place by external manipulation so that either both feet or the head are presented. In cases where the feet are presented, no injury to the arms results. The babies are usually very small, weighing probably two kilograms (4.4 pounds). A very large child will not weigh more than three kilograms (6.6 pounds).

After the birth of the child a hot infusion of garlic sweetened with honey is added to give expulsion to the placenta. Before cutting the cord the baby is covered and allowed to wait until the placenta has been extruded, however long it may take.

To aid in expelling the placenta a cloth about 2 meters long by about 25 cm. wide is wrapped about the abdomen above the uterus. By gradually tightening this cloth a gentle pressure is exerted downward. Meanwhile the patient blows forcibly into a bottle and, with scarcely any exceptions, the placenta and membranes are expelled entire. Hemorrhage is practically unknown. Should there be an excess of bleeding resources are very limited and the patient may die.

After Care—After the placenta and membranes have been expelled, the cord is tied at two fingers' breadth from the baby's body. It is then cut with a sliver of bamboo, and the end is oiled, slated and seared with the flame of a candle. A dressing of warm oil is put on and fastened with a triangular bandage folded twice. For three successive days the cord is seared. It usually drops off on the third day. It is very seldom that a baby's eyes become infected at birth.

The period of close confinement after childbirth lasts three days. The mother is then given a hot bath brewed from herbs and containing sulphur. The bath is supposed to "ripen" or "cook" the milk. The mother may then attend to household duties, such as making tortillas and washing dishes, but she is not allowed to go outdoors until the eighth day. For several days after childbirth, a bandage is worn to prevent malposition of the uterus. The bandage exerts an even pressure except where a knot or roll of cloth has been placed over the uterus to hold it in position. . . .[27]

This is an example of a primitive, yet highly effective technique of obstetrics. Unfortunately we have no such direct testimony concerning other medical and pharmaceutical practices of Latin America's back-country medicine men. As a roving reporter, I can testify, however, that the yerbatero still plays an important role in the primitive administration of public health and that his place is worth noting both for the help which his naïveté gives to the sophisticated microbe invader and for the succor which his simple practicality gives to the suffering native.

Another fifth columnist, with far less to justify it than the yerbatero, is Latin-American water supply.

In the Carnegie Institution medical survey of Yucatan, Dr. George M. Saunders, a member of the International Health Board of the Rockefeller Foundation, listed a brief but particularly pertinent commentary upon this all too common hostelry for microbe tourists in Latin America.

. . . the water supply is derived mainly from these sources: rainwater collected from roofs and from shallow wells. . . . Most of the cisterns are hollowed out of the limestone stratum and are not lined. Consequently, ground-water can seep in through the numerous fissures and cracks in the limestone and can contaminate the rainwater. . . . The greater part of the water used comes from shallow wells which must become contaminated through seepage from the surface.

Very few dwellings in Yucatan have running water, hence very few have water closets. Most of the houses in Progreso have not even a privy, and a corner of the patio, or yard, serves for this purpose. It is quite open to the pigs, fowls, dogs, buzzards and flies. Someone has defined a Yucatan latrine as "two rocks and a buzzard." No wonder that gastro-intestinal infections are prevalent and that most of the people carry one or more kinds of round worms. Flies abound in Progreso in the summer. Swarms of them settle on any food which is exposed during the day time, and that means practically all food in Progreso, for screens are unknown. One has but to sit at noon in any one of the many small restaurants quite open to the street to gain some idea of the fly population. . . .[28]

This is not presented as a typical picture of a typical Latin-American countryside. But it is true for thousands of communities in Latin America. These are the "Grand Hotels," for microbe tourists.

It seems to be the tradition among established diseases in tropical regions to pounce upon the newly arrived who has no immunity. As any medical man knows, the decline of epidemic diseases in the United States and Canada, and the impressively effective results of public health administration, means that the overwhelming majority of North Americans are nonimmunes.

This is a serious problem in the program for hemisphere health. Rather literally the challenge is one of keeping up with the Joneses. When and if the Joneses dash too far ahead of the Gomezs and Ramirezs in public health, relapses are not only probable, but just about inevitable. Each year finds us with more millions of citizens who are completely nonimmune to malaria, diphtheria, typhus, dysentery, and a score of other principal diseases which remain more or less endemic to huge areas of Latin America. With certain exceptions the scarcer these microbe enemies become in the United States the more vulnerable to their attacks are our human immigrants to Latin America, which is to say that by making ourselves healthy we do not prevent our diseases from going elsewhere and, if we follow them, we catch them twice as badly.

Plainly, there is no answer to this disturbing state of affairs other than to regard the health of the Western Hemisphere as a single, indivisible problem north and south, tropical and temperate, together.

As I have already said, and repeat here for emphasis, each month and each day inter-American communication is growing. The proved volume of North American travel to Latin America almost doubles every year. Latin-American travel to the United States also increases proportionately. The airlines alone now carry more inter-American travelers than all shipping lines carried ten years ago.

Before the world exploded into the current war the peak touring season saw about 20,000 of our citizens sailing for Europe each week and about 500 embarking by ship to Latin-American points.

Now that tours to Europe are ended by the war, travel to Latin America, although temporarily in abeyance, is definitely headed toward a tenfold increase. Completion of the more than half finished and very important Pan American Highway could easily double or triple the number of travelers to and from the southern countries in time of peace. But the number of touring microbes which are certain to hitchhike or travel independently along the way will also inevitably increase.

The Pan American Highway is the longest and most significant route of land travel ever projected by mankind. When completed it will link, by highway, the cities of North America with at least seventeen Latin-American capitals. It will lead through Mexico, all the nations of Central America, and will join by ferry routes with the highway systems of Cuba and other Caribbean Islands. It will follow the path of the great Simón Bolívar Highway through Venezuela, Colombia, and Ecuador and, along routes already open, it will skirt the Pacific coastlines of Peru and Chile, cross the Andes to La Paz and, farther south, to Buenos Aires and Montevideo, with an alternate route swinging southward into Patagonia and Magellanes, which is the world's farthest south settlement. The highway's terminus is Rio de Janeiro, via São Paulo and other great coastal cities of Brazil. When completed it will open thousands of heretofore remote communities to the world beyond. And it will sweep through many of the remaining foci of deadly diseases—including typhus, leprosy, tuberculosis, bubonic plague. It will touch many towns and settlements which have contaminated water supplies. It will create some of the most momentous problems in quarantine and warfare against disease ever faced by man.

At this point enters still another paradox in health. It seems distinctly possible that with our help the multiplication of human travel may actually be made to serve as a blockade against the transport of disease. In the modern world it is not so easy as it once was to escape from contagion. Diseases travel with tourists and commercial goods, and alas and frequently, they travel hundreds and thousands of miles farther than they used to. In Latin America today it is well demonstrated that, once the need of it has been made clear, aggressive quarantine measures and thorough public health administration can make the migrations of people a means for eliminating entirely the hitchhiking type of migrant disease-bearing organism.

Such adequate quarantine administration is not yet in existence everywhere. No scientific research is required to show that much of Latin America is still fertile ground for epidemics and that the most obnoxious of all tourists, even excepting those from Long Island City, Greater Brooklyn, Chicago, Cicero, and Hollywood, the lethal organisms which are too small to pay fare and too elusive to be forced to carry passports are still capable of keeping the Western Hemisphere from man's complete and peaceable possession.

Chapter Ten

"FIERCE, DEEP, BLACK
MYSTERIES"

I T is one thing to speak of the Latin American diseases which we know to be the result of infection carried by traveling organisms with which we are familiar. It is quite another to speak of the appallingly long list of those disorders whose causes are still for the most part unknown to us and whose very effects are often so varied and mysterious that they cannot certainly be identified. A layman's round-up of the principal Latin American diseases about which modern medicine knows little, nothing, or not enough, can hardly be complete but neither can it fail to be terrifying. This chapter will serve as an introduction to some of the unconquered evil-doers of the Western Hemisphere.

One of the surprisingly few diseases native to Latin America, and one of the most completely baffling, is that Oroya fever of the highland Andes which, as we have seen, was one of Hideyo Noguchi's chief concerns. Oroya fever is a two-phased malady. According to Zarate's history of the conquest of Peru, it is the disease which decimated Pizarro's army back in 1543. We know that in 1870 it appeared again among workmen who came to build the fabulous railway from Lima to the mountain town from which the disease takes its name.[1]

Oroya seems to be a complex of two distinctly related maladies, one an acute infectious fever frequently ending in death; the other an infectious eruptive disease, lasting two or three months and characterized by successive waves of warts or lesions with pronounced tendencies to ulceration and hemorrhage.[2] The malady usually appears in towns and villages in the narrow, sheltered valleys of the western Andes, at elevations ranging from 3,000 to 9,000 feet.

According to those who have studied the disease, it is caused by a virus supposedly carried by night-flying, bloodsucking flies probably one or more species of the Phlebotomus. As a rule the fever strikes without external indication, causing excruciating pain in the bones and the rapid development of pernicious anemia. The skin becomes waxen and pale yellow. The spleen, liver and lymphatic glands become enlarged. The heart grows flabby. The blood is permeated by peculiar rod-shaped organisms. Red corpuscles rapidly diminish in the blood stream. Frequently the patient grows delirious. Within two or three weeks death takes between a fifth and a half of all sufferers. Except for careful nursing and the attempted destruction of the bloodsucking flies which may carry the disease, modern medicine has no definitely accepted therapy.[3]

The verruga wart, which is definitely, though still inexplicably, associated with the fever, usually lasts two or three months and punishes the sufferer with two types of skin lesions—meliary and nodular, both inclined to ulceration and hemorrhage. Inoculation of a healthy body with the blood from a verruga lesion is likely to produce Oroya fever.[4] The warts usually follow severe pain in the joints, particularly the knees, ankles and wrists. The accompanying fever is usually high. Skin eruptions begin to appear, small wart-like lesions about the size of a small pea, and more rarely, nodular masses as large as a pigeon's egg. The larger eruptions usually appear at the knees or elbows, and come in successive crops throughout a period of two or three months. The small warts are most abundant on the face.

Although severe in adults, Oroya fever is usually mild in children.

There is no proved prophylaxis except good nursing, good feeding and warfare against the guilty insect vector. The verruga-Oroya complex remains principally a mystery [5] for the future to solve.

Another supposedly indigenous ailment is *pinta*, a tropical skin disease. It is, in reality, the work of a group of tropical dematomycoses—fungi which live and multiply in the superficial skin—which produce variously colored patches, frequently of grotesque design and strongly contrasted with the surrounding healthy skin.

Dr. Eduardo Urueta of Colombia defines pinta as an ancient disease chronicled in early Aztec history,[6] but the range of the disease reaches far into the American tropics from Mexico through Central America and Northern South America—particularly Colombia, Venezuela, Brazil, Peru and Chile. It is noteworthy that in each country the disease seems limited to certain sections outside of which it rarely or never occurs.

I first saw pinta while viewing banana properties in the Magdalena Basin of Colombia. It is a startling sight, particularly in the dawning hours after a night out. I saw farm workers and store callers gruesomely splotched with white and dull blue, sometimes with tinges of green. Since that morning on the Magdalena, I have had a chance to observe in the utmost sobriety a great deal of pinta. In a laboratory I have examined about twenty of the fungi which are causative agents and noted the mycelial threads and branches scraped from diseased skins; that the colors of the species range pretty much through the spectrum; blue, violet-black, bright violet, greenish and gray violet, dark gray, bright green, bright red, dull white and jet black.

Quite literally, pinta can make black men white and during the process it can temporarily paint human skins much of the colors of the rainbow. The fungus settles into the epidermis, especially the corneous layer, and in its latter stages it destroys all pigment cells leaving the skin blotched with patches of dull white.

Dr. Eduardo Urueta writes: "I remember a case in our hospital, a man whose abdominal skin, capriciously spotted, formed figures so queer that a tourist who happened to see him expressed regret at not being able to get a handbag made from such a picturesque hide." [7]

Heat and humidity seem to be the conditions required for the life and growth of the pinta parasite. These, together with the uncleanliness and frequent abrasions resulting from rough out-of-doors work, apparently bring the fungi to the skin and open the way for the infection. Insects that are bred in stagnant water, in places where the disease is endemic—especially the sandfly—are thought to be the carriers of the spores. Dr. Urueta takes exception to this belief:

My personal experience induces me to believe that the role of these insects is doubtful, for I have seen foreigners and well-to-do natives remain immune even though they have been exposed many years to the bite of these insects. . . . It is therefore more likely that the slovenliness and the hard work among the manual laborers play the more important role in the contraction of pinta. . . .

Usually the patches start on the forehead, between the brows and spread in this order of frequency, to the hands, feet (in the persons who go barefooted), and sides of the neck. If allowed to go on without treatment the fungus spreads to other uncovered parts of the body. . . .

The chromatic scale of the varieties goes from the yellowish-violet, blue and black, which are the more frequent, to the red, which is less frequently seen here in Colombia, until it reaches the dull white or final stage. The violet is common, the greyish violet variety is still more so. The red variety which is very rare, is met with more among strangers and natives of fair complexion. . . . [8]

Pinta causes neither death nor great pain. It is serious in that it is highly contagious, hard to cure or control, and because it permanently disfigures its victim. Ordinarily it is treated with antiseptic drugs; chief among these is chrysarobin, an orange-yellow powder made from a substance deposited in the wood of a tropical tree, another ancient cure discovered by South American Indian herb doctors and adopted by commercial pharmacy during comparatively recent times. No drug or no doctor, however, can cure the white pinta, which can be hidden only by skillful tattooing.

For generations pinta has been a curse among the Caribs—the somewhat fabulous "black Indians" for whom the Caribbean is named. Lieutenant-Colonel James Cran, of Britain's Royal Army Medical Corps, has estimated that approximately half of all adult Caribs in British Honduras are blotched with pinta, usually beginning with the black or dark blue varieties and finishing up with the white. He has pointed out that among the Caribs the affliction is far more common in women than men, since the women are usually the farmers and gardeners, while the men devote most of their time to the comparatively sanitary labor of fishing.

Personal hygiene and cleanliness of surroundings seem to be the best defense against this strange malady. Throughout most of the American tropics pinta apparently becomes rarer as cleanliness and personal hygiene become more common.

This same generalization applies to several other more or less mysterious diseases of the southern countries. It is true of ainhum, sometimes called "barefoot leprosy," or better defined as "a condition of parasitic origin, the infection taking place probably through the small superficial lesions or wounds which may be found in people going barefoot." [9]

Ainhum is an unpleasant affliction usually resulting in the loss of one or more toes. Arteries leading to the toes develop sclerosis. Festering bands appear about the toes, most commonly the little toe. The bone structure begins to atrophy. The outer skin hardens and shrinks. Presently the little toe remains attached to the foot only by a few fibers of muscle. After a time the toe falls off. The victim feels little or no pain. The only preventative, according to the renowned Costa Rican physician Dr. A. A. Facio, consists of cleanliness and the wearing of stockings and comfortable shoes; a prescription not thoroughly satisfactory for tropical people who are desperately poor and go barefoot from necessity rather than choice.

Preventable poverty and squalor, indeed, are responsible for many of the more serious of Latin-American diseases. Typhus is a formidable example. Typhus still spreads sickness and death throughout the highlands of Mexico (where the malady is called *tabardillo*) and throughout widespread areas of the Andes. Not infrequently cases of Brill's disease, or Murine typhus, appear in the United States, even with some regularity in New York City, where neglect of certain areas permitting an increase in the rat population and of filth among the human might easily result in a mild form of epidemic.

Hirsh notes that the history of typhus belongs to the dark ages of the world, and to the days of famine, war, and wholesale misery which are the modern equivalent of dark ages.[10] He considers it reasonable to suppose that many of the pestilences of ancient times and of the Middle Ages were typhus fever. During the seventeenth, eighteenth and early nineteenth centuries severe epidemics of typhus spread through Europe and the British Isles and time and time again its murderous waves swept through the Americas.

Today medicine is convinced that the disease is spread by body lice which have fed upon infected blood. It is not yet entirely certain whether the virus is transmitted to healthy men by the bite of the louse or by inoculation with its feces.[11] In any case we now know that in the absence of lice the disease can be controlled, as it was in the great Serbian epidemic of 1915. Doctors and nurses run considerable risk of being bitten by infected lice in tending typhus patients. According to E. R. Stitt, however, there is no evidence that the sputum or other discharges of typhus patients can transmit the disease.[12]

Typhus is a violent disease from the outset. Violent headaches, giddiness and nausea are followed by burning fever. Within a fortnight the sufferer is usually either dead or headed for recovery. About the fifth day, red, rashlike eruptions appear on the abdomen, the flanks and chest. Frequently delirium occurs by the end of the first week. Sometimes terrifying hallucinations besiege the sufferer; hallucinations which are apparently responsible for the great number of typhus suicides. Acute circulatory weakness sometimes results in gangrene, usually in the toes. The heart is seriously affected. Severe coughs, bronchitis and bronchopneumonia are common complications. As in black plague, the clouding of the consciousness is commonplace, and, as in plague, the sufferer frequently behaves as if he were very drunk.

Old people usually do not recover. In children the disease is mild. But among adults its death rate ranges from fifteen or twenty to sixty per cent. Since the exact nature of the causative organism of typhus is still in doubt, there is little that can be done to control it other than to eliminate body lice and rats. The field of protective inoculation against typhus is still in the experimental stage.[13]

South American trypanosomiasis, or Chagas's disease, is another serious tropical malady carried to man by mites, ticks, bedbugs, and triatoma (a flying bug which infests stables and pigsties) and perhaps other vermin infesting dogs, cats, armadillos, opossums and probably other animals. The infections are most commonly reported from the South American tropics, particularly Brazil, Venezuela, Peru and northern Argentina. Most trypanosome victims are poor people living in thatched huts.[14] Exceptionally mobile and enormously destructive, the parasite invades many areas of the human body including the lymph nodes, thyroid, heart muscles, ovary, testicles, bone marrow and so on. Acute forms of trypanosomiasis frequently occur in young children, causing them to suffer high and continued fever. Their faces become puffy, thyroids swell, spleens become enlarged. Mortality among the young is very high. Adults usually suffer the chronic types, frequently marked by swollen throat, heart irregularities, sometimes by cerebral afflictions and insanity.

In man, as well as in lower animals, the infection produces its own immunity—how or why nobody knows. There is still very little actually known of the pathology of the disease. The prophylaxis is, as with typhus, a mere matter of destroying or attempting to destroy the vectors. According to Stitt, no curative agent has as yet been proved consistently effective, though certain therapeutics and thyroid extract are being used as remedies.[15]

It might seem that any malady which continues to destroy health and life throughout half-a-million square miles of South America could not long remain a mystery. But medical science remains lamentably ignorant of many other Latin American insect or rodent-carried diseases; even those with perfectly forthright names, such as relapsing fever, also carried by ticks and lice and still common to parts of Central America and north South America; infectious jaundice, or Weil's disease, thought to be transmitted through the infected urine of men or rats; [16] rat-bite fever, extremely painful, marked by successive waves of syphilis-like eruptions and known principally to the West Indies.[17] These are all recognized menaces to the health of the Western Hemisphere, and yet none is adequately understood.

Another mysterious ailment of the American tropics is the disease which results from the cruel blinding filaria parasite, or more formally, *Onchocerca Caecutiens*. About a quarter-century ago this disease was reported from the highland Pacific slope of Guatemala. Research showed that thousands of highland Guatemaltecans (in limited areas as many as ninety-seven per cent of the entire population) suffered nodules upon their scalps, fibroma-like swellings about the size of a walnut and sometimes vivid green in color.

These nodules are commonly associated with chronic eye ailments. Surgeons discovered that nearly blind highland people improved within a few days after the filaria cysts which contain closely coiled worms as much as fifteen inches long, are removed from their scalps. Even though the eye afflictions had failed to respond to other treatment, removal of the nodules appears to restore sight.

It has been found that the worm within the node can be killed by the direct injection of cocaine, carbolic acid, antimony, and various other drugs. The menacing seed of the parasite is, however, apparently present in the blood and accumulates in the tissues. The insect carrier of the disease is thought to be species of coffee fly called *simulium*, or in any case, a daytime arthropod which sucks tissue juices as well as blood.

There are plenty of other tropical filariae and they are all insufficiently known. Among them are several of the most bizarre and lurid entries in all the roster of tropical diseases. One good example is Loa loa, a flesh-worm infection of the region of the eye. Fortunately it is now extremely rare in this hemisphere.

Unfortunately the same cannot be said of *Filaria Bancrofti*, which causes a number of pathological conditions, chief among which is elephantiasis. This organism is still widely prevalent in the West Indies, and much of Central America and South America, as well as Arabia, India, China, the South Pacific Islands, Africa and, alas, our own southern states. The embryo of this filaria is frequently present in the blood stream of persons who show no symptoms of the resulting disease. Conversely people stricken with the most malignant forms, such as elephantiasis, apparently do not always carry the filaria embryo in their blood.

Like the parasites of malaria, yellow fever, and dengue, this particular filaria is mosquito-borne. When one of several species of mosquitoes bites persons having the embryos in their blood, the sheathed embryo of filaria enters the insect's stomach. Bahr has found that if a given mosquito sucks up too many of the embryos at the same time he usually dies—which apparently means that a person whose blood is crowded with filaria embryos may be less of a menace to his fellow man than a person whose blood is only sparsely infected.[18]

Dr. E. R. Stitt explains that upon reaching the mosquito's stomach, the sheath of the embryo becomes fixed in the viscid blood contents and that presently the embryo itself, by active motion, is able to force its way out of the sheath. This escape usually occurs within two hours after ingestion. The free embryo then bores its way through the mosquito's stomach wall, lodges in the thoracic muscles and begins a rapid cycle of development within the insect's body. It was formerly supposed that the larva enters the human body through the puncture made by the mosquito's biting parts, but Bahr has suggested that the larvae really enter the pores of the skin. After getting inside the human host the uninvited guests, now full-grown worms, make their way to the lympathic vessels or glands where the females, duly fertilized by the males, start a new cycle of filaria production.[19]

From the lymph the new embryos then proceed into the blood stream to await the next mosquito. Adult worms may be present in a human body in great numbers and send out thousands of embryos into the blood before the human victim shows any clear evidence of illness. The actual history of the development of filarial infections is not well known. Sometimes the evidence appears in the form of virulent red swellings or as varicosed groin glands. Sometimes the adult filaria cause deep and purulent abscesses in the flesh, the bladder or other organs. "Barbados-leg" is one of the more common manifestations. In this shocking condition the lower legs, calves and ankles swell to almost unbelievable dimensions. Sometimes the elephantiasis occurs in the areas of the breasts or the genitals.

Most of the filarial diseases are equally dreadful and equally little known. Their cure or arrest frequently calls for costly medication and skilled surgery and skin grafting. All of them cry out for relentless attack and ceaseless study.[20]

There are all sorts of visible pests in the tropics; tarantulas and scorpions, giant tropical centipedes, sometimes as many as ten or twelve inches long, venomous snakes, stinging fish and biting ants. None of these can be listed as principal causes of death or sickness in Latin America, or North America. In general the damage done by snakes, scorpions, spiders and their kind is considerably exaggerated, through the brilliant anti-venin research of the Oswaldo Cruz Institute, the Butantan Institute and the Lancetilla Experiment Farm.[21]

The hidden killers are the dangerous ones, the minute organisms whose bodies are inapprehensible, but whose work is definitely visible.

Dysentery is one of the commonest terms in tropical medicine. It means, literally, "difficult intestine" but the "difficulty" has many causes. One of the most justly dreaded forms is amoebic dysentery, which results from invasion of the intestine by a virulent animal parasite called *Entamoeba histolytica*. Bacillary dysentery is a label which covers a huge group of intestinal maladies caused by bacteria. Another vast group of dysenteries results from mechanical irritants or poisonous materials in the digestive track. Still another group is symptomatic of the more advanced stages of many chronic diseases, especially tuberculosis, cancer, nephritis, malaria, heart disease, pellagra and typhoid.

In all, dysentery remains one of the most damaging and baffling of Latin-American afflictions, and one which is still among the first ten causes of death in North America as well. Hippocrates described it and there is good reason to believe that dysentery tormented the peoples of India and Egypt centuries before Christ and that it was carried from the Old World to the New.[22] Most of the little which we know of the symptom complex called dysentery, however, has been learned during the present generation.

Amoebic dysentery exists in greater or less degree in most parts of the tropical world. At present it is one of the chief causes of ill-health in Brazil, Central America and the Philippines. It is well known in our own southern states. Some of the amoebae which live in man are harmless, but the amoeba parasite *Entamoeba histolytica* is no friend to anyone. It is an insidious fifth-columnist, tough enough to bore its way into the intestinal submucosa where it maintains infection by a constant production of offspring.

According to Stitt, the earlier contention that water, fruit, or vegetables from which cultures of amoebae may be grown are sources of the infection must be abandoned.[23] The principal factor in its spread seems to be the highly durable amoebae encysted in human feces. These can be carried by flies, or washed from dried stools into water supplies or carried in blowing dust to lodge upon unprotected foodstuffs.

Once amoebic dysentery is contracted, its course usually shows periods of improvement alternated with recurrence of intense pain and bloody dysenteric stools. Fever rarely appears in the beginning stages. But there is progressive loss in the sufferer's weight and strength. The skin becomes dry. Symptoms of anemia begin to appear. Sometimes bacillary dysentery sets in following the amoebic infection and upsets the applecart of diagnosis. Often there are signs of amoebic ulceration. The large intestine may become perforated. In approximately one case in five, liver abscess appears. Less frequently there may be amoebic abscess of the brain. Dysenteric infections frequently produce arthritis, and ulcerations of the intestines caused by parasite are a common cause of chronic tropical diarrhoeas.[24]

Amoebic dysentery is rarely fatal in its first attack. Its greatest menace lies in its capacity to persist, to alternate latent and active periods, to produce recurring abscesses and otherwise bring about chronic invalidism. Sixty to ninety per cent of liver abscesses occur in conjunction with dysentery. Its most widely accepted cures are emetine and prayer. Some medical authorities oppose the use of emetine, believing prayers perhaps the more effective and certainly the less violent.[25]

Many specifics are on the market: bismuth iodide, yatren, stovarsol, quinine muriate, and others, but no matter what is prescribed, the treatment is tedious and slow. Latin American centers of amoebic infections are usually centers of liver abscess, another serious malady of the Americas to the south.[26]

Grave as it is, amoebic dysentery is not an epidemic disease, although bacillary dysentery frequently is. Unlike the amoebic, the bacillary forms frequently appear outside of the tropics and subtropics; defiant both of boundaries and casual diagnosis. They follow armies and tides of immigration. They attack babies and young children, invade asylums, prisons and barracks. They are enormously contagious since they can be spread by human carriers, by flies, soiled clothing, blown dust, in drinking water and uncooked vegetables.

Bacillary dysentery plagues its victim with intestinal lesions, frequently causing the entire large intestine to turn the grayish red of a lusterless red velvet, dotted with irregular islands of grayish membrane. Bacillary dysentery is particularly virulent in Latin America. Its incubation period is brief, usually from one day to one week. Initial diarrhea is followed by characteristic dysentery stools and by intense pains which tend to center about the umbilicus. There is accompanying high fever. In acute cases the stools become almost pure blood and as numerous as a hundred a day. The pulse quickens and becomes weak as the heart is put under merciless strain. Sometimes arthritis appears as a complication. Sometimes the mucosa becomes gangrenous.[27] Frequently death comes before medication can be made effective. Mortality rates vary widely, from less than two per cent to more than twenty.[28]

Medical researchers have worked and are still working to perfect a successful vaccine. They are making progress, but the goal is not yet reached. The sulfa drugs are finding a place in successful treatment. Meanwhile, successful treatment also requires capable hospitalization, painstaking medication and thorough sanitation, all of which are well beyond the means of the great majority of Latin American sufferers. Dysentery is not a necessary evil, although it has outwitted the medical profession to the point.

No more a necessary evil are the many tropical afflictions of the skin which the Northerner too often thinks of as mere disfigurements. Dr. Aldo Castellani of the London School of Tropical Medicine has pointed out that tropical skin diseases must be classified in at least four groups: the vegetable organisms, bacteria and fungi; the animal organisms, protozoa and metazoa; conditions with physical and chemical causes, and diseases of unknown or doubtful origin.

In the rural tropics of Latin America no one can travel far without observing that various kinds of itch caused by fungus are common. Fungus diseases of the hands and feet, of which our home-grown example is athlete's foot, are far more prevalent south of

Mexico. Medical mycology, however, has made comparatively little progress. For a number of good reasons scientific medicine has tended to focus its research upon bacteria and viruses. Actually, study of the higher forms of fungi which attack man is older than bacteriology. For example, Gruber and Malassez had discovered the fungi of ringworm as early as 1844. But with the illustrious advent of Pasteur, Koch and other great pioneers in bacteriology, medical research among the mycoses and shytoses went into abrupt eclipse. For Latin American medicine, if not for all medicine, this eclipse has been tragic. Authorities such as Castellani estimate that at least twenty per cent more tropical infections are caused by fungi than by bacteria.[29]

In many areas of Latin America ringworm still vies with the notorious dhobie, or washerman's, itch as a foremost tropical example of those vexatious and dangerous fungi which torture human flesh. Skin ulcers, some types of which seem definitely associated with the micro-organisms of plant life, offer a wide field for study. In fact, if not more thoroughly studied, they may become as serious as some of the diseases caused by animal organisms.[30]

Yaws, another disease of skin lesions and flesh sores, is another little known menace to the American tropics. Sometimes called "false syphilis," yaws produces many of the loathesome sores which one sees so frequently in Haiti and other Negro lands of the Caribbean. According to the late Dr. Albert Patterson, former Chief Sanitation Officer of Kenya Colony, East Africa, there is every reason to believe that yaws is acquired either by direct contact with an infected person or by the contamination of skin abrasions by carrier flies. According to Patterson and others, it seems probable that the disease is also spread by ticks, lice, and bedbugs.[31]

Defending people against yaws is inevitably costly and complicated. It involves raising the standards of sanitation, increasing incomes, and bettering living conditions. It requires segregation and the separate study and treatment of each sufferer. Yaws, like so many other tropical maladies, is a consequence of abject poverty. Once acquired, the medication needed to relieve it is costly. Even if the medicine is available, the treatment is usually laborious and painful. The final cure—proved destruction of the last poisoning spirochete—is far from easy.

Yaws remains a disease of many mysteries. Generations of medical men have termed it "syphilis under tropical conditions." At present this definition is largely discarded. Workers of the Rockefeller Institute and others have proved with considerable finality that the organism of yaws is substantially different from that of syphilis.

Perhaps Haiti is this hemisphere's worst victim of yaws. According to Dr. Paul W. Wilson of the United States Navy Medical Corps, the affliction was brought to Haiti more than four centuries ago with the first shipment of African slaves.[32] The havoc of the disease has continued, causing Haiti to be listed (quite erroneously) as the world's most syphilitic island. Haiti's economic loss from yaws has been, and still is, enormous. Particularly in the rural districts, one frequently finds several members of the same family invalid from "crab yaws." Very probably most of the beggars in Haiti, and there are a great many of them, are sufferers from tertiary yaws.

It has been estimated that between a fourth and a third of all Haitians are afflicted by this loathesome disease.[33] Dr. Aldo Castellani has described districts of Ceylon where four-fifths of the inhabitants were cursed with the disease; where commercial and industrial activities have been completely stopped for lack of healthy man-power.[34] Yaws remains among the many front-rank challenges to American medicine, another ruinous tropical disease which has been bred and will continue to thrive in abject poverty unless something is done for Latin-American economy.

Much the same may be said of hookworm, a lingering malady of our own cotton-growing South, and a grim rival of malaria as a tormenter and debilitator of the American tropics. Fortunately, hookworm is one of the better known of parasitic maladies, and as the Rockefeller Foundation has so brilliantly proved, one of the more controllable.

Hookworm is spread by means of human excreta, open privies, contaminated soils and barefeet. In the United States the disease halts growth, saps energy and weakens bodies, but rarely causes death. In the tropics hookworm infections are far more severe and, if no treatment is given, deaths from the disease may be numerous, as many as forty deaths each year per thousand people.[35]

Fortunately hookworm can be cured. In Jamaica a five-year campaign staged by the Jamaica Hookworm Commission, under the joint auspices of the International Health Board of the Rockefeller Foundation and the Government of Jamaica, succeeded in reducing hookworm infection enormously; in some areas from half the total population to less than one-tenth within four years. With still greater progress in this heroic effort, Jamaicans have become healthier; employment has improved; and sickness and deaths from typhoid, malaria, colds and dysentery have diminished.

Dr. E. B. E. Washburn, a North Carolinian recently retired from the tropical staff of the International Health Board, and one of the most lovable of our ambassadors in white, directed Jamaica's epoch-making hookworm campaign. The doctor cherishes a collection of testimonials from Jamaicans who have been cured of the malady. With Dr. Washburn's permission, I should like to quote two:

To the Jamaica Hookworm Campaign, I have five treatments of the hookworm pills and I have been cured at last thank God from that dredful pest. Six of us in my family have been treated and cured. I can tell you doctor every one of us was shameful meagre and horbly crippled, and yet we were fat once. We are all new people now. I am a changed man in every way. Hart stoped to palpetate, giddiness in head ceases, bad feelings all gone, ulcer on foot healed, in fact I can hardly know myself. . . . With three cheers we wish you a great name and a happy Christmas. Robert Lewis and Family.

Dear Dr. Washburn:

I write to complan about the hookworm medsin. It is too strong too stronge and has caus me a lot of trouble. sins I tak the medsin I feel stronge an well in boddie an mind an like work more than before. The which is all very well.

But Dr. Sir a grate change has come over me in other ways. For till I tak the medsin I was mild and of a sweet disposition. An very patient. Now Sir all is chang. So much so that on last Satday when one Jeptha Smith cuss me I box him down too hard and him now threaten to run law wid me.

Sir from your kindness if the aforesaid person run law wid me I respectful ask you to see His Honour for it were no other than the hook Worm medsin make me act in sich a fierce manner.

Dr. Juan Iturbe of Caracas has pointed out that in 1900 no fewer than nine-tenths of all the rural people of Venezuela were afflicted with hookworm. In plazas, patios and barnyards the soil was permeated with hookworm larvae. In 1900, when the United States took over Puerto Rico, that island also suffered from the apparently inescapable tyranny. Since widespread and thorough measures were taken against the malady, the export trade of Puerto Rico has increased tenfold and the death-rate has fallen from forty-two persons per thousand yearly to about twenty. The center of hookworm incidence has shifted to the East Indian tropics. The Netherlands Indies have now replaced Latin America as the world's foremost pestholes of hookworm. In all too much of our own hemisphere, however, the malady remains active. Inter-American defense against the parasite can only be a war of incessant treatment, prevention, and public education. As the great anti-hookworm campaign in Jamaica so brilliantly proved, co-operation and common effort by local health boards, independent physicians, farm owners, school teachers, business men, preachers and public officials is essential. The war against hookworm is not yet won. There is good reason to believe that between the Mason-Dixon Line and the River Plata millions of Americans still suffer from the disease which, although it is no longer to be classed with the deep dark mysteries of medicine, since a method of eradicating it is known, continues to remain a menace because the nature of its threat is in many places still unrecognized.

Yaws is preponderantly a Negro's disease. Tropical sprue is preponderantly a white man's disease. Possibly, sprue isn't a disease at all. Some medical men list it merely as a condition. Others term it a disease of disputed etiology. In any case, sprue is the result of lowered vitality, of disordered digestion, constipation or diarrhea; sallow complexion, lowered blood pressure, persistent loss of weight and, according to autopsy, of diminution in the size of the liver. It usually troubles its victims with nervous irritability and melancholia. Sometimes it causes muscular cramps and undue coldness of hands and feet. Sometimes it produces a brownish pigmentation of the skin. The tongue may become coated and sore, the digestion increasingly irregular, the evidence of anemia more manifest.

Sprue, whatever its pathology, is an insidious bodily decay. Most of its victims are adults, between twenty and forty. More than half are women. The malady occurs more frequently in cities and towns than in open country. It is not necessarily a poor man's affliction. Many of its sufferers are well-to-do. Most of them are engaged in more or less sedentery occupations. School teachers and missionaries and thousands of other white-collared newcomers to the tropics, too many of whom spurn the native foods of Latin America and gorge themselves on canned goods, bread and sweets in the manner of Brooklyn, Staten Island and the Bronx, are among the ranks of sprue victims.

Sprue's menace to the Americas is increasing. In Latin America today it is appearing far beyond the limits of the true tropics, invading rural areas where previously it had been unknown. Its treatment remains as vague as its origin. In general the best cure seems to be improvement in individual diet, with a reduction of commercial sugar, cereals and other carbohydrates. It has been studied with indifferent success. The answer to the problem it creates has not yet been found.

Pellagra, for generations well known in southern Europe, is a name which means little to Americans north of the Mason-Dixon Line. In the South and the southern part of the Middle West, however, it is fairly common. In Latin America it is far more than common. Siler and MacNeal have pointed out that pellagra is never found in cities and towns which have a good sewerage system.[36] It is a dietary disease associated with a deficiency of vitamin B_2. Goldberger of the United States Public Health Service, believing that pellagra is due solely to an unbalanced diet, produced the disease experimentally by feeding a group of prisoners a ration consisting principally of corn-meal, grits, potatoes, fat meats, syrup and sugar —an adaptation of the all too prevalent fare of poor folks down south. By feeding the same group of prisoners a diet rich in milk, eggs, meats and fresh vegetables the disease was arrested and in some instances cured.[37]

Dr. William Deeks of Canada and the Panama Canal Zone, whose brilliant and colorful career has already been described, had announced his belief in the nutritional origin of pellagra as early as 1904.[38] McCollum and Funk, two more great North American nutritionists, confirmed Deeks's assumption, but McCollum changed his dictum to state that, although an improper diet is a predisposing factor in the production of pellagra, some kind of infection is the exciting cause.[39] Many investigators continue to agree, though the "exciting cause" remains in dispute.

Memorable testimony has been offered by Dr. R. McCarrison, a British Army Surgeon stationed in a remote region of the Himalayas. Dr. McCarrison became convinced that lowered resistance resulting from an unbalanced diet predisposes man to numerous infections, pellagra included. During fifteen years of service among the rugged, well-fed and long-lived Himalayans, Dr. McCarrison performed more than 6,000 major operations. He stated that during all that time he had never seen a case of gastric ulcer, asthenic dyspepsia, appendicitis, colitis, or cancer. He ascribed this almost miraculous freedom from abdominal diseases to the use of good natural foods—milk, eggs, grain fruits and leafy vegetables.[40] The surgeon in far-off India did not claim that improper diet is the only cause of pellagra, but determinedly proved that pellagra is merely one of many ruinous infections which wait to invade an inadequately nourished body.

The diagnosis of early stage pellagra remains difficult. It is distinctly possible that thousands, even millions of Americans, from Missouri south to Cape Horn have pellagra and don't know it. Some of its victims recover. Many of them live, whether recovered or not. Any Latin-American wanderer, however, is likely to become unhappily acquainted with the advanced type of pellagra: a distressing complex of fever, sore tongues and mouths, eruptions on feet and hands, colitis, ulcers and diarrhea. Prolonged cases are likely to mean a lingering painful death, since the pellagra-ridden system frequently becomes unable to assimilate food and leaves the victim to die of starvation.

In the Panama Canal Zone, between 1915 and 1925, according to autopsies performed by the Board of Health Laboratory, deaths from pellagra approximately equaled those from typhoid. The same records indicate that most pellagra victims are adults and that a majority are women.[41] Pellagra records are far from complete, but the disease remains of outstanding concern to our ambassadors in white and to the American people generally, for there is ample evidence that only well-nourished people can stand against it or a score of other similarly debilitating diseases which continue to spread sickness, despair and death wherever in the Americas inadequate nourishment prevails.

This statement is not easily contradicted. Bad food is still one of the worst enemies of the Americas, in fact of most of the world. Ironically, the occasional famines which apparently harassed Latin America during pre-Columbian times are reproduced far more destructively by the infiltration of inadequate commercial preparations which, because they are modern, and much advertised, often give the impression of being the last word in food values. From the constant use of these arise multitudes of diseases, many still little known; but all real and all destructive.

In Latin America, as anywhere else, improvement of diet is handicapped by the conservative forces of tradition, by commercial exploitation of worthless foods, by human laziness, and by apathy and ignorance. Diet is conditioned by the practical and variable business of agriculture, which in turn is dependent upon factors of climate, topography and economy. Although Latin America is the largest and richest frontier in the world today, its agricultural resources are barely tapped. With enlightened ownership and sound direction, its enormously fertile soil, its varied and favorable climates could unquestionably provide a superb fare for the people dependent on it. In the Americas diseases caused by malnutrition should be nonexistent since there is, potentially, enough of the right kind of food for everyone. Such diseases are, however, real and commonplace. Much has already been done to overcome the tragic paradox. Much more waits doing.

Important as nutrition is to Latin-American health, there are plenty of serious diseases south of Mexico which are not definable in terms of diet. Leprosy is one of the most important of these. Throughout the American tropics and throughout most of the world leprosy has, it is true, tended to become increasingly rare. Vaccines are proving at least partially effective. Throughout Latin America leprosy, with its repulsive red swellings, its ulcerated hands and ears, its withered flesh and thickened skin, is being fought. Methodical treatment lessens its terrors. One after another Latin-American governments have established refuges for lepers. It is true that, when left for ten or more years without treatment, leprosy is still practically incurable, but when treatment is begun within six months of contraction, current records prove there is an excellent chance for successful arrest of the disease.[42]

There are many types of leprosy. Some remain more or less mysterious. The bacilli of leprosy, like those of tuberculosis, often lie dormant for years, then awake to intensely active life. In Latin American and other tropics there seems to be a notable similarity between the problems of leprosy and those of tuberculosis, although the latter, not the former, are now of foremost concern.

Both leprosy and tuberculosis are most frequently contracted in the course of prolonged contact, particularly in over-crowded, ill-ventilated, unsanitary quarters. In both diseases the greatest risk of contagion is during babyhood or childhood. The late Sir Arthur Newsholme has said: "That tuberculosis is more readily acquired than leprosy appears certain. . . . But the fact that leprosy has disappeared from most temperate countries during historic times is not without bearing on the possibility of a similar disappearance of tuberculosis. . . ." [43]

Tuberculosis is known to be accentuated by malnutrition. "No satisfying evidence," says Newsholme, "has been advanced to prove that inadequate food has any influence on the origin of leprosy, though this may be so. . . . [44] Like tuberculosis, leprosy is lingering and chronic frequently with long latent intervals. In Latin America, like tuberculosis, it usually occurs among poor people, badly housed and little learned in hygiene and sanitation. Like malaria and tuberculosis its links of infection can be gradually worn down, though perhaps not entirely obliterated. [45]

Yet as leprosy tends to recede from Latin America, tuberculosis shows an alarming increase. Broadly stated, tuberculosis is today the deadliest of tropical diseases. For the past third-century medical statisticians have pointed out that tuberculosis is on the increase throughout much of the tropical world; and that its occurrence within the tropics is not so much a result of the climate as it is the habits of its people and the conditions under which they live. The dark mystery of Latin-American tuberculosis is not the disease itself, not its causation organisms, nor its treatment, but the state of being of our less fortunate southern neighbors. Solve that mystery and you go a long way toward solving the problem of the American tropics.

The common citizen's ability to resist tuberculosis is far less in most of Central and South America than in North America. There is no doubt of that. Apparently the essential defense lies in better sanitation and hygiene, better housing, and, perhaps most important, better diet. Our southern neighbors are working heroically to bring these defenses to the front line. They have built and staffed dozens of public sanitariums, many of outstanding excellence. They have assembled staffs of renowned clinicians. But below our Southern border the situation remains almost as if the problems of tuberculosis had never been touched at all.

Clinically, the progress of the disease is usually more rapid and virulent in the tropics than in temperate climates. The final, fatal stage frequently and quickly follows primary lesions of the lungs. In general, tuberculosis of the bone, joints and skin is less common in Latin America than in the United States. But the pulmonary form is in its element among the humble people of the Southern Americas.

Dr. William M. James, colorful veteran of the Panama Canal Zone, gives one of the best possible summaries of the problem: . . . "With us tuberculosis causes almost always 100 percent mortality. The most I have been able to do in Panama is to keep patients alive long enough to get them out of the country. . . . Our cases cannot follow our proper treatment. There are economic reasons for this which are absolutely beyond the control of the physician (bad housing, improper nourishment, ec.).

"From the point of view of the clinician to whom patients come every week with every sign of incipient or advanced tuberculosis, and with a positive sputum, the clinician knowing immediately that these patients in all probability will be dead within two or three years, in spite of anything that he can do to help them,—this is one of the most distressing things occurring in practice. The patients themselves seem to look on a positive diagnosis with mingled resignation and despair, and place their trust in God rather than in any medical treatment. . . ." [46]

Could there be any more eloquent statement than that of the helplessness of medical men within the working range of private medicine? The remedy is primarily not with medicine at all, but rather in the field of international economics.

In temperate climates people who believe themselves in good health usually are. In the tropics a man may go about his work (or his rest) and live his usual life for years. Yet if examined he may be found to harbor malaria, syphilis, filiariasis and perhaps several other major infections. What he dies of is, ironically enough, frequently something else—tuberculosis, typhoid, dysentery or some other disease entirely beyond the scope of the original diagnosis.

Large numbers of Latin-American ailments are relapsing. Their victims may be gravely ill in June, apparently recovered in July, and again desperately sick in August. Certain races or communities show persistent immunity to certain diseases, and inexplicable susceptibility to others. Time and time again lowered vitality caused from malnutrition baffles the most expert diagnosis. These are among the mysteries.

In most temperate countries the widening gap between pure medicine and surgery is noticeable. In general, Latin-American surgery is not notably different from that of North America. It must deal with only a few surgical conditions which are definitely peculiar to the tropics. Speaking generally, however, Latin-American medicine and surgery decline to be separated. Outside of the principal cities specialists and specialized equipment are usually lacking and the doctor, like the cherished country doctors of our own childhood, must stand by himself in his ability to fill the patients' needs, whether spiritual, medical, or surgical.

The path of Latin-American medicine remains dark, but far less dark than it was a century ago or even a decade ago. Great work has been done, greater work is being done by the many thousands of

Latin America's eminent physicians, surgeons, researchers and technicians. Great work has also been done by our own ambassadors in white. Nevertheless, the darkness is still there. Millions of our southern neighbors are dying in its shadow. Countless other millions, feeling its presence, are helpless, suffering, unable to work, unable by the fruits of their labor either to contribute toward the work that is yet to be done, or even to feed themselves and their families.

Chapter Eleven

DAMN THE MOSQUITOES!

THE immortal Sam Weller of *The Pickwick Papers* once remarked upon the scarcity of people who had actually seen a dead donkey. He might have mentioned another extremely rare character—one who had never seen a mosquito.

All continents of the earth, most islands inhabited and uninhabited, be they equatorial, temperate or arctic, are plagued by one or many of the some seven hundred different existing species of that insect pest. If all mosquitoes were like the male, the breed would not have such a bad name. Unfortunately for man and beast, most female mosquitoes, regardless of species, are genuine vampires, able to suck blood by puncturing the skin of living creatures. In consequence of this bloodthirstiness, and for reasons to be shown later, mosquitoes are not only a nuisance, they are also a particularly deadly enemy of mankind.

There are probably between twenty and thirty kinds of mosquitoes which carry human diseases. The exact total is not agreed upon, though many students of mosquitoes believe it may prove several times the current estimate. There is good reason to believe that certain species of mosquitoes are in a state of mutation or transition, possibly with expanding capacities to carry diseases. For example, the *Anopheles gambiae,* thought to have been imported from Africa to Brazil, has shown a heretofore unsuspected capacity for carrying the more virulent types of malaria.

We have noticed, too, that other species of mosquitoes, particularly the *Stegomyia,* or *Aëdes aegypti,* carry yellow fever, one of the most terrible diseases suffered by man. In preparation for hard fighting in hot countries, the United States Army is now vaccinating our fighting men against yellow fever. But unless our entire population is vaccinated, or unless all foci of the disease can be eliminated, yellow fever remains a potential menace of the United States and an active menace of several hundred thousand square miles of South America.

Until every last thing about a disease has been discovered and laid bare it cannot make much sense to say that that disease is conquered. Granted that there is today no evidence that yellow fever exists in the United States, it may be rational to assume that the stegomyia mosquito is practically nonexistent in the region. If, however, you do not positively know (and no one does) that the yellow fever organism cannot adapt itself to dissemination by other types of mosquito, and if you do not surely know that the same organism cannot maintain itself in the blood of other than jungle animals (which no one does know), certainly you cannot say that yellow fever will never again be a menace to Temperate Zone America. We do not know these necessary things and we must assume that yellow fever is still a menace to the North Americans as it proved to be to Noguchi, who knew everything any man ever learned about the disease and still could not avoid dying of it. The insect carrier of the organism of yellow fever, as well as the organism itself, appears to be groping about in search of new worlds to conquer and new ways of conquering them.

Yellow fever and malaria are by no means the only mosquito-borne diseases. Among the others are dengue, or breakbone fever, the conditions resulting from various filaria infections and from such things as heart worms, which deal death to horses, dogs, and other animals. That certain types of sleeping sickness and other serious diseases also may be carried by mosquitoes is probable, though not yet established. Some facts about mosquitoes, however, are beyond question. It is undeniable, for example, that they are a nuisance, capable of ruining a summer vacation. It is certainly true that they bite and bother in every section of the United States, on all continents of the earth from the equator to the Arctic Circle and beyond, and pretty much everywhere else except Bali, Samoa, and perhaps some of the Hawaiian Islands. On the whole the mosquito remains an enigma with which those still toddling sciences called entomology and bacteriology are not yet able to cope.

A human being is likely to talk of the particular kind of mosquito which has caused him the most trouble. In the New York area we speak of New Jersey mosquitoes; in New England (outside of Maine), of Maine mosquitoes; in the Midwest, of Great Lakes mosquitoes, and so on. This is entirely appropriate. "Mosquito" is Spanish for "little fly"—which is a masterly understatement of its social, economic, and medical significance. It is noteworthy though not surprising that one of the great mosquito-study centers of the world now belongs to the New Jersey State Agricultural Experiment Station at New Brunswick. The keeper of this renowned mosquito house is Dr. Thomas Headlee, state entomologist for New Jersey and professor of entomology at Rutgers. Dr. Headlee's work has demonstrated that mosquito-control measures are most effective when centered upon the aquatic stages of the insect's life cycle.

Mosquito eggs are laid in water or in places where water will shortly appear—in "rafts," or floating batches. As a general rule, one healthy female can provide from one hundred to four hundred eggs. From the eggs emerge schools of tiny aquatic creatures, light-colored cylindrically shaped larvae, usually about a quarter inch long, and equipped with a sort of tufted propeller. These larvae get their food from minute water plants. Most people are familiar with them as wiggle-tails or wrigglers. The larvae, being air-breathers, must stay close to the surface of the water. Usually the tail serves as breathing tube. For this and other reasons, any sort of air-obstructing film on the water can suffocate them. Mosquito larvae body are affected by many types of poison and they are easily drowned by floods or heavy rainfall. Minnows, fish, frogs, and other water predators feed greedily upon them as they wriggle about helplessly near the surface.

In nature the mortality among mosquito larvae is numerically enormous. Unfortunately it is not one hundred per cent. After about a week, or two weeks, or at most three, those which survive the attacks of their natural enemies undergo metamorphosis and become pupae. This transition rarely requires more than three days. Viewed by microscope or even by the naked eye the pupa is a nightmarish creature, a misshapen hobgoblin like some comic-strip fiend. It is more than half head, a great grotesque, hooded head, with a tiny, reptilelike abdomen. Like the larva, the pupa also breathes air, taking oxygen through two tiny horns protruding from the top of the head. This means that the pupa must remain continuously suspended from the surface and that during its brief existence it is even more vulnerable to destruction than the larva.

The final metamorphosis is equally astonishing. After about three days the pupal skin cracks and rises to float on the surface as a minute floating raft. In this raft rides the newly born mosquito, sodden but voracious. The creature has only to wait until its wings are dry to rise and fly away in search of food.

The male mosquito is a mild-mannered vegetarian. His piercing mechanism is too feeble to puncture the skins and hides of animals and it therefore must spend a somewhat namby-pamby career poking at flowers and pollen and getting its taste of life in the raw by mating with the bloodsucking and forever publicized female.

The female is relentlessly carnivorous during most of her adult life. After a few hours spent in learning to fly she begins her criminal career in search of blood. If none is about, she will stab plants and suck their sap instead, but she prefers blood and her special dish is human blood. Her tactics are comparable to those of a combat air-plane. Guided by some little-known but usually unerring sense, the mosquito locates her victim; seeking out human beings where human beings are to be found, otherwise taking almost any animal victim whose hair she can manage to part—monkey, rabbit, horse, or cow. Having located her quarry, the mosquito hovers for landing. The enormous rapidity of her wing-flapping results in a telltale buzz or hum, a sound which I am sure I do not need to describe. In opening flight and in combat dives the mosquito is silent. Stealthily she settles upon the prey and unlimbers her proboscis, which is equipped with four knifelike mandibles, two of them having jagged, saw-tooth termini. The mosquito settles, cuts and drills through the victim's skin. Ordinarily about two seconds are required for puncturing human epidermis—considerably longer for drilling through the tougher hide of horses and cattle.

The mandibles are not long enough to cut into any principal vein, even in a human being. This fact does not stump the vampire. She stings and spits, injecting from her salivary glands a fluid irritant which causes the blood she cannot quite reach to rush to the area attacked. It is this spitting habit which gives the mosquito its ability to transmit disease. When the injection is made and the blood drawn to it, she proceeds to siphon out the blood, a process ordinarily re-quiring from thirty to ninety seconds. In drawing the blood, she may load herself up with any disease organisms it contains—organ-isms which may eventually cause her own death. Fatal or not, the combination of spitting and sucking within vein areas—spitting an irritant, perhaps an albuminous protein substance, and sucking fresh blood—establishes the possibility of contagion. The mosquito's next victim may get not only an irritating bite but also an injection of disease-producing germs.

The capacity to attract mosquitoes is still not understood. Some people appear to be seductive to the "little flies"; others are appar-ently repulsive to them. During the earlier phases of the famed cleanup of the Panama Canal Zone, William Gorgas noted that certain human beings were virtually immune to mosquito bites; also that where mosquitoes feasted upon the blood of horses they would sometimes torture one horse incessantly and leave a dozen others unbothered.

Human immunity to mosquito bites is usually temporary and frequently misleading. Sometimes would-be immunity is merely the incapacity to react to the spittle which the mosquito shoots through the skin. Sometimes persons who have believed themselves invulnerable discover suddenly that mosquitoes have taken a liking to them.

The many still unsolved mysteries of mosquito life remain mysteries because of the great size and variety of the mosquito family. In New Jersey and other research centers of the United States, principal attention is given to the common nuisance types of mosquitoes which infest most temperate areas, particularly along the coast. Some of these breed in salt waters, though more of them begin life in stagnant fresh water. This has resulted in such sanitation measures as the wholesale spraying with larvicides, the systematic draining of standing water, and the cleanup of rubbish and water receptacles. It has also given rise to careful study of the many species of mosquitoes which can be identified by natural markings, such as wing designs, antenna length, coloring and striping of the body, legs and hair-tufts, or by characteristic biting positions, techniques of flight, types of larvae, and patterns of egg deposits.

The social as well as the pathological importance of the mosquito is enormous. Reporting in the New York *Times,* Harry M. Davis tells how Governor William Bradford of Plymouth Plantation complained of

faint-hearted members of the Pilgrim band who returned to London complaining among other things, about being "anoyed with muskeetos."

To this the Governor could only reply: "They are too delicate and unfitte to begine new-plantations and collonies, that cannot enduer the biting of muskeeto; we would wish such to keep at home till at least they be muskeeto proofe." [1]

The prevailing mosquito war in the New York-New Jersey areas is at best mildly indicative of the sort of measures which would have to be taken to produce comparable results in the wider stretches of the warmer Americas. New Jersey has about 300,000 acres of salt marsh, separated from the open sea by sand bars and therefore particularly menacing as mosquito breeding grounds. The state has drained about half of this area with ditches (totaling about 10,000 miles at the end of 1941). Near New York City and in the vicinity of the Pulaski Skyway, several thousand acres of mosquito marshes have been filled with excavated earth. Suffolk County, Long Island, has provided money and direction for draining about 70,000 acres of mosquito-breeding swamps. New York City, much of which is lowland and full of potential mosquito traps, has also constructed thousands of miles of ditches, dikes, and pipe drains. In upland areas the great city's sanitation department has painstakingly removed or attended to such mosquito breeding places as cesspools, standing ponds, and garden pools.

The New Jersey State Experiment Station researchers, under the direction of Dr. Headlee, continue to develop mosquito-killing sprays and larvicides. One of these is crude oil mixed with the highly toxic extract of the pyrethrum plant. This product, called "New Jersey Larvacide," is now being spread by the millions of gallons over pools, marshes, swamps, and ponds throughout the New York-New Jersey countrysides and various other Atlantic coast areas.

Dr. Headlee and his assistants have developed a number of mosquito traps, some consisting of light bulbs, to lure the bloodsuckers, and electric fans, which draw the mosquitoes into bottles full of cyanide vapor. The catches of these traps are counted and classified as to species; in this way the seriousness of the mosquito menace in a given area is accurately estimated. If a trap catches fewer than a dozen biting mosquitoes in one night, the mosquito problem in that particular area is of no real importance. But if a night's catch numbers hundreds or thousands, that is another and more serious story. The New Brunswick center continues to experiment with control devices which may ultimately help extend mosquito fighting far down the Atlantic seaboard, and perhaps eventually over most of our southern states, where malaria is still uncurbed. Airplane spraying, machine ditching of lowlands and actual or potential swamp areas, application of infra-red and other destructive light rays and, more important, capable public education regarding mosquito dangers throughout this country are among other significant elements in our growing domestic campaign against the mosquito.

For good reason mosquitoes are less dreaded in the United States than in most of Latin America. Nevertheless, our nonchalance in the face of this disease-bearing pest would not continue to exist if the public were better informed about the actual danger. There is much to be told, even though the whole tragic story of mosquito-borne diseases is not yet completely written or known.

There can be no question of the menace to the entire Western Hemisphere of the disease-bearing mosquito. It is certain that anopheline mosquitoes continue to distribute malaria parasites to tens of millions of people. Joseph A. Le Prince, whom I have already introduced as the first great sanitary engineer for the Panama Canal and a pre-eminent authority on mosquito fighting and the control of mosquito-borne diseases, had this to say about the situation:

The writer was recently occupied with mosquito control measures on the coastal plain of Mexico, and noted that many of our petroleum corporations are so busy obtaining oil that they take practically no precaution to control malaria, even where half or more than half of their labor force are affected by malaria. Petroleum companies' financial losses from this cause are probably ten times the cost of what the preventive measures would be. Until a few years ago, there was a similar condition in some of our own southern states.

One of our problems, therefore, is to learn how to prevent business corporations from wasting their own funds. . . . It is not unusual for men of good executive ability to consider applied sanitation a non-essential. Possibly it is true that sanitarians are often poor sales-men . . . and therefore no doubt that, with a few brilliant excep-tions, we have failed to impress on the minds of our public, and upon those who develop natural resources, that uncontrolled malaria means financial loss.

We do not achieve that state of malaria control which we should obtain, because we fail to make the public want it and work for it. The desire for freedom from malaria *can* be created. . . . It takes time, hard work, and enthusiasm to bring it about, but it *can* be done. Our people have not yet caught the idea that they are paying the bill exacted by malaria and getting nothing in return. . . .

In the United States we find that the public pays screen manufac-turers about $25,000,000 a year for mosquito screen-wire to protect their homes. But this protection is only partial. Too many buildings that are screened either are not effectively screened, or else the screening is not effectively maintained. The financial investment is made, but owing to neglect or lack of interest, the screening is too often ineffective. . . .

In areas where malaria prevails, Anopheles that gain access to screened buildings can be found on the screens in the early morning, and again at dusk, at which time it is easy to destroy them. Even in buildings which are not screened the gorged Anopheles resting on the walls are easy to kill with a fly swatter. This systematic destruc-tion can be achieved even in the homes of the very poor . . . and where the procedure is systematically carried out, it has a tremendous influence on preventing malaria transmission.[2]

Le Prince stressed the importance of closer study of the vital habits, likes, and dislikes of mosquitoes and urged the strategy of building artificial ponds and puddles to lure mosquitoes to deposit their eggs, then to destroy the larvae with poison. He pointed out that fish and minnows are probably the most effective natural enemy of mosquitoes and that stocking streams and ponds with fish has proved one of the best possible means of destroying mosquito larvae —easier and cheaper than the use of artificial larvicides, longer last-ing and more effective.

For the past third of a century the United States Public Health Service has worked toward complete malaria control in the United States and, although at least one-third of our own country is still plagued by malaria-carrying mosquitoes, hundreds of antimalaria campaigns have actually been carried on within national boundaries, principally in the South.

In the majority of instances, these have not been projects of county, municipal, or state governments. Instead they have been paid for by local businessmen who were convinced that mosquito fighting is good business. Our Federal Health Service has shown a high degree of competence in convincing local citizens of the continuing need for self-protection from disease-carrying mosquitoes. The late Dr. Henry R. Carter of the United States Public Health Service, dean of tropical medicine in the United States, summarized the strategy with typical directness:

We have attained outstanding success by going to small towns where there are large factories—as at Crystal City, Missouri, and Electric Mills, Mississippi—and getting the business men to understand that it will pay them to do anti-malaria work. . . . We don't speak of the elimination of malaria, but if you can reduce its prevalence from fifty percent down to five percent, or even to two percent in a year—and that can be done—you control the disease. If we can get a place in which the business men are interested in having work done, and if the doctors we send there know the facts about malaria, we can nearly always raise sufficient funds locally for malaria control work; and the work has always been successful from a financial point of view. In the South of the United States many business men are in the habit of spending $100,000 to get $150,000, but the ordinary municipality does not like to spend $100,000 no matter what the returns are. Go to the business man himself and in ninety-nine cases out of a hundred you will be able to secure money for malaria work.[3]

In the United States and in other American lands, railroads, hydroelectric plants, and many other utilities and enterprises spend time and money to combat malarial conditions which frequently accompany building and construction work. As mosquito fighting progresses, the quantity of man-made malaria also tends to increase through such institutions as farm irrigation, highway culverts, seepage dams, and water reservoirs. In 1924 Dr. Carter declared, "The present generation will see malaria pretty fairly under control, but I think never eliminated in the United States." [4]

Dr. Seale Harris, the former president of the Southern Medical Association and medical consultant to Gorgas, Pershing, Woodrow Wilson, and others during the First World War, mentions as a significant instance the malaria-control work of the Tennessee Coal and Iron Company of Birmingham, Alabama; a subsidiary of the United States Steel Corporation.

The firm employed 35,000 people and provided for the medical care of 100,000 people—employees and their families in the district. About 1912 George Crawford, the president of this company, made a trip to Panama and the Canal Zone. While there he was impressed, he told me, by the fact that the laborers of the Canal Zone appeared to be in better physical condition than those he had known in Bethlehem, Pennsylvania, and in Alabama. He therefore decided it would be good business for the Tennessee Coal and Iron Company to spend some money to prevent disease among their employees. He secured the services of Dr. Lloyd Nolan of the Canal Zone staff. During the first year of Dr. Nolan's work there were more than 2,000 cases of malaria among employees of the Company. In less than five years . . . among 90,000 to 100,000 employees and their families—there were fewer than 150 cases. [5]

Control of the dangerous *Anopheles* involves keen observation, painstaking study of mosquitoes, and skilled diplomacy in dealing with the afflicted people. Accessibility of mosquitoes to dwellings or to places where men work is another foremost consideration in waging mosquito warfare. The presence of mosquitoes in the environment of men is governed by many factors of climate and geography: the strength and prevailing direction of the wind, the amount of rainfall, the temperature and ratio of shade and sunshine. Frequently mountains or hills serve as barriers to mosquitoes and other insect life. For example, in the Cordilleras of Colombia I have been in valley villages which were pestholes of malaria and yet have found the next valley apparently free of both mosquitoes and malaria.

Under certain conditions mosquitoes may travel over great distances. In Guatemala, not long ago, I was lodging in a high mountain village about twenty miles from Guatemala City. Ordinarily mosquitoes are practically unknown in the village and the entire countryside about it. One stormy night a hurricane swung far up the valley of the Motagua River. Next morning the mountain village—almost two miles above sea level and a mile and a quarter higher than the common habitat of *Anopheles*—was plagued by swarming thousands of the creatures. Abruptly the winged hitchhikers vanished. In another week there was hardly a mosquito to be seen, heard, or felt in the entire village. But they had left their calling cards. Malaria broke out. Within another week the local doctor reported thirty cases among the seven hundred citizens of the town. Mosquito tourists must have visited the village before, for human carriers were present, able to offer the disease for transfer to others. Extremely few, if any, of the Indian villagers ever travel beyond the sanctuary of their mountains. Since they do not go to malaria, the disease must have come to them—via tourist mosquitoes.

The "direction trap" is a particularly ingenious device for mosquito control. It consists of one or more strips of window glass coated on both sides by a sticky material such as a mixture of resin and castor oil. The pieces of glass are propped or suspended in an open house or a shaded outdoor location which has proved attractive to mosquitoes. Each piece of glass is set to face a particular direction.

The strategy is to determine simply and accurately the dominant direction of mosquito flight. When two pieces of glass with sticky surfaces are set up, one facing north and south, the other set east and west, or at right angles to the first, and if next morning several anopheles are caught on the north side of the first plate and only a few on the south side, and if no mosquitoes have adhered to the sticky surfaces facing east and west, the evidence is positive that the principal flight of mosquitoes is from the north. If approximately the same number of mosquitoes are found on the east face of the second piece of glass as those adhered to the surface which faces northward, indications are that the principal direction of mosquito migration is from the northeast. Obviously, wind direction or other weather conditions might cause variation, but the testimony of direction traps is usually extremely reliable. Once the trap has given its evidence the mosquito fighter proceeds in the direction indicated and, locating the hidden breeding place, probably within five hundred yards of the location of the trap, is enabled to destroy the existing larvae.

In several areas of the American tropics, particularly the Canal Zone and the banana-growing regions of Central America, where mosquitoes too frequently carry malaria, mosquito catching has become a skilled profession. Boys are best at the trade—youths between twelve and sixteen. Frequently they are paid standard wages to make daily rounds of homes, warehouses, and barracks. Their working tools are rudimentary—fly swatters, spray guns, and sometimes glass tubes or cups with bottom linings of cotton saturated with chloroform or some other asphyxiating agent. Carried on persistently, this work proves highly effective—usually more effective than the same money spent for pills and powders or larvicides and sprays.

For where malaria exists and anopheles mosquitoes are heavily entrenched, men cannot be protected merely by swallowing quinine. The following episode, told by Dr. William M. James, now of Herrick Clinic in Panama, a veteran warrior against mosquito-borne diseases, will illustrate the point:

Perhaps ten or twelve times a year we are consulted in Panama by parties that are going to Darien, probably one of the greatest hotbeds of malaria to be found anywhere in the world. These people have been advised elsewhere, merely to take with them pills and capsules. They make the trip without any physician, go into the bush where all the natives are infected by malaria, and within four or five days members of the party succumb to fever. They cannot hold quinine on the stomach, and in a short time they come back to Panama ready for the cemetery. When one has seen these conditions . . . and has lost personal friends, he is particularly impressed by the fact that no one should go out into a heavily infected district without a competent physician in the party, nor trust to taking quinine by oral methods.[6]

Dr. Arthur McCormack, former president of the Kentucky State Board of Health and assistant to Gorgas in Panama, described how mosquitoes were caught in the hard-fought canal-building days:

Upon arriving at Panama . . . I was fortunate enough to find a couple of mosquitoes in my house. . . . I telephoned down to the sanitary inspector. . . . In a few minutes a truck came up with the sanitary inspector and four or five laborers in it; and they spread themselves through that house looking for mosquitoes. And they knew just where to look. With their flashlights casting their beams behind everything that cast a shadow, they went everywhere.

And in a very short time they found these two mosquitoes . . . caught them in a test-tube with a little chloroform cotton in it, and, with a magnifying glass, soon found what kind of a mosquito each was. They would then know whether it had bred in the house or whether it had come in the house from the outside. This happened to be a kind of mosquito that flew against the wind, and always bred in shallow wet places on the ground. That meant there was such a place somewhere near my house. . . . The sanitary inspector brought a map of the neighborhood, and knowing the direction of the wind for the preceding few days, he knew they had come from a certain direction.

So a search was made in that direction, and on the following day a leak in a water pipe revealed the place where the mosquitoes had bred. . . . We can understand very readily . . . from the perfection of that organization, why the death rate of Panama is half that of the ten best rates in the United States; and the rate of sickness in Panama is about one twenty-fifth of that in this country.[7]

It is probable that from twenty to thirty species of mosquitoes actually transmit some form or other of human diseases. This figure is still only a guess; continued research may double it, or treble it. We are comparatively certain that in terms of the enormous adaptability of mosquitoes to land areas throughout most of the world, their complete destruction is impossible. This means that an effective fight against mosquito-borne diseases must require the working union of preventive and curative medicine; of field sanitation, public hygiene; highly practical insectology, continued research, and unceasing work.

With a never-lessening toll of sickness, debility, and death, malaria remains far in the lead as the number-one mosquito-borne disease. It is now common scientific agreement that mosquitoes which carry the zygotes of this malignant blood parasite are invariably the females of the genus *Anopheles*.

Dr. Francis M. Root, medical entomologist at Johns Hopkins, pointed out the extensive evidence indicating that mosquito genera are still undergoing notable evolution; and that many apparent species are not yet well enough known or "solidified" to encourage dogmatic classification. Also, the relation of the various anopheline species to the actual transmission of malaria calls for more and better study. At least five species of anopheline mosquitoes found in the Americas are known to be important carriers of malaria. At least eight more species are proved to be susceptible to malaria infection; and four species, or more, are suspected of transmitting the disease, although their implication is not yet verified.[8]

Johns Hopkins laboratory experiments in the dissection of malaria-bearing mosquitoes indicate that the percentages of anopheline mosquitoes infected with malaria vary enormously by species; also that a given species of mosquito, depending upon location and human carriers, can carry all three types of malaria—tertian, estivo-autumnal, and quartan. Infection ratios produced by laboratory methods range from 5 per cent to 85 per cent, depending upon the species; while natural infections vary from zero to one-fourth of 1 per cent, to a maximum of 1.47 per cent for North American species and to an apparent world high of 5 per cent for one South American type, the mosquito *Anopheles bellator*.

Presumably only the bloodsucking female mosquito can carry disease; and even among the most menacing *Anopheles* rarely more than one female mosquito in a hundred actually carries the organisms which afflict man with malaria. Moreover, the mosquito is not particularly easy to infect. In the Canal Zone, Dr. Samuel T. Darling devised an ingenious system for weighing the mosquito before and after feeding, and of counting malaria "crescents" in the human blood upon which the mosquito fed. His experiment proved that it takes from twenty-five to fifty gametocytes of malaria to infect one mosquito, and suggests that, although human population can and frequently does become virtually one hundred per cent malaria-ridden, in the mosquitoes the ability to spread and propagate the malady is a minority phenomenon.

A Temperate Zone locality rarely harbors more than three or four mosquito species in great abundance. For example, if you are in New Jersey and a mosquito bites you, the chances are that it is the *Culex solicitans,* the common gray mosquito which breeds in marshes of the Atlantic coast. The chances are, too, that aside from being irritating, the bite of this *Culex* will prove comparatively harmless.

This particular species breeds in salt water. Hundreds of other species cannot endure salt water. Some require brackish water; others, fresh water. Some breed freely in polluted, muddy water; some can live only in fresh, clean water. Some types of mosquitoes, like some types of people, insist upon living and breeding in cities or suburbs. Others can survive only in remote rural regions. Some appear to revel in cold climates, such as Iceland, northern Canada, Alaska, and Scotland. Others die if removed more than a few miles from the equatorial tropics. Few if any of the far-north mosquitoes are disease carriers. *Aëdes aegypti,* and other yellow fever carriers, are preponderantly mosquitoes of the tropics or subtropics, though in summer they can be transported far north. The *Anopheles,* carriers of malaria, range widely over nearly eighty degrees of latitude. In this hemisphere they are found at their evil trade from the Argen-

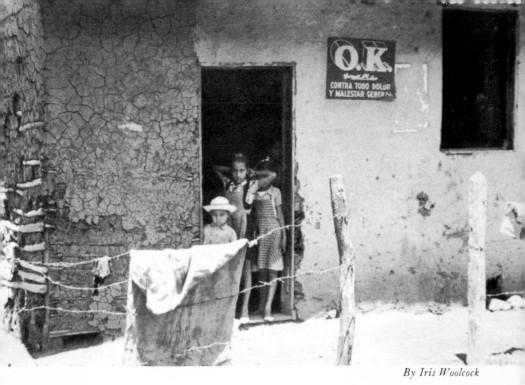

Healthy children make healthy adults.

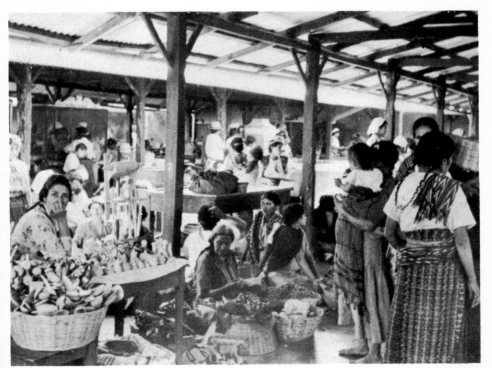

Indian market in Antigua, Guatemala.

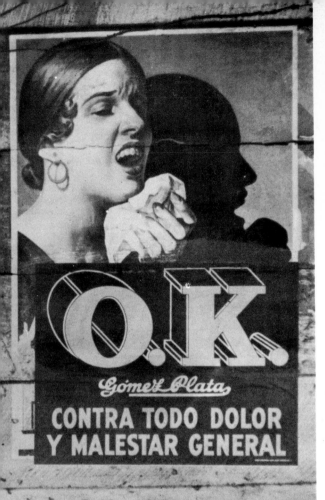

By Iris Woolcock
Latin America is also harassed with patent medicines.

By Thomas D. Mulhern, Agricultural Experiment Station, New Brunswick, N. J.
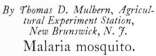
Malaria mosquito.

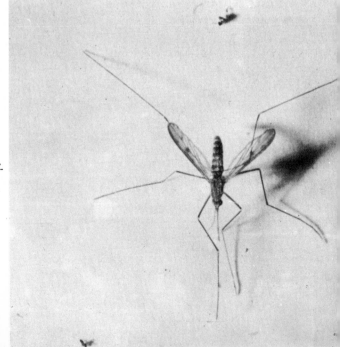

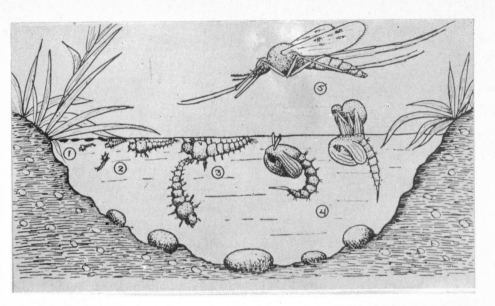

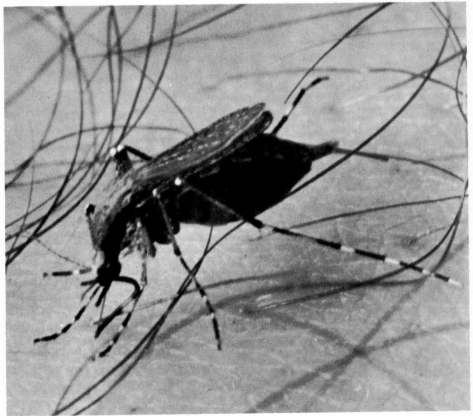

(Upper) Life history of a malarial mosquito.

(Lower) Aedes Sollicitans, common salt marsh mosquito.

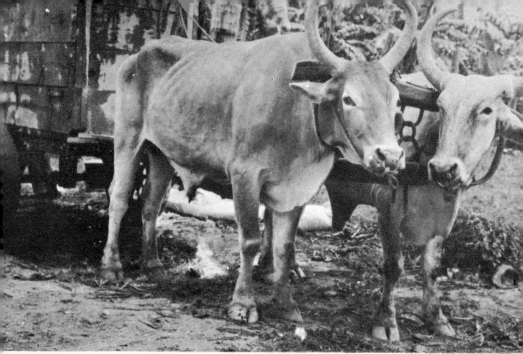

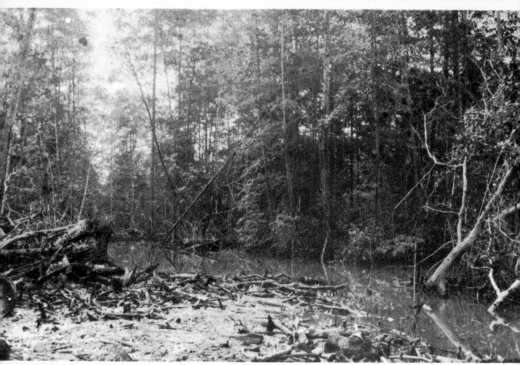

By C. M. Wilson
(Upper) Jamaica model of oxdrawn spray rig.

By C. M. Wilson
(Lower) Typical tropical jungle, Costa Rica.

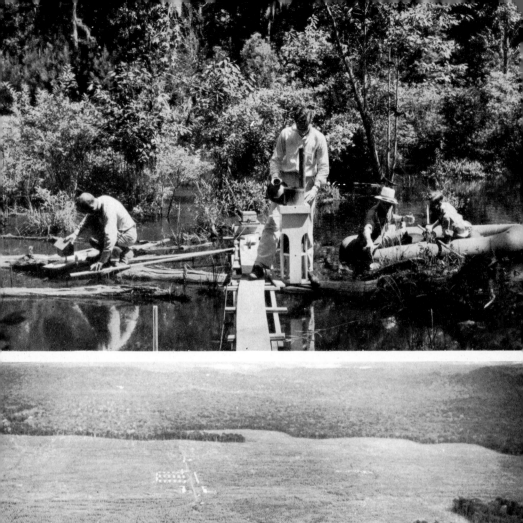

Courtesy of United States Public Health Service
(Upper) Mosquito observation station, latest model.

By Iris Woolcock
(Lower) The best banana country is usually mosquito country.

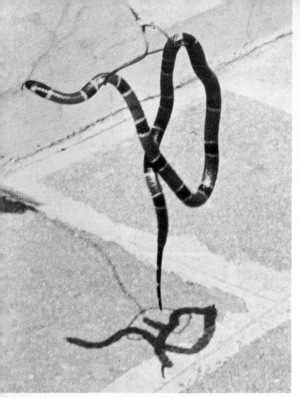

By *Iris Woolcock*
Shadow of trouble, the tropical
corral snake.

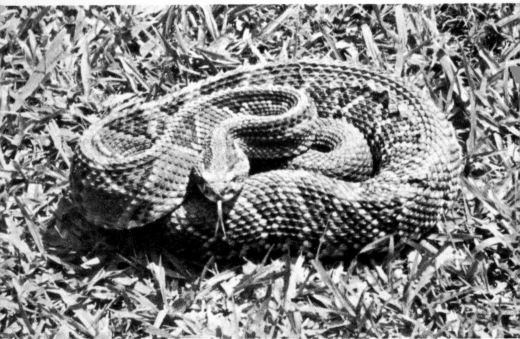

By *Iris Woolcoc*

The mankilling Bothrops, deadly snake of the American tropics.

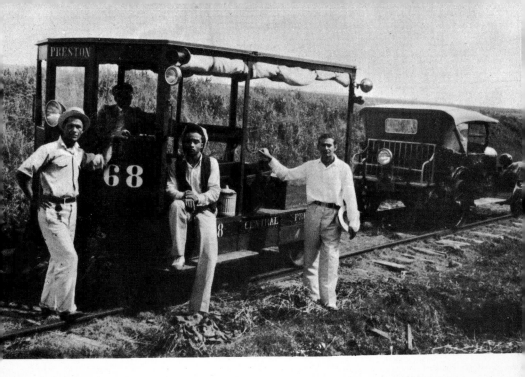

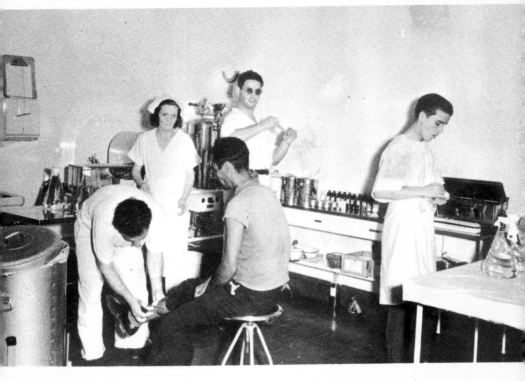

By C. M. Wilson
(Upper) United Fruit Company's field sanitation patrol in Rural Cuba.

By Iris Woolcock
(Lower) First aid for banana land injuries at Golfito, Costa Rica.

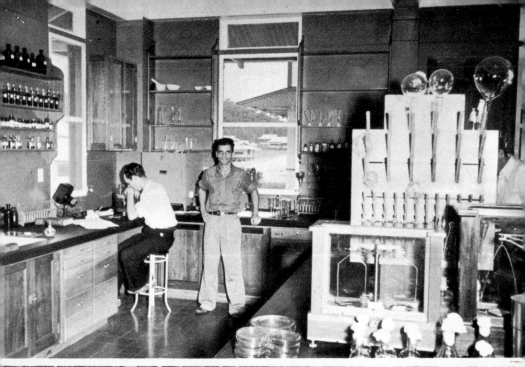

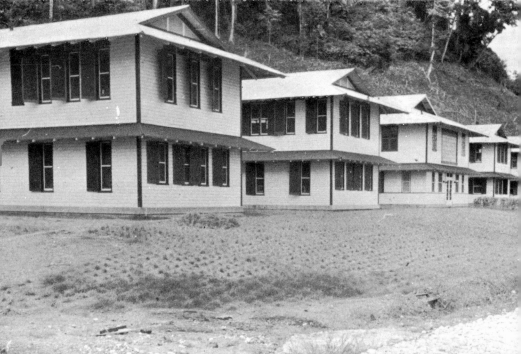

By Iris Woolcock
(Upper) Bloodtesting in United Fruit Company laboratory.

By Iris Woolcock
(Lower) Newest 200-bed hospital of the United Fruit Company at
Golfito, Costa Rica.

tine northward to New England. In the other hemisphere the north and south range of the *Anopheles* is even greater. Though most heavily concentrated within thirty degrees of latitude—north and south—and most heavily centered in India, the malaria carriers of the Old World ply and propagate as far north as southern England, Wales, and southern Scandinavia. The *Anopheles* is predominantly rural—probably because its larvae prefer algae and grass to protect their watery cradle.

To identify mosquitoes on the wing is no easy task. Usually the larvae are more readily distinguishable than adult mosquitoes. For the larvae vary greatly in size, shape, and habitual position. Those of the malaria mosquitoes lie horizontal to and in contact with the surface of the water, while the more common *Culex* larvae rest vertically—with heads down and tails touching the surface. The *Anopheles* larva is long and slender; the *Culex* short and chunky. Unfortunately, larvae of disease-carrying mosquitoes are usually more astute than those of the ordinary bloodsuckers. Both *Anopheles* and *Aëdes aegypti* larvae dive and seek shelter if they detect sounds or shadows on the water. The *Culex* larva does not seem to protect itself in this manner.

Luckily there is one vital condition common to all mosquitoes. Their eggs must hatch in water. Some types lay eggs in places free of water, but if the eggs hatch they must be covered with water or very closely accessible to water. Thus, defense against mosquitoes becomes plainly a matter of watching and treating water. Rather strangely, the *Aëdes aegypti* prefers man-made containers of water for breeding places—especially containers made of wood and cement rather than those made of metal. Strangely too, as Dr. Carter pointed out, its progeny actually have a much better chance of reaching maturity in their chosen breeding places than those used as a last resort, when preferred localities are not available. After a third of a century of experience in mosquito fighting, in Peru, Mexico, Yucutan, Central America, Panama, Colombia, and other American lands harassed by yellow fever, Dr. Carter strongly recommended the practice of encouraging mosquitoes to breed in preferred locations so that men might promptly and effectively destroy the larvae.[9] He stated his findings:

> Does the provision of suitable breeding places, of easy access to the mosquito of which we are trying to rid ourselves, seem a paradox? I have been asked whether I wished to encourage mosquitoes to breed? We don't care whether they breed or not *provided there be no production*. . . . We are not trying to control the breeding, but the production of adult mosquitoes. By themselves mosquito eggs, larvae and pupae are absolutely innocuous and, if breeding is stopped short of this final development into the imago, which alone is offensive, we are satisfied.[10]

Such is the new practice of mosquito baiting. It is now common knowledge that pregnant female mosquitoes can be attracted to water that contains sugar. The larvae do not thrive on sweetened water. Obviously this is one of the instances—extremely rare in lower life forms, and, alas, extremely common among human beings—in which the maternal instinct is its own worst enemy.

Dr. Aristides Agramonte reported an ingenious method for the destruction of yellow-fever larvae in Santiago de Cuba, a city where most of the drinking water must still be taken from cisterns and reservoirs, which, as already indicated, provide excellent breeding places for *Aëdes aegypti*. Dr. Agramonte offered the simple expedient of placing in each receptacle one or more live fishes—of the Gambusia variety—which, without affecting the purity or palatability of the water, happily and continuously destroy any larvae developing within their reach.

"By the use of fish," said Dr. Carter, "or of oiling, or by emptying water containers at proper intervals, we can, in general, sufficiently control the production of the yellow fever mosquito and yet allow the mosquito access to its preferential breeding places. . . . These methods involve no risk of driving the mosquitoes to unusual breeding places, the control of which may be difficult or even impossible."[11]

Like other contemporary warfare, mosquito fighting is, at least in part, a combat by finesse. Under compulsion, mosquitoes, like men, change their daily habits and routines. A warfare that takes no account of this fact may prove more disastrous than no defense at all.

Not long ago at Saltpond, on the Gold Coast of West Africa, one of the many lingering strongholds of yellow fever, and at Parahyha, also a yellow fever focus, Dr. John Carr, of the International Health Board, noted that, by natural inclination, yellow-fever mosquitoes do not breed in open puddles. A research worker placed moist sand in a basin, packed the sand tightly against the side of the basin and poured water into the hollow sand. He then placed a screened cage containing *Aëdes aegypti* over the basin. The mosquities proceeded to deposit their eggs on the wet sand just above the edge of the water. Strangely enough, these eggs developed larvae which promptly wriggled down to the water, where they proceeded to live and to flourish.

On hearing of the experiment, the research director promptly ordered the experimenting doctor to destroy all adult mosquitoes thus produced. He saw in this one simple, even trivial experiment a possible compulsion development of a strain of yellow-fever mosquito which could change its habits sufficiently to breed in puddles of water enclosed by sand, thus enabling forthcoming generations of *Aëdes aegypti* to learn the heretofore unpopular trick of depositing eggs in sand—beyond destruction by fish or water predators, or by motion of water, yet near enough to water so that the newly hatched larvae might live and flourish. Such a happening, abetted by man, the future victim, might thus serve to re-establish yellow fever in a region from which the former habits of the local brand of *Aëdes aegypti* had excluded it.

Man's fight against mosquitoes may very well be the most beneficial warfare in the world today. For the warfare for health is just and noble, and the enemy is enemy to the core. It is a war that complements other wars. When military activities reach more and more deeply into the tropics, the protection of fighting men from mosquito-borne diseases is as important as any other strategic plan. In the present conflict we have succeeded, to date, better than our enemies. British troops in Africa have been protected against yellow fever with vaccines perfected and manufactured in the United States. German troops in Africa have suffered and died of yellow fever. There is no complete protection against malaria. But in the Far East the soldiers of Japan have reportedly suffered far more from malaria than soldiers of the United Nations. As this book is written the United States Army Medical Corps reports that a majority of Japanese prisoners are stricken with malaria. The winning or losing of the mosquito war may yet decide the destiny of mankind and the fate of the democratic way of life.

Chapter Twelve

BANANA MEDICINE

FROM mosquitoes to bananas is no great stretch, inasmuch as the production of bananas is, to a considerable extent, dependent upon the subjugation of mosquitoes. The banana is not just a tropical fruit; not on a New York fruit stand, at any rate. It is a symbol of the union of tropical luxuriance with industrial enterprise. It is more than that.

The jewels that sparkle at the throat of a beautiful woman, the power of a locomotive or steamship in motion are no farther removed from the lusterless lumps of carbon in which they had their origin than is the banana on a New York breakfast table from the cluster in which it grew among the heavy shadows of a Caribbean farm. For the banana, although it is a crop like any of our northern fruits, has in its culture elements which if required of a northern grower would cause him to abandon his farm as rapidly as possible.

In Aroostook County, Maine, a man may grow potatoes without any serious consequences to himself, without impairing his health. In Iowa he may grow corn and, with ordinary luck, never have to see a doctor. In fact, the Iowa farmer and the Maine potato grower may even, when their crops are in, find themselves in better health than their customers in the nation's cities.

In North America, crop lands are for the most part lands of health and hope in spite of civilized curses like tuberculosis. Even in the South, cotton may be harvested without too much danger from hookworm, malaria, or malnutrition. Good banana land, however, is usually a good producer of a primary crop of disease which must be killed off before the fruit will grow. The same can be said of good rubber land, good cocoa or chocolate land, spice land, indigo land, sugar land. In the flood plains, river valleys, and watery jungles of Latin America lie the undeveloped agricultural resources of the Western Hemisphere. There also is the hemisphere's greatest concentration of disease-producing organisms, malignant fungi, and other venomous forms of life.

Behind every bunch of bananas stands a man, and that man cannot be a sick man. As early as the sixteenth century, as recorded by the historian Antonio de Herrera, the Spaniards of New Spain learned that sick men cannot work. As recently as half a century ago many a banana grower hired hundreds of laborers in the often futile hope that ten out of every hundred might remain healthy enough to be of some productive use.

Minor Cooper Keith, when at the age of twenty-three he joined his three brothers and an uncle in accepting a contract to build the first railroad across the republic of Costa Rica, knew plenty about gradients, fills, crossties, and Johnson bars but he knew nothing about jungles. He was a man of enterprise and energy; having a job to do, he set out to do it. He spent the first months of 1871 recruiting a force of seven hundred laborers. Without other preparation than arming the men with tools and machetes he set them to clearing the jungle from the vicinity of what is now Port Limón, only ten degrees north of the equator. Keith soon learned that labor in Costa Rica was something very different from work in his native Brooklyn. Most of his seven hundred employees promptly and agonizingly died of tropical fevers. Baffled as well as shocked, he recruited more laborers and kept at the work of railroad building until what he and his brothers had set out to do had been accomplished.

Minor Keith never forgot what that railroad line cost in human life and human disability. Counted in that cost were his three brothers, who died of malaria, and counted, too, was the anguish it caused him to see them and others suffer. He himself, being fortunate enough to survive both malaria and yellow fever, learned what must be done to make tropical work possible. That he learned well is evidenced by the fact that he remained to develop the region opened up by his pioneering. Near Port Limón, in 1873, he set out an experimental plantation of bananas which turned out to be successful and provided the focal point for a great industrial empire of railroads, steamship lines, plantations, and jungle commissaries.

In 1899 Keith persuaded Andrew W. Preston, tired-voiced former commission-house clerk who had built up a large New England outlet in the Boston Fruit Company, to merge with the Keith interests and other tropical properties. Thus the great United Fruit Company was born.

From his own tragic experience Keith knew that Northerners could work successfully in the tropics, but he also knew that such work, like a successful battle, required a great deal of preliminary skirmishing and barrage laying. He convinced Preston that there was no use trying to do business in Latin America at all unless you first conquered the local health problem. The United Fruit Company has not forgotten this principle of its founder. The company would not be in business today if it had. What adherence to the principle involves will be seen from a glance at the newest of the company's tropical divisions on the Pacific coast of Costa Rica, one of many fragments of a great tropical farming front extending from Cuba and Honduras to Colombia and from the Atlantic to the Pacific.

The company's medical activities in the west coast of Costa Rica date from 1937. They were a carefully planned preliminary to the opening up and development as a banana-producing center of a new and hitherto untenanted wilderness. In January of 1937 a dispensary car in charge of a pharmacist was sent over the existing line to the Pacific port of Puntarenas. This point was to be headquarters for a series of beneficial raids by river launch through the areas marked out for development—some of the wildest jungle lands in all Central America. In July of that year a temporary dispensary was opened at Puntarenas. In November, still keeping ahead of the main working body, dispensaries were opened at the prospective banana plantation centers of Parrita and Pozo. Within a few months the labor force in the section had grown from a mere handful of pioneers to an army of some 4,000 workmen. Front-line dispensary treatments were provided for slight accidents and illness. Serious cases were invalided back to hospitals in Port Limón or Puntarenas. The scouting force in the outpost line undertook to make malaria surveys. These, together with the work of field sanitation services, kept sickness reasonably well under control during the early stages of the advance of the banana men.

Pioneering of this sort continued through August, 1938, by which time approximately 2,000 native laborers were at work on the jungle site which has now become the banana town of Parrita. The next step was to build and open a temporary hospital at this outpost. By the end of 1938 there were as many as 4,500 employees in the new division. The temporary hospital took care of a daily average of twenty patients and its dispensary treated a 24-hour average of eighty. Other outposts of the jungle development, in the form of local field dispensaries at Quepos and Puerto Cortés, also treated the sick and injured.

Meanwhile, the number of workers consolidating their positions in Costa Rica's newest banana front climbed from a year's average of about 2,600 in 1938 to 8,005 during 1939. The division's load of medical and sanitary work grew in proportion under the direction of two experienced sanitary inspectors. During 1939 another temporary hospital was opened at the outlying banana center of Palmar. Then, rapidly but carefully, the two permanent hospitals of the division were rushed to completion. Until they were ready, the more serious cases from the front line were transported by plane to the company hospital at Puerto Armueilles.

These two hospitals, the newest of the United Fruit Company's string, are located at the newly developed Pacific seaports of Quepos and Golfito, Costa Rica. They are tangible evidence of the importance to the company of its medical work. Three years after the first machete was laid against the jungle growth of the Golfito region, a modern 200-bed hospital, the company's largest, opened its doors and its arms to the employees of the district, their friends and relations. Today the Golfito Hospital is one of the best-equipped medical centers in Latin America.

The exterior of the huge frame building, its broad roofs of galvanized iron, the carefully graded lawns surrounding it, the hillside view of blue bay and glittering Pacific, for all their pleasing, simple atmosphere, give little hint of the efficiency and functional beauty of the interior and equipment.

On entering, the visitor might think he was in the Grand Central Palace, New York, at any exhibition of the very latest in hospital furnishing. Air conditioning, trim and effective tubular lighting, batteries of stainless steel cabinets, superlatively modern kitchens, clinic rooms and laundry, make one forget the jungle outside. Here are the best, heaviest, and newest of X-ray devices; operating room impressively accoutered; huge stocks of surgical and pharmaceutical goods; sparkling and much-gadgeted laboratories; well-fitted wards and corridors of private rooms, pleasing and variable color schemes, modern metal furniture; an exquisite choice of decoration throughout—tapestries, seat covers, and room walls painstakingly matched and blended.

Earlier traditions of the plain and colorless tropical hospital are blasted at Golfito. This hospital at the same time perpetuates the old health principles of Minor Keith and introduces a new era in banana medicine. It is a public monument to be envied by any city in the world.

Modern as it is, the hospital also illustrates the conventional patterns, the real, practical nature of banana medicine. It is a place of men who go into untenanted jungles, as much a part of their equipment as machete and sombrero. It is a supporting column for the pioneers who pave the way for fruitful plantations and new agrarian frontiers.

The exemplary institutions of Golfito and Quepos, however, are merely a link in the chain of medical service which the United Fruit Company has recognized and made the world recognize are essential to the development and use of tropical lands, as much a part of the Latin-American picture as the technology of the blast furnace, which turns useless ore to something usable, is to the North American steel industry.

From its modest but resolute beginning in 1899, the United Fruit Company's medical department has grown until it now comprises a line of fifteen base hospitals and medical centers stretching through three oceans over a semicircle of more than 2,000 miles from Banes and Preston, in Eastern Cuba, to Santa Marta, in Colombia, the longest and largest chain of corporate hospitals in the American tropics.

From its beginning the building up of this great chain has involved much more than the mere erecting and equipping of hospitals and dispensaries and the employment of doctors and nurses. Tropical health is total health or nothing. Its maintenance has committed the company to an interminable and costly program of field sanitation; of regular and emergency treatment of employee dependents and private citizens in neighboring villages and farming areas; of incessant vigilance, relentless war against common epidemics. It means unending effort in public vaccination, inoculation, and blood testing. It calls for the establishment and maintenance of water and sewerage systems, garbage collection and disposal, regular medical inspection of work camps and commissaries. It involves dozens of other costly public health enterprises of the sort we in the United States receive and accept as matters of course.

Good health is good business anywhere, but in the tropics good health has to be bought. This investment in health is prerequisite to all other investments. A kindergarten child knows that sick men can produce little wealth, that dead men produce no wealth at all, that sickness is cumulative as well as contagious.

A great many prominent North American business leaders apparently cannot grasp this simple fact. The histories of many *yanqui* ventures in Latin-American railroad building, mining, logging, and petroleum recovery have proved that it is not widely understood. Not many years ago North Americans and Europeans in Latin America complacently planned their work on the basis of employing five hundred local laborers in the hope that as many as fifty might be able to work on a given day. That was the case in the first futile attempt to build a Panama Canal. It was true of the building of the Panama Railroad. It has long been at the bottom of such tropical realities as the daily funeral train and the community burying dump where interments are too frequent and hurried for easy recording.

The United Fruit Company does not conduct its medical department as a charity. On the contrary, being the world's largest banana company, it is interested in profits. The Western Hemisphere's largest combine of farms (bananas, sugar, cocoa, abacá, and other crops); the owner or lessee-operator of thousands of miles of railroads, of two shipping lines, a radiotelegraph system, and the employer of about seventy thousand national citizens of Central America, South America, and the West Indies is not giving anything away. The company does not pretend that its increasing efforts to maintain common health in the American tropics are to be classed as philanthropy.

To a certain extent there is a humanitarian urge behind it, for it is carried on largely by the toil, enterprise, experience, and skill of doctors, nurses, dispensers, and technicians who have little time or firsthand experience with the culture of bananas, sugar or cocoa, or the technique of operating railroads, shipping lines and radiotelegraph systems. Good health is an enlightened and durable policy, as

Messrs. Keith and Preston agreed more than forty years ago. It is also good business.

What kind of business banana medicine is, may be gathered from some interesting figures: During 1941 medical department employees of the United Fruit Company totaled 876; 66 were physicians, 79 nurses, 54 office workers, 25 technicians, 60 dispensers, druggists and pharmacists, 351 ward and kitchen operating employees, 97 laundry personnel, 103 sanitary workers and yardmen, and 41 were engaged in miscellaneous tasks. In addition to the employees of the medical units of United Fruit's twelve tropical divisions, there are twelve physicians who are normally assigned to passenger ships of the Great White Fleet and nine physicians stationed in ports of the United States.

During 1939, a typical year, the company's medical force handled a total of 594,660 dispensary treatments and 326,406 hospital days. On a per-employee basis, that is about four times the work load of New York City hospitals. The average daily number of patients in United Fruit Company hospitals is about 900. Average daily dispensary treatments are about 1,370.

The company built its first hospital in Panama during 1900. The others followed in rapid succession as new lands were opened up. East Coast Panama Hospital opened in 1900; East Coast Costa Rica, 1904; Banes, Cuba (a sugar-growing division), 1906; Preston, Cuba (also a sugar division), 1908; East Coast Guatemala, 1909; Santa Marta, Colombia, 1914; Tela, Honduras, 1914; Kingston, Jamaica, 1919; Truxillo, Honduras, 1921; West Coast Panama, 1929; La Lima, Honduras, 1930; West Coast Guatemala, 1937; Quepos, West Coast Costa Rica, 1940; Golfito, West Coast Costa Rica, 1941. We have already seen that in opening each new division a dispensary, or temporary hospital, has to be provided to attend the first working force of jungle fighters. Before a new banana-growing division is really on its feet, a permanent hospital must be built, equipped, and staffed. Throughout the far-spread banana front the volume of hospital service and the scope of field sanitation continues to increase as production increases. A majority of the physicians and surgeons employed are natives or citizens of the respective countries in which banana hospitals have been established. Many of the nurses, pharmacists, and technicians also are natives of localities served.

In Jamaica, where the prewar employed personnel of the United Fruit Company was about 8,000, federalized crown colony hospital services are supplemented with a medical dispensary service. Malaria control has always been an important part of the Jamaica service. During the two years 1938 and 1939 only one malaria death was reported from the entire Jamaica roster.

The medical department of the Chiriqui Division in South Coast Panama, with headquarters at Puerto Armuelles, employs three physicians, three nurses and a total staff of 95 to administer medical care and sanitation for about 3,700 employees, including the personnel of the banana port of Armuelles. Located in the isolated Chiriqui jungle, this particular division is exposed to a terrific barrage of malaria infection. Yet the Chiriqui hospital admissions for that disease are now only about 60 per thousand employees per year. The theoretic expectation is at least 300 per thousand.

The combined medical departments of the two active Honduran divisions, with a central hospital at Tela, compose one of the largest co-ordinated medical establishments in the American tropics, providing medical services to about 9,000 regular employees. For more than a third of a century the medical department of the East Coast Costa Rica Division with headquarters at Puerto Limón, has served a medical haven for the population of the entire middle tropics. Besides the medical and sanitation services maintained for company personnel, this hospital has provided accommodation for tens of thousands of noncompany Costa Ricans.

In the Colombian division, the medical activities of the United Fruit Company are carried on in collaboration with the *Centro Mixto de Salud,* a socialized medical system operated by the government of Colombia to assume responsibility for the medical care of workers and their dependents. The Fruit Company, however, maintains its own hospital center at Santa Marta. In Guatemala the company's Quirigua Hospital is one of the best known in Central America. Its superintendent is Dr. Neil P. Macphail, graduate of the University of Aberdeen and one of the most celebrated physicians of the American tropics.

The practice of banana medicine offers proof of Le Prince's renowned proverb, that the sanitarian's enthusiasm must outlast his boots. It is basically an open-country task; a job for field crews who wade swamps and wear themselves out hacking at grass and bushes; who go forth into the jungle to meet sickness before sickness comes from the jungle to attack men; who meet all kinds of venomous jungle creatures whose bite is far worse than their bark.

There are death-dealing snakes in the American tropics; not so many as writers of fiction like to assume but enough to create a considerable medical problem. Most of the Central American man-killers are of the genus *Bothrops*.

Among the more formidable of these is the *cascabel*, or tropical rattlesnake, usually found in the foothills and pasture lands of the interior. The cascabel's bite is one of the deadliest known. The action of its poison is neurotoxic. Saving the life of its victim frequently requires use of the specific serum *Antivenin cascabel* to neutralize the venom.

The *barba amarilla* or *fer-de-lance* is one of the most common and dangerous reptiles of banana lands. It is a small-headed, dark-spiraled snake, which moves and strikes with amazing swiftness. The barba is one of five species of *Bothrops* common in many parts of Latin America. Bites of all members of the genus are treated with the same specific antivenin. The barba is a big snake, growing to a length of nine feet. Its venom is particularly deadly, destroying the red blood cells and the walls of blood vessels. It has been known to bring death in half an hour or less.

The following case records, taken from files of the United Fruit Company's hospital at Santa Marta, Colombia, suggest that the barba's bit is not always fatal, even when treated with the most primitive of first-aid measures:

A.E. was bitten about 3:00 P.M., Feb. 12, 1929, on a sugar-cane farm in Mamatoco, about six miles from Santa Marta. He was hunting among banana plants and sugar-cane, and when he tried to draw back a branch of a tree, the snake jumped at his face. He attempted to defend himself with his left hand, and was bitten on the dorsal surface between the thumb and index finger. The snake was approximately four cuartas (32 inches) in length and bears the local name of *Boquidorada* (gold mouth) although it is also called *barba amarilla*. He was sure that the snake was empty, as he opened it to get the gall-bladder.

First-Aid Measures—The patient stated that immediately after he was bitten, he felt faint and vomited. He therefore tied his arm with a tourniquet, and swallowed bile of the same snake; bile of the *guatinaja* (a small animal of the opossum family); contra-cruceta (a plant which the Indians use for snake bite) *Curarina* (a patent medicine), and about twelve ounces of rum. He declared that he improved after his self-treatment and went home. He had dinner at 5:00 P.M. and said that he felt well until a pregnant woman came to see him; and from that moment he was very sick, had an extremely high fever and vomited blood.

Hospital Admission—The patient arrived at the Clinic at 2:00 P.M., February 13.

Treatment—At 2:00 P.M. on February 13, the patient was given 10 cc of Mulford's antibothropic serum. No other measures were taken except to release the tourniquet and allow the patient to rest. Shortly after the antivenin was injected, he became unconscious and vomited more blood. Next day the patient felt much better. He improved rapidly thereafter until entirely well.[1]

There are many other poisonous snakes in Latin America, though luckily most of them are comparatively rare. One is the hog-nosed snake, or *Bothrops brachystoma*, smallest in size of its murderous tribe; sometimes less than a foot in length at maturity, yet one of the deadliest of all venom bearers. Its tiny mouth divides a sort of piglike snout and the plump, brownish-gray body tapers into a tiny whiplike tail.

Another of the impious *Bothrops* is the *tamagas verde*, a slender brilliant green snake which lives in trees and low bushes, avoids the ground, and strikes its prey from behind barricades of dense foliage. Tamagas verde is distinctly a jungle snake and, because of its fleetness and tree-climbing skill, is rarely captured. Its bite, particularly if untreated, is capable of causing death.

Still another of the death dealers is the *timbo* or *mano de piedra*, or more formally, *Bothrops nummifiera*. It is a chunky, crease-backed snake with a wedge-shaped head and a tail that tapers to a shoelace stub. Unlike the green tamagas, it is distinctly a ground snake. Dappled greenish brown, its usual habitat is the brown dry foothills of the interior.

Bothrops schlegelii, commonly called the viper or eyelash viper, is appropriately named. The reptile is horribly ugly and each of its eyes is protected by two hard spiky scales. This viper is small, rarely more than two feet in length, usually less. Its coarse diamond-shaped scales are camouflaged in a sort of olive drab. It lives in trees and bushes, frequently in palms, and its bites are almost invariably directed toward the heads, shoulders, and arms of men going through the bush. It is rarely seen, almost never captured.

Perhaps more frequent, though no better known, are the bushmasters, or *mapanas*, local names for the *Lachesis mutus*, a justly feared venom bearer of the tropics. Probably the most common of all and most easily identified is the *micrurus*, or coral snake, a slender swift-moving reptile, marked by wide, jet-black body bands each bordered by two narrow bands of yellow.

For centuries and for rational as well as fanciful reasons, Latin Americans have lived in dread of venomous snakes. It seems to be certain that poisonous snakes are more common in banana lands than in any other densely inhabited section of the American tropics with the possible exception of interior Brazil. The obligations of banana medicine, therefore, include effective antidotes and treatments for snake bite. Pure and tested antivenins must be acquired regularly and kept on hand.

For this reason, the United Fruit Company, co-operating with the Museum of Comparative Zoology at Harvard and the Mulford Biological Laboratories of Philadelphia, established a snake farm at Lancetilla, the seat of the renowned experimental gardens near Tela, Honduras. Here poisonous snakes were collected from many parts of the western tropics and their venoms regularly extracted. From these venoms the Antivenin Institute of America formerly supervised the production and distribution of commercial antivenins; this duty is now being taken over by commercial pharmocology.

Wherever men work in tropical Latin America similar work is carried on, especially in the Instituto Butantan of Brazil.

Reliable estimates of the numbers of people bitten by poisonous snakes of the American tropics are hard to find. To James S. Cudlipp, veteran assistant to the general manager of the United Fruit Company's medical department, I am indebted for this noteworthy information: During a typical three-year period, only 104 alleged or verified instances of snake bite occurred among 150,000 residents of Ceneral America and the West Indies—a yearly total of some 23 casualties per hundred thousand persons.

Most of the sufferers are rural laborers. Among the 104 victims of venomous snakes there were only seven deaths— for a mortality rate of 1⁶⁄₁₀ per hundred thousand. It seems likely that only two of the seven deaths were unavoidable. In three instances records were incomplete or indecisive and did not conclusively prove that death actually resulted from snake bites. Two of the death may have resulted from incorrect first-aid measures. The problem of venomous snakes appears to be considerably more serious in Brazil and other South American lands than it is in Central America or the Caribbean islands.

In any event, persistent hospital direction, education in first-aid practices, and continued research in the development of better anti-venins are combining to make the dread of tropical snakes rather more an interesting bit of folklore than a morbid reality. Again the rule that the lower the degree of visibility the greater the menace of the enemy seems to hold good. In the same jungle the microscopic filaria is more deadly than the deadliest serpent.

Knife and arrow wounds are among other dramatic entries in the logbooks of banana medicine. Fortunately, these rather unnecessary instances of mayhem are becoming less numerous as the southern frontiers come more closely within the scope of law and order. Arrow wounds and spear wounds, comparatively common a generation ago, are rare nowadays and virtually limited to the Indian borderlands of jungle states like Ecuador.

Tending the machete or knife wound, however, remains no easy matter. The machete, working knife of the American tropics, remains indispensable, the standard tool for clearing bush and chopping firewood, for mowing undying weeds and grass, for slicing bread, carving meat, slaughtering fowls and pigs, for personal manicure and sometimes, alas, for fighting.

Usually the machete wound is an unfortunate by-product of payday. Work brings paydays; paydays bring cash; cash buys rum, and rum motivates fights. Whether deliberate or accidental, machete wounds represent the moments of too great stress in an otherwise orderly society. Usually, as already remarked, they are the result of overindulgence in the demon rum; frequently they are delivered by otherwise peaceable and gentle citizens. In any case they demand considerable medical and surgical skill and so are one of the problems of industrial medicine in the tropics.

One night in a South Coast Panama banana outpost, I met a middle-aged *mestizo* staggering along a grassy pathway leading to the United Fruit Company hospital. It was bright moonlight and I saw that the *hombre's* shirt was drenched with blood. I overtook him and, when he stumbled, I helped him to his feet.

He was about to faint. He said that he had been stabbed with a machete about an hour before—at a dance. He was gasping with pain and begging for water. His skin was cold and clammy and his pulse was weak. Also, there was a gaping hole in his upper abdomen.

At the hospital a white-clad doctor answered my ring. He summoned an attendant and led the way to the clinic. There he hurriedly undressed the wounded man and made an examination. The wound was ragged and deep and the blade which had inflicted it had obviously been twisted about in cruel vengeance. With each labored breath, stomach contents oozed from the wound. The surgeon voted an immediate operation, began to apply anesthetic, then opened the abdomen through a median-line incision. A profuse hemorrhage, which had already filled most of the abdominal cavity with blood, issued from a wound in the left lobe of the liver, which the machete had penetrated.

The surgeon packed the liver wound and checked its bleeding. Next he found that the anterior wall of the stomach had been cut through, spilling gastric contents into the abdominal cavity. He closed that wound with two layers of sutures, then irrigated the inner abdomen with warm salt water, inserted drains in both flanks, closed the incision and put his patient to bed. After a few days the sufferer was stricken with bronchopneumonia, but in spite of all complications he recovered. Within a month he was able to sit up. Within another month he was back at work, harvesting bananas.

A more remarkable instance of machete surgery was reported by Dr. B. M. Phelps, surgeon of a United Fruit Company hospital at Puerto Castilla, Honduras. A youth was carried to the hospital two days after a not very heroic knife brawl. A razor-sharp machete had chopped away most of his face. His nose had fallen to his chin. The cut extended almost to the anterior part of the jaw. The entire facial structure, including antrum, nose, right superior maxilla, and palate had been cut through. The knife had sliced down through the end of the tongue and finished its descent by wounding the right shoulder.

The surgeon administered anesthesia and proceeded to close the wound in layers, using chromic catgut and beginning with the mouth. He took scrupulous care in closing the cavity linings and preserving the exact anatomical relationship of the damaged parts, and gave careful attention to all superficial wound infections.

Three weeks later the surgeon again examined his patient. The scar of the mouth wound was barely perceptible. Both nostrils were open. Percussion over the maxillary sinuses was not painful. The upper teeth and jaw were firm. True, there was a complete anesthesia of the nose, of the upper lips, and of the areas at the angle of the mouth, but the patient could be discharged as cured. He continues to harvest bananas.

The scope of banana medicine includes not only tropical medicine and surgery, but cosmopolitan medicine as well. It continues to recognize that malaria is the most important preventable disease with which employers of labor have to deal throughout the majority of the American tropics; that most malaria of banana lands is of those pernicious types, the control of which is only realized with the utmost difficulty. After malaria come hookworm and dysentery, with their inevitable aftermath of anemia, pneumonia, and the many other diseases of debility. Also important are the pernicious effects of malnutrition.

Treatment of the worst forms of malaria is relatively complex. Each patient can and frequently does become a separate problem as difficult to handle as if the disease he suffers from was unknown. One malaria sufferer may require a mere ten minutes of treatment time in a dispensary; another ten years of hospitalization. The malaria sufferer may walk briskly on his own feet or he may be carried in unconscious and limp. Frequently he is incapable of taking medication by mouth or retaining it in his stomach. Quinine must be injected into his blood, muscle tissues, or rectum. In any case, quinine supplemented by atabrine is the number-one ally of banana medicine; the one drug for controlling the asexual cycle of the malaria parasite, checking clinical malaria, preventing relapse and halting the formation of the deadly gametocytes in human blood. Without quinine and atabrine there is good reason to believe we should have no bananas.

Besides being the foremost destroyer of man's energy in the tropics, malaria is the worst enemy of tropical childhood. In general the malaria rate among children is approximately double that of adults. In hot countries, children wear few or no clothes. Their body surfaces are almost constantly exposed to mosquitoes. They lack the adult's resistance. Frequently they are not conscious of malaria symptoms. They merely lie down during the earlier periods of paroxysm. They are rarely bedfast, and not easily subject to mass treatment. Without treatment they remain the principal reservoir of malaria-contaminated human blood.

For this and other good reasons, if it is to be effective, banana medicine cannot consider age, sex, or local boundaries. It is an exacting, costly venture in mass medication. Figuratively, the control of malaria and of most other infectious diseases is an equilateral triangle. One side is the source of infection; another side is the mode of transmission; the third side is the susceptibility of a given population. To break any one of the three sides causes the triangle to collapse and stops the progress of the disease. Banana medicine has learned, however, that, although in tropical lands the chances are a thousand to one that no side of the fateful malaria triangle can ever be completely broken, all sides must be tirelessly, ceaselessly attacked.

That is why in banana lands one hears a great deal about the "mosquito index." That is why the sanitary inspector and his squads of helpers are a staple fixture of every great banana center.

In most divisions of the United Fruit Company, the sanitary inspector turns in daily reports stating which plantations and labor camps have been visited; describing the water areas inspected and treated; stating whether or not mosquito larvae were found, the type of larvae and the quantity of mosquito breeding as evidenced by the average number of larvae in each "dip," and a listing of the amount of larvicide and oil used during the day's work.

Inevitably the problems of mosquito fighting and open-field sanitation change with place and season. But in all the history of malaria fighting on the far-flung banana frontier, I know of no instance more typical than that of the Chiriqui Land Company, a comparatively new division of the United Fruit Company which operates banana plantations, railroads, and the port of Armuelles on the remote southwest coast of Panama.

The latitude of the Chiriqui lands, a little more than eight degrees north of the equator, is approximately that of the Orinoco Basin in Venezuela. Puerto Armuelles, headquarters of the division, is located on the shore of a crescent-shaped bay of the Pacific. Inland from the port, to the north one can see the 11,000-foot purplish volcano of Chiriqui. Before the coming of bananas, the countryside was one vast green growth of dense jungle, partly drained by swift rivers, partly standing in swamps. The few inhabitants were Spaniards, mestizos, and occasional Chiriqui Indians who had drifted down from the highlands. Malaria was endemic, and very nearly universal.

The Fruit Company began its preliminary construction of railways, bridges, and docks. The jungle population was rapidly augmented by newcomers from the United States, Nicaragua, Costa Rica, and the West Indies. The felling of trees bared streams and earth to the sunlight. Multitudes of fresh breeding places for mosquitoes appeared. Railroad construction increased the hazards of stagnant water. While the pioneering was in full blast, Dr. Herbert C. Clark, now superintendent of the Gorgas Memorial Hospital, then director of laboratories and preventive medicine for the United Fruit Company, conducted a malaria survey which indicated that more than a third of all people in the area were infected and that the malaria rate at headquarters was nearly 60 per cent.

Labor turnover was rapid. Sanitation workers were blocked by surrounding jungles. Lack of fresh meats, fruits, and vegetables gave rise to many dietary ailments. The native people lived principally in open manaca palm shacks. There was little or no law enforcement. Backwoods medicine peddlers tramped through the new colonies, encouraging laborers to avoid quinine and to buy worthless nostrums instead.

Despite all this, bridges, railroad, warehouses, and modern farm villages were completed and put to use. Native police were recruited. Good foods were imported and home gardens established. A pioneer medical department began methodical blood surveys of all workers, distributed free quinine, and directed the screening of all homes. A sanitation squad went into action, treating standing water with oil or Paris green, mowing grass and bush. The engineer force began construction of hundreds of miles of drainage canals. Farm overseers and work bosses assembled workers for blood tests and treatments. Quinine and plasmochin were given to all workers, the latter to render the asexual form of malaria parasites sterile, thus making the carrier noninfectious to mosquitoes for several days. A malaria record was made for every citizen of the division. The tip of the worker's ring finger was cleansed with alcohol, several drops of blood extracted with a Hagedorn needle and the smear placed on a numbered microscope slide. All slides were painstakingly examined by laboratory technicians. Positive findings were recorded in red ink opposite the subject's name.

From these records a treatment list was made. A member of the medical department, assisted by the local dispenser, attended to individual treatment.

Thirty grains of quinine daily was the usual prophylaxis. Babies and children were given a quinine sulphate powder suspended in a honeylike syrup. With the syrup each child received a bar of sweet chocolate. As final treatment all patients were given a two weeks' supply of tonic. Within one year the occurrence of malaria in Chiriqui had dropped from 35.6 per cent of the division census to 20.4 per cent; in eighteen months to about 8 per cent. That is banana medicine at work.

Banana-land warfare against malaria continues to prove that the public enemy number one of the American tropics can be halved and quartered, if not entirely destroyed. During 1939 in the two Cuban divisions of the United Fruit Company, hospital admissions for malaria averaged only one per thousand employees. That was probably the most effective malaria control ever attained in the American tropics or subtropics. Unfortunately, the recent migration southward brought about by the necessity of building defense outposts, especially in connection with the refitting of the Guantanamo Naval Base, having brought in new, nonimmune blood, finds Cuba once more a victim of epidemic malaria which proves, among other things, that in hot countries it is far easier to arouse that sleeping dog, the organism of malaria, than it is to lull it to sleep in the first place.

Common diseases of temperate climates sometimes exhibit strangely intensified characteristics in the tropics. Lobar pneumonia is an example. In Central America pneumonia deaths are rarely fewer than a fourth of all cases reported; sometimes as high as 65 per cent. In the United States pneumonia kills rich and poor pretty much without fear or favor. In the tropics, and apparently in most of Latin America, pneumonia is mostly a disease of the poor. It follows ruthlessly in the wake of malaria, hookworm, anemia, and the diseases incident to habitual poverty. Prompt diagnosis, immediate hospitalization, and good nursing care are essential for its control. Throughout the banana regions pneumonia, vulturelike, watches the course of other mightier killers. As the activities of banana medicine cut down the prevalence of disease in general, the susceptibility to pneumonia is also fortunately decreased.

The same is generally true of beriberi, a nutritional disease common in most of Latin America and still too little understood. Regardless of country, as already pointed out, beriberi is likely to be found in areas where the poor man's fare lacks green vegetables and shows too great a proportion of white bread, rice, and beans. Time and time again the management of the Cuban sugar divisions and various banana divisions of the United Fruit Company has halted the disease outside of hospital walls, merely by donating garden plots and distributing free vegetable seed among their workers. In the tropics and out, subsistence gardens are among the best of all medicines.

Banana lands, like all others, are bothered with syphilis, which follows its usual treacherous course: cerebrospinal syphilis bringing violent headaches, crippling, and alexia of speech. Syphilis of the bladder is often found, as are syphilitic leg ulcers and occasionally syphilis of the skull.

In the banana tropics are also found many conditions and maladies not so well known, in spite of their widespread occurrence. One of these is night blindness, a condition reported a third of a century ago by United Fruit's Dr. Neil P. Macphail. In Guatemala, Dr. Macphail noted that railroad workers, brought to the United Fruit Company hospitals for malaria treatment, complained that when night came they found themselves stone-blind.

Medical literature offered little information about this condition. One text described it as a functional disease, somewhat similar to snow blindness, an affliction suffered by people who are continually exposed to bright sunshine. According to this text, removal of the cause was the only treatment.

Dr. Macphail noted that night blindness tends to follow a history of alcoholism and malarial infection, but he doubted that these facts were decisive. In daytime the patients' eyesight seemed normal: no refractive errors, congenital defects, or other flaws. Yet the patients swore that they became blind with the arrival of twilight. Dr. Macphail pondered and experimented. He learned that the local railroad gangs were fed an extremely poor diet, which provided meat only once a week, included no milk or green vegetables, and allowed only corncakes, or tortillas, beans, rice, and coffee with sugar. Their three daily meals were practically identical.

Dr. Macphail directed that all patients complaining of night blindness should be given milk to drink. Recoveries became more rapid. There was evidence that the condition is merely another affliction resulting from bad diet. Macphail began to supplement a well-balanced hospital ration with still larger quantities of milk and to add issues of cod-liver oil. Within a few days, ten at most and five as an average time, the railroad workers recovered the ability to see at night.

It should be apparent to the reader by this time that the medical enterprise of a tropical commercial organization like the United Fruit Company is not merely a matter of attacking and conquering such obvious scourges as yellow fever and malaria. It involves a constant surveillance of all health matters. Various common eye ailments, for instance, considered mild and relatively unimportant in temperate climates, become grave liabilities in the tropics. The common refractive errors of eyesight seem to be comparatively rare in banana lands. The United Fruit Company's carefully studied use of safety devices and precautions in machine shops and in building, railroad, and plantation operation has greatly reduced the incidence of eye injuries. Throughout most banana lands, however, "sore eyes"—acute catarrhal conjunctivitis—remains rather commonplace, frequently taking fourth or fifth place in the list of diseases treated by the Fruit Company's tropical hospitals and clinics.

Catarrhal conjunctivitis is a bacillus disease, usually resulting from the presence of Koch-Weeks bacillus, and sometimes pneumococci. It responds readily to simple treatment, but without treatment the malady becomes painful, destructive, and very contagious. Also there is sun blindness, more formally named follicular conjunctivitis, also requiring prompt and careful treatment, good food, and abundant fresh air. Trachoma sometimes appears. Medical authorities point out that this disease is apparently being brought to Central America by Syrian immigrants, from whom the malady sometimes is passed to native people.

Quinine blindness, or amblyopia, a by-product of malaria, is comparatively rare. It is not real blindness, but a concentric contraction which tends to allow good central but poor marginal vision. It is usually controllable by prescribing suitable glasses. Pterygium, supposedly influenced by heat, brilliant sunshine and dust, is the result of a growth that harasses the pupillary area and the cornea. When well established, skillful surgery is its only cure.

In the banana regions which, without a working population, would have to revert to jungle, all diseases are, in a sense, occupational diseases. This is true of the many varieties of ulcer which are found in all banana centers. Ulcers of the feet and lower legs are most prevalent. Some are fungoid ulcers, usually curable by antiseptic dressings or skin grafts. Others result from syphilis, from tubercular conditions, and from various other underlying complexities which demand constant study and painstaking diagnosis.

United Fruit Company physicians are frequently confronted with freak diseases which cannot easily be identified or cured. Recklinghausen's disease is a good example. Here is a typical hospital entry:

History—W.I.M., colored Jamaican, aged 38 years, presented himself to determine whether or not his physical condition warranted his employment for service on the United Fruit Company's engineering staff. He had been married for six years and had three healthy children. He stated that he . . . had never suffered any serious disease, nor experienced any disability nor loss of time from work as a result of illness. From birth he had marks, molds and small swellings on his body; and the growths gradually increased in size, but caused no pain or inconvenience. He gave no history of venereal infection. . . .

There were a few scattered moles on the trunk. The skin, beginning at a point two inches below the umbilicus and extending downward almost to the knees, showed a dark bluish pigmentary stain. This pigmentation encircled the body; and numerous large and small moles appeared here and there through the diffuse discoloration. There were a few small tumors in the skin, ranging from the size of a large pea to that of a hen's egg; and four large tumors about the size of a grapefruit (one on the left side above the iliac crest, and three on the buttocks) which were irregular, wrinkled, foldlike masses hanging down from a base as large, fleshy growths which could be easily raised by the hand. They felt soft and boggy; and were painless to such an extent that the patient experienced no discomfort either when sitting or lying on them. From the knees downward, the skin was discolored in patches and dotted with numerous moles. . . .[2]

The list of minor diseases which to banana medicine are major human problems is painfully long. There are such misfortunes as Baelz's disease, characterized by a dilation of the mucous glands of the lips, which is highly resistant to cure; arsenical dermatitis, a severe skin rash which sometimes results from exposure to arsenical sprays or solutions; tumors, lumbago, and stomach ulcers; and a score of complications of obstetrical cases. The company staff must use its X-ray and surgical skill to attend the various neglected fractures which are unfortunately frequent among our poorer southern neighbors; arms, hands, or legs left distorted and useless when broken bones were either left to set themselves or were improperly set before the advent of organized medicine.

Since its founding in 1900, the work range of the United Fruit Company's medical department has shown a continuous widening. It continues to face most diseases and disease problems common to the United States and a great many others which are variously common to the American tropics. It must determinedly preach and practice preventive medicine, since in the tropics curative medicine is not in itself sufficient.

In the tropics, as elsewhere, preventive medicine merges into the new social science of sanitation. Accordingly, banana medicine links itself to sanitation, as a string of cars to a locomotive. Throughout its half century of inter-American farming and transportation, the United Fruit Company has invested millions of dollars in the provision and improvement of adequate water systems. Its work has proved, among other things, that when good water is available tropical Americans are glad to make use of it; that wherever water facilities permit bathing and laundering, most tropical Americans are eager to keep themselves and their clothes clean.

As a rule towns and farm settlements of the banana realms are fed by pipe lines radiating from central plants at which water supplies are purified. The peril of using surface water in the tropics has necessitated the boring of hundreds of pipe-driven wells beyond the depth of possible contamination. Latrines and sewers are kept at the greatest possible distance from water sources. Stagnant ponds and pools which cannot be drained are treated with chemicals or oil and are stocked with larvae-eating fish. The hazards of man-made foci for mosquito breeding must be constantly attended.

Wherever possible, work camps and homes are located on "turtleback" lands where the ground drains in all directions. Otherwise artificial drainage is required. Unnecessary faucets and other water outlets must be avoided. Family washing centers, a fundamental element of Latin-American life, also require careful drainage and regular inspection. On banana plantations the overseer is responsible for daily inspection of the plantation work camp; of living quarters, kitchens, drains, and latrines. It is a part of his job to seek out sick people and direct them to the nearest hospital or clinic. Professional sanitary inspectors are employed to supervise all activities and conditions affecting the health and comfort of the banana-growing community; mess halls, *cantinas*, commissaries, labor *barracones*, and other living quarters; as well as dairies, stables, and slaughterhouses.

Sanitation can never be enforced by individual effort or by proclamation, or by the mere passage of laws. Hygiene, sanitation, and malaria control are all taught in plantation schools and by means of pamphlets, motion pictures, lectures, and open-forum discussions. A veteran sanitary inspector for the United Fruit Company explained: "The maximum results in sanitation can be obtained only by the voluntary co-operation of every resident. To enlist such co-operation should be the ultimate aim of the sanitary inspector. If he will approach the workers in a cheerful and considerate manner, manifest a real interest in their health and welfare, minister to the sick to the best of his ability, and in other ways show that he is working in their behalf, he will soon gain their confidence and respect and receive their co-operation."

All the activities of a great company engaged in productive business in the American tropics are, it is obvious, dependent upon measures for blending into a constructive whole a great many diverse elements, from climate, topography, racial characteristics, and folklore to the combatant forces of disease and medicine. What the United Fruit Company has done to make its work possible is, in miniature, what could, even what must, be done for tropical America as a whole. The company's example—while it is not the only corporation to engage in large-scale medical activity—is significant because it is the most complex and enlightened.

The story of the United Fruit Company's medical department is doubly significant. The company not only has made its own operations possible; it has provided a pattern for North American operations in Latin America. It acknowledges and fulfills an obligation essential to any organization attempting to develop tropical wealth. This attainment stands in sharp contrast to those of many United States concerns which live, or seek to live, by exploiting Latin-American resources.

Unfortunately, many United States businesses have willfully avoided the responsibility of maintaining or helping maintain good health in their operating areas within Latin America. Time and time again United States petroleum companies (also British and Dutch petroleum companies) have taken over working locations in South America, imported labor and recruited local workers, drained regions of their resources as rapidly and greedily as possible, and when the resources were exhausted, pulled up stakes and left behind them permanent points of contagion. Such procedure is not only venal and cruel, it is stupid, and Latin-American nations cannot stand it much longer.

It is true that the entire blame for creation of the nuisance areas of disease which so often linger in Latin-American countrysides after oil fields or mines or lumbering centers have been abandoned is not always attributable to any deliberate antisocial intention on the part of United States business interests. The contributing conditions have

often been tolerated by shortsighted or otherwise incompetent public officials of the victim nations. Frequently the trouble has resulted
from careless or incompetent planning on the part of the exploiter.
Often the short-term exploitation practiced by various Yankee petroleum companies, or surface mining companies, or timber buyers
makes it next to impossible to plan and to maintain the careful
sanitation so essential to good health in the tropics.

It is true that at least five United States petroleum companies in
the course of their South American operations have spent generously
to build and equip hospitals and to employ capable medical staffs,
but unfortunately without providing for field sanitation, drainage,
mosquito combat, water purification, and other preventive measures
essential in hot countries. The net result is that base hospitals are
perenially crowded and medical effort becomes a matter of slow
and costly cure instead of comparatively quick and inexpensive prevention. Here again outlying work areas are too frequently abandoned to remain as dangerous sources of contagion. However generous medical appropriations may be, health maintenance under
such circumstances becomes an impossibility.

All that is required is planning and a clear understanding of hot-
country sanitation. It is evident that the road to contagion, like the
road to hell, can be paved with the most noble intentions. To some
measure the situation is being remedied. Good life in the Americas
demands that it be remedied completely. Today the fact is undeniable that business concerns which are too poor or not sufficiently
inventive to protect the health of their Latin-American employees
and adjacent peoples are not qualified to engage in work in a region
where sanitation and health service are the condition of survival.
Many vast areas of Latin America remain to be developed for the
benefit of the people of the Western Hemisphere. They can be
brought to productive use only by the application of those principles
which made possible the construction of the Panama Canal and the
continuing success of the United Fruit Company.

Chapter Thirteen

WANTED: ANOTHER
WALTER REED

WE need another Walter Reed, or, better, several more. We urgently need a multiple reincarnation of William Crawford Gorgas, who was probably the greatest sanitarian the world has ever known. We are in desperate need of more Carlos Finlays—young men of medicine who can fill the boots of that illustrious "Pasteur of Cuba."

More of the same—*mas de lo mismo,* as our southern neighbors say. We need more ambassadors in white. We need them because mosquito-borne diseases are still among the greatest menaces to this hemisphere—as murderous as Axis dictators, and potentially about as disrupting to trade and society. We need them because many other epidemic and infectious diseases continue to undermine hemisphere solidarity, to disrupt and impede progress toward the good life in Latin America. We need them because many of these menacing diseases are still mysteries, and because those which are not are not sufficiently understood.

Malaria remains an active menace to the Americas. I have already mentioned that, according to the United States Public Health Service, there are today not less than four million chronic cases in our own South. Public health reports throughout Latin America indicate that malaria parasites molest the blood streams of millions and tens of millions of fellow Americans. We do not know exactly how many Americans die of malaria, but British authorities estimate the world total of malaria deaths as four million yearly. But we do know that malaria is a poisoning stain which continues to work in a huge area from our Mason-Dixon line southward far into the Argentine.

We also know that yellow fever is a continuing threat. School texts, Broadway drama, and Hollywood to the contrary, yellowjack is not beaten. After five centuries the mosquito-carried malady which dealt havoc so many times to American seaports and coastlines still infests large areas of inland Brazil, Colombia, and perhaps other regions of continental South America. According to indisputable authority, yellow fever is still on the loose, riding the wings of more than one type of mosquito vector.

For confirmation read the newest report of the Rockefeller Foundation, which outlines the current news of yellow fever. At present millions of doses of yellow fever vaccine are being supplied by our laboratories to the United States Army, the United States Public Health Service, and the British government. At the request of the latter about 250,000 doses of the vaccine have been sent to the Sudan, where in 1940 a virulent outbreak of yellowjack occurred in the Nubian Mountains of Anglo-Egypt. British authorities report this outbreak as indigenous and say that the guilty carrier is the same *Stegomyia,* or *Aëdes aegypti,* mosquito with which Walter Reed, his Yellow Fever Board associates, and their illustrious fact-finding predecessor, Carlos Finlay of Havana, worked in Cuba at the turn of the century.

During the First World War era, yellow fever, so prematurely erased, as conquered, from the list of dangerous diseases, flared up fiercely in many tropical lands: in Suez, Mesopotamia, and Iraq; in the Belgian Congo, along the middle Nile and the British Gold Coast of West Africa. During the same calamitous era it was reported in numerous South American areas—from Rio to Barranquilla and Guayaquil. It swung northward into Central America, perilously near to our own boundaries. During 1918 it swept both Atlantic and Pacific coasts of Guatemala. On the Pacific coast the epidemic lasted for eight months and the mortality rate was reported as being approximately half of all cases.[1] Earlier, during 1916, Guatemalan troops on the northern frontier of Huehuetenango had died of yellowjack.

During 1938, in the Carnegie Institution publication entitled *A Medical Survey of the Republic of Guatemala*, Dr. George Cheever Shattuck summarized the status of yellowjack in Central America:

Very recently, tests to show the presence of resistance of yellow fever have been performed in parts of Guatemala and elsewhere in Central America. These tests have shown that there are resistant individuals in El Salvador, Guatemala, British Honduras, Honduras, Nicaragua, Costa Rica and Panama. Apparently there were epidemics of yellow fever in Guatemala in 1910, 1918 and 1924; and in 1924, yellow fever occurred in epidemic form in El Salvador and British Honduras as well (Sawyer, Bauer and Whitman, 1937). It is now 13 years since there has been a recognized epidemic of yellow fever in any part of Central America. However, we cannot feel sure that yellow fever will not occur in Guatemala.[2]

Other authorities would now extend the uncertainty to much of the American tropics and subtropics.

During 1925, so far as I can discover, only three cases of yellow fever were reported in the Western Hemisphere. But during 1936 an outbreak of the malady was reported in certain areas of Brazil, Colombia, and Venezuela, which apparently do not harbor the *Aëdes aegypti* mosquito. Since 1934 there has been reason to believe that other species of mosquitoes carry yellow fever. During 1940, Rockefeller medical workers presented some astonishing and alarming information. Their recent field and laboratory studies revealed that more than one species of mosquito—probably as many as fourteen species—actually carry yellow fever and that many jungle animals carry the virus in their blood.

According to several authorized spokesmen of the Rockefeller Foundation, the new studies of yellow fever lead to the following conclusions:

Yellow fever is primarily a disease of jungle animals. The classical form involving transmission from man to man by the *Aëdes aegypti* mosquito is more of a secondary cycle depending largely upon conditions of population concentration and mosquito breeding created by man himself.

Transmission of jungle yellow fever appears to be by jungle mosquitoes from animal to animal.

. . . The virus continues to circulate in the blood of susceptible animals for three or four days and does not subsequently reappear. Mosquitoes, however, once infected, tend to harbor the virus for the remainder of their lives, which may be several months under favorable conditions.[3]

Rockefeller authorities point out that the most immediately effective way to control yellow fever is to vaccinate all people who live in or visit infected jungle areas. Obviously, that is a formidable undertaking. Most jungle people are still unacquainted with the principles of vaccination. There are appalling problems in isolation—thousands of square miles of South America without highways, railroads, or any other land communications. Much of all Latin-American jungle land is lacking in qualified doctors. Vast areas are without police or administration centers.

But thanks largely to the work of the Rockefeller Foundation there is now a workable vaccine for yellow fever—"Virus 17-D." By the end of 1938 the Brazilian government had vaccinated more than a million of its citizens against yellow fever, and by the end of 1942 this total may have reached two million. Colombia is following suit. Other Western Hemisphere nations have been studying the problem of public vaccination. The task is difficult. In warm countries, or warm weather, mosquitoes can travel wherever men can, and yellowjack moves faster than preventive medicine.

However effective, vaccine alone cannot halt yellowjack. Quarantine and ceaseless medical vigilance are essential, all the more so because the *Aëdes aegypti* mosquito is reported prevalent in some areas of this hemisphere where there is as yet no record of yellow fever.

They call the 1942-style yellowjack "jungle yellow fever." Clinically it seems to be substantially the same yellowjack which blocked Spain's road to a successful American empire and punished North America with a two-century succession of epidemics, some of which closed great seaports, blacked out proud fleets, and cost millions in trade and hundreds of thousands of lives. During previous onslaughts yellow fever was preponderantly a city and seaport disease. Apparently the new jungle yellow fever, like malaria, is preponderantly a rural disease. This adds difficulties and complexities to the control work. But it does not alter the truth that yellowjack is on the wing, within eight or ten hours by plane from our shores, or that the most crucial war of this hemisphere is still a mosquito war.

The terrifying epidemics of yellow fever which used to decimate populations and tie up the trade of our great port cities were presumably carried by slow-moving ships. The quarantine board of British Jamaica set up what some authorities believe to be the first competent airplane quarantine against yellowjack. Jamaican authorities require that all commercial planes landing in their ports be thoroughly sprayed with insecticide before leaving a port of possible infestation and again within half an hour of arrival in Jamaica. All landing passengers from reported yellow fever areas are placed under medical observation for a period of six days, the so-called "infective period." If no active symptoms appear within that time the arriving passengers are termed safe entrants.

In terms of hemisphere welfare this item is important. The presence of yellow fever is reliably reported within many South American and African areas which are upon or readily accessible to inter-American air routes. Aviation quarantine is one of the still troublesome problems which our much-needed new generation of Reeds, Gorgases, and Finlays must solve, and emphasizes the imperative need of an inter-American front for effectively combating mosquito-borne diseases—a need which was pointed out by Gorgas forty years ago.

Yellow fever, which ordinarily kills about one-fourth of its victims, develops its own immunity. That is not the case with malaria, which can, and usually does, besiege the same person time and time again. Perhaps 65 per cent of all cases are recurrent. There are three or four specific forms of malaria. Particularly within the American tropics the most ruinous form is blackwater fever, a malady which ravages liver and bladder cells and causes startling discoloration of urine.

The etiology of blackwater is somewhat controversial, but the malady occurs virtually everywhere that malaria of malignant or advanced types is prevalent—throughout most of the quarter billion square miles of South and Central America which are plagued with malaria, and within our own southern states, particularly Arkansas, Mississippi, Alabama, Texas, Georgia, Florida, and South Carolina.

Blackwater's occurrence and rate of spread seem directly responsive to bad housing, poor clothing, malnutrition or poor diet, and abrupt migrations of people, all of which are increasingly common to Latin America, now so very hard hit by losses of European trade. Blackwater usually deals death to about one-fourth of all its sufferers. Debility injuries are much higher. The latter, alas, are common to all types of malaria. Direct mortality resulting from "chills and fever," or the elementary types of malaria, averages less than one per cent in temperate climates and between two and ten per cent in the tropics. But it is impossible to compute the ultimate fatalities; for most malaria deaths result from "complications," since a malaria-weakened system is open to easy attack by many maladies, contagious and otherwise. The International Health Board has estimated that not less than one-third of all sickness in Latin America is now directly attributable to malaria.

Today the menace of malaria is one of the most uncompromising enemies of inter-American solvency and progress. Repeatedly during the past quarter century, accredited blood-testing projects in widely divergent areas of the American tropics and subtropics have proved that from one-third to two-thirds of all native people carry malaria zygotes in their blood streams.

The inter-American malaria menace is still far from being solved. In an article entitled "Sanidad en el Paraguay" published in the July, 1941, issue of the official *Boletin de la Oficina Sanitaria Panamericana,* Dr. Ricardo Odriosola, of the Public Health Ministry of Paraguay, terms the current prevalence of malaria in his country a "national calamity." The following significant, if localized, report on recent blood tests in exceptionally well-sanitized areas of lowland Guatemala—between Puerto Barrios and Zacapa—is compiled by Dr. Neil P. Macphail, veteran superintendent of the great Quirigua Hospital of Guatemala. During April, 1941, blood samples taken in three labor camps under Dr. Macphail's supervision showed minimum percentages of malaria as 6.8 per cent, 8.1 per cent, and 4.4 per cent respectively. During July, 1941, surveys of the same three labor camps showed the following positive reactions—13.5 per cent, 14.6 per cent, and 15.4 per cent, or in three months an average increase in malaria occurrence of more than 200 per cent.[4]

You need not be a doctor of medicine or a student of tropical disease to be certain of the frequency of malaria in this hemisphere. You can study official health statistics or make a brief observation trip into the American tropics or into our own deep South. If you visit petroleum camps in northern South America or mining properties in Central America and the Andes valleys, you will be reminded that fighting malaria costs money. It diminishes private and corporation profits. It takes time, and the work and expense are continuous. Managers of fly-by-night promotional enterprises in

Latin America and in our own South have repeatedly sought to avoid the expense and bother of mosquito fighting, of blood tests for employees, treatment of malaria-infested workers, and other precautions essential to control of the disease. In Colombia not long ago, I visited a petroleum field where the manager boasted that only the pumps could work. Practically all workmen were down with malaria or related diseases. The foreman felt benevolently thankful that the chills and fever had not taken over until the pumps had been installed.

I have seen mining operations which malaria had closed before the first ore veins were tapped. Unfortunately, such observations are too easily made in too much of present-day Latin America. Consider, for instance, the Mexican government's expropriation of United States, British, and Dutch oil properties within Mexico. Anyone familiar with the situation in Mexico knows that a considerable number of the affected corporations had in the course of their operations made no real effort to control infectious diseases. In many areas of Mexico an oil field is still synonymous with a pestilential malaria center—needlessly created and criminally neglected.

This book is not a study of the expropriation of petroleum properties. When and if the straight story of Mexico's act is written, this writer willingly bets his hat and shoes that the subject of malaria will provide an important chapter. Without invitation or extra charge, I respectfully suggest that, had the money which United States, British, and Dutch petroleum companies spent on propaganda designed to whitewash themselves and smear Mexico been spent on intelligent sanitation, health administration, and fair play generally —there might never have been any expropriation.

Throughout much of Latin America today public health departments or ministries, operating and investment companies, and local independent medical services join in waging gallant war against the continuing mosquito plague. As already noted, the United Fruit

Company's forty-year and thirteen-nation fight against malaria is a brilliant example.

Everywhere today preventive measures are being taken. Yet the malaria war, like many other wars against disease in this hemisphere, is not yet won. Even partial victory cannot be had without still greater effort and better leadership, more money and more efficient co-ordination of forces. At the next Pan American Sanitary Conference, to be held in Rio de Janeiro during 1942, the Malaria Committee of the Pan American Sanitary Bureau promises to report its "continental scale" studies of inter-American malaria problems. These studies can be of the greatest importance.

The treatment of human carriers of disease presents some of the most difficult problems in medicine. The necessary handling of human carriers can readily violate constitutional law and the most hallowed of traditions. In spite of the risk, several Latin-American governments, such as Brazil, Costa Rica, Guatemala, Panama, and others, have launched admirable campaigns to reduce the numbers of human carriers of malaria within their boundaries. The benefits of field sanitation in one country can be marred or largely obliterated by the absence of effort in an adjoining country. Boundary lines in the Americas can be the boundaries of death and ruin. Our new generation of ambassadors in white is well aware of this problem. It will be for next year's Walter Reeds, with the help of American statesmen and diplomats, to solve.

There is one specific for malaria, once it has become a human disease and not a mosquito-borne threat; and the possession or want of that specific may mean the difference between disaster and victory. World supplies of quinine, greatest of therapeutics, are short and threatened with exhaustion. There is no real substitute, natural or synthetic. The quinine molecule, one of the most complex ever studied by chemists, has baffled the best industrial scientists of Germany, France, Britain, and the United States. Hundreds of efforts to fabricate a synthetic quinine have failed.

Modern medicine has learned that quinine does not cure all forms

of malaria; that against the advanced forms of the parasite, the drug
is of limited benefit. Unless active parasites are present in the blood,
quinine is of little or no help in blackwater fever.

Nobody knows just how or why quinine kills the malaria parasite.
As a matter of fact, the organism will thrive in a solution of quinine
and water. Obviously quinine itself does not do the killing, though
it apparently provokes the human system to do the job. Nevertheless, quinine remains the number-one curative agent for malarial
infections. It is most effective while eruption of the blood cells is
still impending.

But quinine can also cure or eventually overcome malaria in most
of its styles up to and sometimes including the sexual stages of the
parasites. It is an invaluable preventive. Newly developed quinine
complement drugs, such as atabrine and plasmochin, are effective
against the far-advanced forms of malaria. Even so, they are most
commonly administered with quinine. Thus throughout the world
quinine remains the staple defense against malaria; the standard
prophylaxis and the standard curative; the best gauge of man's survival and progress within the tropics.

The pharmacology of quinine began about three centuries ago,
after the Count of Chinchon sailed from Spain to become Vice-
roy of Peru. At Lima the count's wife was stricken by malaria. A
local citizen recommended a potion which local Indians brewed from
a native bark. The countess drank the bitter dram and recovered.
Jesuit missionaries began to collect the bark and to spread its story
throughout their fraternity. By 1750 the virtues of "Peruvian" or
"Jesuits'" bark were well known to the medical world, even though
the facts about malaria were not.

The bark comes from species of the *Cinchona* tree, which is native
to the north Andean foothills. It is another invaluable American
crop which has been snatched away from the Americas. For a century and a quarter the Andes held an easy monopoly upon production of the bark. But the Indians stripped off the prize, killed the

native trees, and failed to replace them. And a century ago the more productive varieties of the wild tree were becoming extinct.

In 1859, the British government commissioned Sir Clements Markham to lead an expedition into the Andes wilds, collect cinchona seed, and consider the possibility of growing the tree in India. British experimental plantings in India, Ceylon, and other tropical parts of the empire did not succeed, but by 1880 Dutch botanists, vastly superior to the British, had successfully adapted the tree to plantations in Java and Sumatra. Today these rich but troubled islands hold a rigid monopoly upon the production of quinine, much to the disadvantage of the Americas and mankind.

As the blight of the Axis War blackens the Eastern tropics, approximately 125 Dutch-dominated plantations of Java and Sumatra continue to produce 98 per cent of the world's annual supply of some twenty million pounds of cinchona bark. Enlightened practical botany, superb plantation management, and multitudes of native coolie laborers (standard farm wage of the Netherlands Indies is nineteen cents per day), plus abundant crown subsidies, have combined to establish what used to be an American crop 13,000 miles from its homeland.

The Netherlands had the quinine supply and, until recently, except for a few futile antitrust suits in United States courts, we have done nothing about it. Virtually all our current quinine supply came from the Dutch tropics; barely one per cent from this hemisphere. For a third of a century the eleven members of the Kina Bureau of Amsterdam had ruled not only the production of quinine, but its manufacture, distribution, and world price. Repeatedly between 1920 and 1935 the Health Committee of the League of Nations informed the Netherlands that at least 90 per cent of all malaria sufferers could not afford quinine at Kina Bureau prices. Repeatedly the Kina Bureau answered that her Majesty's tropical planters would not produce cinchona unless they were assured "reasonable" profits, and that only the Dutch cartel has been able to provide a world pharmacy with a dependable quinine supply—admittedly for those who can pay "good" prices.

League of Nations statisticians countered with the assertion that the annual operating profits of cinchona plantations averaged about 36 per cent between 1920 and 1935, and that profits between 1900 and 1920 had been even greater. Net profits of the Sedep Cinchona Plantation, the largest in Java, with an annual harvest of about 400,000 pounds of bark, were reported as from 40 to 60 per cent, while those of still richer plantations, in which Dutch royalty reputedly has investments, have been as high as 600 per cent yearly.

Today Hitler holds Amsterdam and the Kina Bureau. The Netherlands Indies are held by Japan. Retail quinine prices are skyrocketing to new highs of $1.50 to $2 per refined ounce. (Nine-tenths of all malaria sufferers probably couldn't afford it at 40 to 60 cents an ounce.) The amounts available to the Americas are pitifully limited.

The Department of Agriculture admits "there is every evidence" that quinine is "now out of reach of the poorer classes of this hemisphere. . . ." [5] Unfortunately malaria is not. It continues to sow havoc among the poorer classes, reducing their life span, their solvency, and their working efficiency, increasing infant mortality, planting wretchedness and distress throughout three-quarters of this hemisphere. Repeated flare-ups of blackwater fever are reported in eleven American republics between Mexico and Paraguay.

At last our government is considering possibilities of redeveloping here the desperately needed cinchona crop. In Puerto Rico our Department of Agriculture is establishing a cinchona experiment station. In Guatemala and Bolivia small acreages of cinchona trees are actually in bearing. It is reported that a small supply of quinine can be acquired in Colombia. The story of the quinine monopoly epitomizes the worst abuses of international trade, the cruelty of undisciplined capital, and the utter disregard of human suffering and the essential needs of human beings by greedy exploiters. Dutch and British capital have much to answer for in this connection.

It becomes more and more apparent that our new generation of Reeds, Gorgases, and Finlays must include plant breeders, horticulturists, farmers, merchants, and statesmen who can establish a solvent cinchona industry within this hemisphere and make it strong enough to yield and distribute a plentiful supply of quinine at prices which the masses of Americans and the less wealthy governments of this hemisphere can afford to pay. As a student of cinchona, I believe it possible to produce refined quinine at ten cents per ounce. Such production could not pay 60 or 600 per cent dividends. It could not produce titles or help fill up international society pages and gossip columns, but it could keep men from dying. It could help restore health to millions of Americans. It could make ours a stronger and better hemisphere.

Gradually our hemisphere defense against mosquito-borne diseases has begun to assume a tactical pattern. At present the Rockefeller Foundation is its greatest research arm. From a standpoint of United States enterprise, the Cuba-to-Colombia chain of fifteen base hospitals and field sanitation headquarters built and maintained by the United Fruit Company of Boston is its greatest administrative arm.

Other distinguished progress in malaria control is, however, being made in many parts of Latin America. The recent work of the Guatemala Public Health Service is a noteworthy example. Dr. Maria Giaquinto Mira, malariologist for that service, has provided a particularly interesting report on the subject. His introductory paragraph is worth several readings:

Malaria constitutes, without doubt, one of the sanitary problems of greatest importance for the Republic. Guatemala is essentially an agricultural country and this is especially true of the tropical zones of the coast, the north and the south. . . . It is necessary to provide a constant supply of effective laborers to continue the agricultural production and the prosperity of the country, and it is necessary to protect workers effectively against malaria, which decimates the population, reduces the activity and energy of the workers, depresses intelligence of the children, and diminishes fecundity. From times immemorial, malaria has represented one of the greatest dangers to the inhabitants of the agricultural areas but, until recently, the real importance of the problem has not been appreciated.[6]

Dr. Mira and his assistant opened the campaign in 1929, and after General Jorge Ubico had become president of Guatemala, they were capably assisted by the Guatemala government.

They began their campaign with a careful survey of population. Roughly two-thirds of all Guatemalans—at least 1,400,000—are Indians. Most of the remainder are of Spanish origin with considerable Indian and immigrant mixtures and a more recent minority of Negroes, Caribs, Chinese, and other Asiatics. The population is rather easily divided into rural and urban. Harvestime sees considerable domestic migration, principally from Indian-populated highlands to the larger farms, most of which are in valleys or lowlands.[7]

At Geneva, during 1928, the Malaria Commission of the League of Nations Comité de Hygiène had recommended organization of a special malaria section for each national health department. Guatemala's Director General of Health promptly accepted the recommendation. Dr. Mira became head of Guatemala's Malaria Section.

Dr. Mira faced a host of problems inevitable to malaria fighting. Vital statistics rarely convey the real importance of the disease, since most malaria deaths result from subsequent complications. Moreover, it is almost impossible to compute the exact amount of malarial sickness, since thousands of sufferers in Guatemala, as elsewhere throughout Latin America, are beyond easy reach of hospitals or practicing physicians.

Dr. Mira first undertook to locate epidemic areas. He directed his first investigation toward children under twelve. Young children are more readily accessible for examination, they are usually not migrants, and according to good medical testimony they may be considered the reservoir of malaria virus.

Dr. Mira next directed the study and classification of all species of anopheline mosquitoes native or resident in Guatemala. He discovered seven species; one, the *Anopheles hectoris*, had never before been classified. His mosquito research proved also that certain types of *Anopheles*, such as the *albimanus*, common to hot humid lowlands, has adapted itself to cool dry mountains and plateaus. Dr. Mira further demonstrated that certain species of Anopheles are distinctly house dwellers, while others usually come out of neighboring forests and jungles to attack man.

Of the twenty-nine departments of Guatemala, the Mira investigations proved that thirteen were undoubtedly strongholds of endemic malaria, that eight probably were, and that only one was free from the destructive virus. He found that migration of labor from highlands to lowlands was not only oiling the fires of lowland malaria, but the return of the workers was serving to establish many chronic malaria centers in the mountains.

Much of the more healthful land of Guatemala is poor, while the less healthful lands are enormously fertile. But Guatemala could bear the cost of attempted malaria annihilation, as practiced, for example, in the Panama Canal Zone. As an opening wedge, Dr. Mira established four experimental antimalarial stations, choosing as sites the widely separated settlements of Puerto Barrios, on the Caribbean; Puerto de San José, on the Pacific; and the inland communities of Nueva Santa Rosa and Monjas.

Each first-class station is directed by an experienced physician, two assistants, and a working force to carry on open-country destruction of mosquito breeding places. Before opening these stations, Guatemala's principal malaria fighter held a school for his workers. The personnel of each station began a census of malaria within its particular locality, calling at all homes and examining the blood of all residents, clearing blood samples from a central laboratory, all without cost to the patient. The laboratory chief advised the station director by telegraph of each positive blood sample, so that the director could begin treatment promptly. Meanwhile sanitation crews were dispatched to destroy mosquito larvae within several thousand yards of the outer limit of each experimental area.

Within two years, or by the end of 1931, malaria occurrence within the areas of the four experiment stations had fallen by 70 to 80 per cent. Meanwhile the station staffs began to help fight malaria epidemics throughout Guatemala. They learned that quinine was frequently not available where malaria epidemics were taking place; that diluted or poor quality quinine was being sold by peddlers, and that in many places the prices were exorbitant.

So the Guatemala government established an office charged with buying quinine (wherever possible from Guatemala producers) and selling it at minimum cost to the Antimalaria Section or to licensed druggists. This helped stabilize quinine prices.

After its painstaking experiment period, Guatemala's war against malaria carries on. Hospital treatments have increased from a few hundred cases to more than forty thousand yearly. Antimalaria stations have been extended to all quarters of the republic. The work has yielded magnificent dividends in health, and is one of the significant social experiments in the American tropics today.

For constructive research and practical field sanitation, modern tropical medicine still seeks foresight from hindsight. Its classic precedents are the attainments of our two great ambassadors in white—Walter Reed and William Gorgas.

Guatemala's stand against malaria is a highlight in current public health administration. But its effectiveness has only served to prove that we need vastly more detailed and comprehensive observation of mosquito vectors. We need more capable classifications of non-immunes among human subjects. We need more information about the mosquito-borne diseases; more understanding of the parasitic lives which create them; better knowledge of constructive prophylaxis. Definitely we need many more Reeds, Lazears, Finlays, Carrolls, Deeks, Noguchis, and Carters. For meeting the fast-increasing inter-American problems in field sanitation, we also need more Gorgases, Rosses, and Macphails; distinguished men of medicine who have so ably proved that successful defense of hemisphere health requires diplomacy, gentle persuasion, good business sense, and enlightened education along with accurate, diligent medical science; also that homes must be entered, personal habits must be changed, boundaries and racial lines forgotten; that the hungry must be fed, the sick attended, and above all, that red tape must often be ruthlessly slashed.

The new generation of Reeds and Gorgases need not fear that it will lack worlds to conquer. In Panama, Gorgas and his men cleaned up about 500 square miles of the Canal strip. Their successors face comparable toils throughout a quarter billion square miles of this hemisphere. They face the continuing fact that human migration offers a vast problem in the control of diseases; and that pills, powders and vaccines per se cannot make men healthy or sufficiently resistant to pestilence. It is a safe bet that nine-tenths of all malaria carriers and all other malaria victims throughout Latin America and our own South are too poor to be adequately nourished and clothed. Since they are preponderantly rural, agricultural conditions must be stubbornly improved before these Americans can have health.

Good agriculture and solvent trade remain the most effective of all mortal prescriptions. Today and tomorrow, our essential ambassadors in white do not all need to be men of medicine. Some of them will be, and must be, aggressive socially minded businessmen, traders, salesmen, and statesmen. Men and women who fight inter-American poverty are also fighting the greatest disease scourge of the Americas. In my own study of the medical literature of malaria I can find no more pertinent comment than Bentley's notation that "with general improvement in agriculture and better utilization of the land malaria tends to disappear," owing "perhaps as much to physical improvement and greater resistance of the people as to the incidental destruction of mosquito breeding places." [8]

Recent news from Latin America clearly indicates that we can anticipate cordial co-operation from the governments to the south. As never before, these governments realize the menace of mosquito-borne diseases to the whole hemisphere. Records of legislation from a dozen Latin-American capitals prove it.

Latin-American leadership today seems well aware that the great ravisher of the Mayans, the Incas, the Aztecs, and the Quiches has survived the centuries and stands today more dangerous than ever before. During recent months the Latin-American press has repeatedly and eloquently urged that defense against malaria is an essential step in any enduring hemisphere defense; that tomorrow's hope for victory against the ruinous Pan-American plague of today rests upon stubborn campaigns for mass education in hygiene, agriculture, and marketing; and also upon vast expansion and improvement of public clinics and sanitation facilities throughout Latin America.

This defense requires money and talent in large quantities. Latin America looks to the United States for part of the money and part of the talent. From this nation has gone out an illustrious procession of medical men now known and revered throughout the Americas. The stories of these ambassadors are and will remain a pattern of brave experiment, stubborn research, and invincible determination. The scope of the great work done in inter-American health defense is best measured by the men of medicine who have given their lives and their skills to make it possible. The measure of the future, with its success or failure, will be in the lives of those followers of Reed, Gorgas, Finlay, and the others who take up the battle where death forced their great predecessors to leave it.

Chapter Fourteen

LOOKING FORWARD

O N January 15, 1942, a memorable conference convened in the great Palacio Tiradentes of Rio de Janeiro. Less than six weeks before, at Pearl Harbor, the first active indication of danger to the Western Hemisphere had materialized out of the Pacific skies and struck at all the Americas. The world was watching the Rio conference, its fingers ready to count the emerging ostriches. But in addition to direct political results, the world got something which few observers were expecting.

Sumner Welles, acting Secretary of State for the United States, provided the memorable note. He told the conference that the attainment of political solidarity was not the only purpose of its deliberations.

"My government," he said, "believes that we must begin now to execute plans vital to the human defense of the hemisphere, for the improvement of health and sanitary conditions, the provision and maintenance of adequate supplies of food, milk, and water, and the effective control of insect-borne and communicable diseases.

"The United States is prepared to participate in and to encourage complementary agreements among the American republics for dealing with these problems of health and sanitation by provision, according to the abilities of the countries involved, of funds, raw materials, and services. . . ."[1]

Mr. Welles's declaration was of the greatest significance, not simply because it helped to consolidate the interests of the Latin-American governments and to express our own support of them, but even more because it emphasized for North Americans our unavoidable dependence upon Latin-American sanitation and general health. Today we are engaged in enterprise in South America on a scale never before conceived—a military as well as commercial enterprise. Because this is the case the North American people cannot help seeing that Latin America, where we must maintain garrisons and even, perhaps, field armies, is all too capable of giving our troop and our construction enterprise contingents the negative benefit of all its contagions, its polluted water supplies, its mosquito-ridden jungles, its fly-blown borderlands, its polluted milk and food. We are going to have to extract enormous quantities of rubber from the greatest focus of tropical disease in the world—the Amazon Basin—and if we do not plan for defense of the health of those who must do the work, we shall lose, as the French lost the Panama Canal, not only this endeavor but ourselves and our Latin-American friends as well.

Mr. Welles's recognition of this fact makes one of the most admirable, one of the clearest and frankest statements of intention in Pan-American history. What is much more important, this statement has not remained a mere statement. It is materializing into an active beneficial program. Early in March, 1942, the United States sent to Ecuador "an important scientific and technical mission" to assist in constructing a base "vital to the defense of the Western Hemisphere."

Dispatching this mission was also the beginning of an extensive, urgent endeavor to improve sanitary conditions in areas deemed to be of supreme importance to the successful defense of the Latin-American countries. Our government is today employing sanitarians and other specialists to undertake drainage projects, water supply and other essential health requirements in at least six Latin-American countries—Colombia, Ecuador, Peru, Uruguay, Brazil, and Venezuela.

In the near future other southern republics may be added to this list. The initial program is concerned primarily with the building of hospitals and improvement of health conditions in the areas adjacent to defense bases and in all South American coastal regions. The program of defense sanitation is being planned by the United States government in collaboration with certain Latin-American government which will in most cases help bear the cost of the work.

The specific details are still insufficient. But plainly enough the program is a significant if sadly belated step in the right direction. It is hardly necessary to repeat here the burning obvious certainty that our government should have launched such programs five, ten, twenty, or fifty years ago; or that once more we have been dully apathetic and stupidly lazy and greedy in our official evasion of the life-and-death obligations of good neighbors.

Better late than never. It is not quite too late to recognize and wipe out the result of our generations of ignorance and neglect. Does anyone ask, what business is it of ours? Listen!

It takes money to keep a family healthy. It takes millions more to keep a continent of families healthy. Where is family or national income to come from if not from trade? Trade with whom? No longer, if the Western Hemisphere is to live, with Europe or Japan. For better or for worse, in war and in peace the United States is the greatest trading force in the Western Hemisphere. In the past we have cruelly, stupidly, and greedily neglected trade with our southern neighbors. Year after year the citizens of the United States and our press and radio have permitted Washington lobbies and Congressional farm blocs to swing legislative blackjacks (with the supposed approval of the people of the United States) against all or any part of Latin America—for the apparent benefit of minor commercial interests in the United States and to the unheeded detriment of our southern neighbors and our own citizens.

Through smug apathy and deplorable incompetence on the part of our government, because of greedy, collusive, and undeterred intrigue on the part of many of our largest and richest industrial firms, we have permitted invaluable sources of rubber, tin, quinine, copra, palm oils, and at least twenty other immensely valuable resources of the American tropics to be lifted from Latin America and established in British, Dutch, and other impotently defended and poorly controlled territories of the Far East—Malaya, Java, Sumatra, Borneo, Ceylon, and other far-off corners of creation which our enemies, the Japanese, have now appropriated or are in process of appropriating.

The seven million acres of Malayan and Netherlands Indies rubber orchards were planted from the seed and stock of Brazilian Hevea which were lifted easily from the helpless hands of an earlier South America.

The United States has played its part in this plundering. Prewar statistics published by the highly reliable Office of Foreign Agricultural Relations of the United States Department of Agriculture show that during 1938 we were importing about twenty deficit crops, virtually all of which can be grown in Latin America, many of which originated in that region. Yet we were importing more than 94 per cent of all these deficits from the Far Eastern tropics, principally from Malaya, Ceylon, and the Netherlands Indies, for average distances of 10,000 miles or more, over shipping lanes which any navy man knew we could not competently defend.

A blind Chinaman—almost any blind Chinaman—could have told us of the menace and the villainous might of Japan. But even during 1941 we were buying more than 96 per cent of all our absolutely essential rubber supply from Malaya and the Netherlands Indies, leaving the vast indigenous rubber resources of Latin America to be engulfed and lost in the jungle. From 1937 through 1939 our total import of Latin-American rubber averaged 7,889 long tons per year in contrast with about 500,000 long tons from the Far East, where rubber estate profits were reportedly ranging from 18 to 60 per cent per annum.

From 1937 through 1939 we were importing about 350,000,000 pounds of tapioca, or cassava, per year. This is another great staple crop of the American tropics. But we were importing only about 3.5 per cent from all Latin America, and the rest from the other hemisphere, principally from British colonies.

Indispensable tung oil, made from the nut of an Oriental tree, can be had today from much of the American subtropical region. We have been importing a yearly average of 120,350,000 pounds, of which an average of 1,336 pounds worth $94 per year came from all Latin America. The peanut is another tremendously important crop that is indigenous to the American tropics. Immediately before the war, we were importing an average of 25,770,000 pounds yearly from the Orient, principally from Japan, and none from Latin America. The cashew nut also is an important crop of the American tropics. We were importing $5,000 worth per year from Latin America and $4,000,000 worth per year from British tropics.

We were buying about 325,000,000 pounds of palm oil per year from the other hemisphere and none from the world's greatest reservoir of oil-bearing palms, the American tropics. Coconut oil is essential to the colossal cosmetic and toilet soap industries of the United States. From 1937 through 1939 we imported over 346,-000,000 pounds per year, buying the generous average of about 53 pounds, or $5 worth, from all Latin America, which, in terms of native groves of coconut (most of which remain unharvested), is the greatest coconut region in the world.

The vanilla plant is native to Mexico, our closest southern neighbor, yet for the past twenty years we have been buying 97 per cent of our requirement from Madagascar. When Mexico pleads for a chance to re-establish its vanilla crop, our vanilla dealers shake their heads gravely and deluge the market with synthetic substitutes.

Deaf to the counsel of our own medical men, we have been dividing our budget for the purchase of quinine, made from the bark of the originally South American cinchona tree lifted by rather scurvy means from the Andean foothills to the Netherlands Indies and Japan, as follows: East Indies, $735,411 per year; all Latin America, $2,605.[2]

This list could be continued by the page, so conspicuous for the past twenty years or more has been our commercial snobbery toward Latin America.

The point, however, is clear. The apathy, shortsightedness, corruption, and greed of United States business and prewar United States government, which permitted and encouraged the literal removal of vital resources from Latin America to a tyrant-driven East, have also permitted and encouraged uncounted hundreds of contagions and epidemics and unrecorded millions of avoidable deaths to sweep through the jungles, valleys, plains, and mountains of Latin America.

Let us remember that every time a western senator snaps his galluses and roars condemnation of Argentine beef growers or Brazilian cotton growers he is strengthening the forces of disease—pathological and moral. He is damaging all of us, and all of the free world.

Every dollar in bona fide trade which we can give to Latin America, and every Latin-American job that results from this trade, now builds for a stronger and more healthy hemisphere of which we are a part. Our trade with Latin America is now increasing more rapidly than ever before. Since 1938 it has increased almost fourfold. It deserves at least one more multiplication by four, for each of its digits spells longer life and better health for millions of Americans.

Before we can right this wrong and undo the damage we have done to ourselves we must win this war. The life-or-death struggle continues to sweep southward. In the Eastern tropics we and our allies have suffered tremendous defeats. They must be changed to victories. Latin America is already a theater of war. Our soldiers, marines, and sailors are already fighting in many tropical lands and waters. They must be, and to a gratifying extent they are being, protected from tropical diseases. In the Philippines our Army Medical Corps reports that the majority of Japanese prisoners captured by the forces of General Douglas MacArthur have been suffering from malaria. In these instances our enemies did not have quinine and many of them do have malaria.

In North Africa British fighting forces have been safeguarded against yellow fever by vaccines developed and manufactured in the United States. At least in part they have been protected against malaria by means of atebrine, plasmochin, and other therapeutics also made in the United States. It is reported that German forces in North Africa have suffered extensively from malaria and probably from yellow fever. Our own armed forces are being vaccinated against yellow fever, and against typhoid, paratyphoid, and other diseases still common or prevalent in tropical lands. Diligent and capable work is under way to save our fighting men from malaria.

As our war sweeps ever more deeply into the tropics, however, the defense of our forces against all principal cosmopolitan and tropical diseases—which are the chief health menaces of Latin America—becomes more and more essential to our victory and survival. Competent protection of fighting men from disease demands the competent protection of civilians. Literally and figuratively winning the health war of Latin America is the first step in winning the world war, which we must win, and the attainment of any peace which can enable our victory to endure.

Ambassadors in white are soldiers essential to the growth and the life of all Latin-American enterprises.

Today we look belatedly to the south for at least part of our rubber supply, upon which the survival of our nation may also depend. The huge domesticated acreages of hevea, or tree rubber, of the Netherlands Indies and British Malaya, which until recently supplied more than 96 per cent of all rubber manufactured and consumed in the United States, have now fallen to our enemies. Our government and our manufacturers are working frantically to develop an annual domestic output of at least 400,000 tons of synthetic rubber. Even this ambitious figure, which is seven or eight times the estimated synthetic rubber manufacture of Germany or Russia, is still not enough to supply military needs, much less civilian needs.

And the goal of 400,000 to 700,000 tons of synthetic rubber per year is still in the realm of daydreaming and wishful thinking. Rubber experts of our Department of Commerce estimate that, in all, United States factories may produce somewhere between 40,000 and 100,000 tons of synthetic rubber during 1942. Beyond 1942 all estimates must be mere guesswork.

The American tropics are actually the botanical homelands of all the great rubber-bearing plants. Brazil introduced rubber to the world. Improved Brazilian hevea trees have, as I have said, been responsible for the vast rubber wealth of Malaya and the Netherlands Indies and the commanding majority of mankind's contemporary rubber supply. But hevea trees still grow wild in the forests and jungles of the vast Amazon Basin—an estimated 300,000,000 trees.[3]

The possible recovery of wild hevea is a ray of light in the sudden blackness of our rubber picture. Our common war and our common determination to win demand that we have wild rubber from the Amazon Basin. Yet in order to have it we must also fight the man-killing diseases of the Amazon Basin. Sick *seringueros*, or jungle rubber tappers, cannot long continue to recover rubber and bring it to market. Millions of producing hevea trees are scattered throughout the widespread yellow fever belt of Brazil. They are also scattered through hundreds of thousands of square miles of mosquito-infested lands which are among the world's most deplorable foci of malaria. They grow in tropical regions still mercilessly ravaged by bacillary and amoebic dysenteries, by typhoid and paratyphoid, virulent fevers, yaws, tuberculosis, and many other formidable diseases. The essential recovery of Latin-American sources of wild rubber requires that people be better protected from their pathogenic enemies.

The Latin-American petroleum industry is similarly threatened and hampered by disease. At this time, when oil and engine fuels are vital to our struggle for victory, it is well to remember that Venezuela ranks third among the petroleum-producing nations of the world. At its present rate of increase it may soon be second or even first. During 1941, according to the National Geographic Society, we imported more than 30,000,000 barrels of petroleum from Venezuela,[4] which was more than half the entire production of the Netherlands Indies.

During 1917 Venezuela's recovery of petroleum was barely 120,000 barrels. During 1939 it was more than 200,000,000 barrels, or three and one-half times the production of the Netherlands Indies. Today petroleum is more than three-fourths of all Venezuelan exports and is supplying the fuel for thousands of United States, Dutch, and British fighter planes and bombers.

Colombian oil production too is important. But the use of the wealth of South American petroleum by the forces of democracy is dependent upon the maintenance of better sanitation and better health conditions for workers in the oil-producing districts. Venezuela's great oil fields of the Lake Maracaibo areas are still in or near permanent centers of disastrous disease. So are the extremely promising new fields of the Orinoco Valley.

The same situation applies to many other Latin-American resources which are more or less essential to solvent hemisphere trade and American survival. Most of our tin now comes from Andean areas where altogether too many people are avoidably sick. The same applies to chicle lands, to Latin-American mining areas of iron, micas, nitrates, and manganese; to Latin-American sources of hemp fibers, and essential drugs, pharmaceuticals, and other products. In a hundred instances the feat of helping our southern neighbors in their crusades against disease is more than good business, more than good-neighborliness. It is now indispensable to American survival.

Although not enough North Americans realize this, many Latin Americans have realized it. For years the governments of the Spanish-speaking Americas and Brazil have been well aware of the ever-increasing need of larger and more versatile medical staffs; for thousands and tens of thousands of doctors, nurses, surgeons, laboratory and hospital technicians; for sanitarians, medical administrators, and educators.

As we have already pointed out, our southern neighbors actually had public hospitals and generations of distinguished physicians long before there was a United States, centuries before there were medical schools north of the Rio Grande. The medical tradition of Latin America is an illustrious one. But through the centuries the exercise of this tradition has been hampered by insurmountable obstacles resulting from climate and isolation, bitter poverty, high illiteracy, and impoverished treasuries.

There are many by-products of these problems, some of which are also the result of local nationalism. For instance, the laws of most Latin-American countries have attempted to protect their citizen physicians by limiting and in some instances prohibiting the licensing of doctors from other countries. Unfortunately many Latin Americans still fear a wholesale invasion by physicians, surgeons, and dentists from the United States.

In the United States as a whole, our licensing boards have been extremely generous, perhaps too generous in granting the privileges of medical practice to almost unlimited numbers of alien or refugee physicians, principally from continental Europe. Many officials and opinion-shapers of the southern republics still see the many and overcrowded medical schools of the United States as a threat to the financial solvency of Latin-American medical education and medical practice.

Such fears are neither completely justified nor easily brushed aside. It is worth remembering that in many Latin-American countries medical licensing rules are used as a spur to public support of medical colleges and research institutes within home boundaries. Also that in South America, as in North America, medical education is comparatively costly. For small, poor countries it is a tremendous drain and responsibility. Although Latin America is terribly in need of country doctors, extremely few medical immigrants from the United States, Canada, Europe, Great Britain, or anywhere else are disposed to enter rural practice. The leaders of the southern republics know this. Some go so far as to specify by contract that national citizens attending medical schools or institutes must pledge themselves to begin their medical practice in the country.

We know that these and other problems of exchanging medical talent between the twenty-one American nations can be met and solved. Already several United States business firms that operate in Latin America have succeeded in establishing tropical medical departments made up of a few hand-picked physicians, surgeons, nurses, and other medical specialists from the United States, supplemented by a greater number of physicians and other medical workers who are citizens and licensees of the particular country in which they are employed. The United Fruit Company and the Standard Oil Company of New Jersey are notable instances of United States firms which have succeeded in perfecting tropical health programs.

The Rockefeller Foundation and its International Health Board, the Carnegie Institution, the medical schools and faculties of Harvard, Tulane, Johns Hopkins, and South Carolina are among United States institutions which have already proved themselves highly successful in capable and reasonably tactful medical endeavors in Latin America. The work of Walter Reed and his associates at Camp Lazear, the enormously successful Latin-American crusades of William C. Gorgas, and the amiable work trips of Noguchi to Venezuela and Brazil are good instances of successful co-operation between English-speaking and Spanish- and Portuguese-speaking Americans.

Such co-operation is now more than ever important. In the United States we have the world's greatest centers of medical education, administration, and research. We have outstanding developments in technical equipment and laboratory facilities. But it is for us to remember that the Latin-American medical man also holds great advantages—of environment, experience, understanding of local problems, and viewpoint.

South of the border the United States physician quickly learns this. He usually begins work without understanding the language or the environment. He faces continuous difficulties in diagnosis owing in part to the fact that the Temperate Zone normal is not the tropical normal. He faces the inevitable tropical quandary of disease superimposed upon other diseases with symptoms that are ironically baffling.

He is in a place, or places, where medicine and surgery are not yet and perhaps never can be clearly separated; where specialists are comparatively scarce and where specialized equipment is frequently either uncommon or nonexistent. He finds that effective surgery demands preliminary treatment of the many conditions or diseases which cause lowered resistance. He discovers that the need for surgery is frequently merely a symptom, or a complication of an underlying pathological condition.

Surgical cases are likely to be very different from the sort which have given North American and European authorities the bulk of their experience. In the tropics appendicitis, for instance, is all too likely to be just a complication of malaria.

In the American tropics the medical *norteamericano* usually discovers that he cannot be a successful surgeon until he has become a superb physician. He must study anew and increase his vigilance against infection. He is harassed by bacteria which cannot be avoided simply by the use of rubber gloves or standard antisepsis. Air-borne infection of operative wounds is unhappily frequent. Skin disinfection is difficult. Most sterilizing agents deteriorate quickly. Infections are unusually hard to treat. Delirium and coma are commonplace.

We learn from geography texts that the Torrid, or tropical, Zone is that part of the earth's surface which extends both north and south from the equator to the respective and imaginary tropics of Cancer and Capricorn—which are 23° 28′ 40″ north and south latitude. Within these tropics lies the greater part of Latin America. The subtropics extend to about 35 degrees of latitude north and south to include most of the remainder of South America, the rest of the Caribbean lands, and a substantial part of the United States.

But latitude is not the real denominator of tropical climate. Ocean currents, prevalent winds, and rainfall are usually more decisive. In the American tropics there are at least three distinct climate areas: the equatorial lowlands, where year-round average temperatures vary from 80 to 84 degrees Fahrenheit; the trade-wind belts, considerably cooler; and the mountains, which are sometimes above frost lines or snow. Latin-American rainfalls vary from 240 inches per year at Puerto Bello, Panama, to almost absolute desert, as in Chile, Mexico, or Colombia. All told, tropical climate is a paradox, an everlasting hodgepodge in which a mile of horizontal distance or a quarter mile vertical can establish a hundred new climatic problems, all adding to the toils and contradictions of practical medicine.[5]

Latin-American medical talent is indispensable to the crucial struggle for Pan-American health and solvency. So are North American talent and resources. One of the brightest omens in the Western Hemisphere today is the fact that more and more Americans, laymen and doctors alike, have begun to appreciate these very obvious truths. More widespread and dynamic appreciation is in order, for actual accomplishments in practical medical co-operation between the American nations are still inconspicuous, considering the crying human needs which exist.

Now, fortunately, American governments are officially acknowl-

edging the obligation to defend public health throughout this hemisphere. The first official and inter-American acknowledgment of this
sort came from the Fifth International Conference of American
States held in 1923 at Santiago de Chile. That conference recommended the creation of full-time public health departments for all
American governments; the stabilization of quarantine laws; the
enactment and enforcement of pure-food and drug laws throughout
the hemisphere; a standard Pan-American sanitary code and many
other significant reforms.

Since 1926 four inter-American conferences of national directors
of health have been held at Washington. The last, during 1940, included official representatives from all American republics, also
Canada and the Guianas. That meeting gave particular attention to
the control of malaria and other common menaces to Pan-American
health. It recommended the drastic extension of public education in
nutrition, the establishment or re-establishment of public school
gardens, and it undertook some still sorely needed studies of vitamin
standards and national food problems.

The Pan American Sanitary Bureau, which is associated with the
Pan American Union, has likewise grown into an important clear-
inghouse and recording headquarters for medical and public health
workers and public health officials from all nations of this hemisphere. During 1942, Rio de Janeiro is acting as host to a Pan
American Sanitary Conference and to the Inter-American Conference
on Sanitary Engineering. In 1945 Rio will again be the scene of a
Pan-American conference on leprosy control.

It is not always easy to evaluate conferences. But it is evident that
the medical delegation, or study group, is becoming a more and more
frequent entry in the fast-expanding fields of inter-American enterprise and that fraternity in work and community of interest usually
result when medical men from many nations come together and
talk over their work, problems, findings, and hopes.

The gathering on common ground of medicos from the many
American nations is significant also from a standpoint of the recom-

mendations and resolutions proposed and rejected or accepted. Current Pan-American health department resolutions now call for better public health training, for greater accent upon preventive medicine; for civil service status for public health workers, for better collection of vital statistics, better conservation and protection of water resources, and for co-ordinated combat against particular diseases which are now rapidly increasing in many American lands, such as malaria, tuberculosis, and infantile paralysis.

The opportunities for successful medical co-operation between American nations are growing rapidly. Indeed the great medical success stories of today, and most likely of tomorrow, cannot be separated or isolated one from the other. The continuing epic of this hemisphere's struggle for health reaches far back into the pre-Columbian Americas. It has been an epic of individuals and of groups who seek to serve the multitudes. The great stories of our own ambassadors in white have been and inevitably will be merged into the lives, the needs, and the fortunes, good and bad, of Latin Americans.

For many reasons, as I have already suggested, Undersecretary Welles's statement: "My government believes that we must begin now to execute plans vital to the human defense of the hemisphere, for the improvement of health and sanitary conditions, the provision and maintenance of adequate supplies of food, milk, and water, and the effective control of insect-borne and communicable diseases" is one of the most important in the history of American statecraft.

It is a gracious admission that the United States, however belatedly, now recognizes that plans and actions to defend the Western Hemisphere from disease are part of our job as well as our southern neighbors' jobs. It prefixes the supremely important fact that we are now officially and as a united nation getting down to work.

Temporarily, at least, the work is part of our gigantic war effort. But in no other war has our nation chosen to undertake the human defense of this entire hemisphere, in which and with which our nation must survive or perish. The defense of hemisphere health cannot be effected overnight, or in one year or ten. It is a long-term battle which we can and must win.

However slight our beginning may be, it is promising. Our nation has finally recognized a salient truth which other American nations have known, pondered, and toiled with for generations and centuries. We are the strongest of American nations. In medicine we are also the most powerful. We are undertaking a noble task in the company of neighbors, many of whom are our allies in the greatest of wars. Today a thousand old difficulties can be quickly solved; a thousand previous barriers can be promptly brushed aside; a thousand locked doors wait to be opened.

The inter-American will to effect the human defense of this hemisphere is the fundamental way of effecting it. The resources and good faith of the United States are already pledged to defending the hemisphere. Without exception the Latin-American countries have officially expressed their desire and willingness to co-operate in the endeavor; whenever possible, to provide part of the needed money and personnel. The records show that the southern republics have been proportionately far more generous in public health expenditures than we have. Since 1900 the grand total of Latin-American government appropriations for health administration has increased almost twentyfold, that of Mexico more than a hundredfold. During the thirties, while our federal grants to the United States Public Health Services averaged less than one-eightieth of one per cent of the total costs of federal government, health appropriations of several Latin-American governments reached a maximum of almost half the annual receipts of their respective national treasuries.

That Latin-American governments will appropriate money and resources for safeguarding public health when or as long as money and resources are available is beyond question. Any Latin-American official, political or otherwise, who intentionally seeks to thwart such appropriations would prove himself an uncommonly bad politician as well as an antisocial imbecile. Few Latin-American *politicos* are either bad politicians or imbeciles. On the whole their political standards and ethics are easily on a par with those in the United States.

Time and time again it has been proved that when a mayor of, say, New York City invites or tolerates insubordination, corruption, and bribery in his police department or fire department he is rapidly and effectively cutting his own political throat. Similarly, a Latin-American president who allows incompetence and neglect in his department of public health, or who allows incompetent dissipation of public health money, is on his way out or down. Further, the medical profession holds an extremely important place in the political as well as the social and economic life of the southern republics. For more than a century past the doctor president has been a frequent phenomenon in Latin America. Medical men continue to play important roles in the public life of the southern nations, which is a plain indication of the fact that, in public health, Latin-American leadership has been and still is doing its best with the means at hand. Co-operation by the United States in the "human defense" of Latin America is excellent war strategy. It is a practical beginning and an admirable investment in the essential tools which our southern neighbors can use to carry on their great and indispensable combat against disease. Those United States business firms and institutions which have already sponsored or created capable medical and sanitary establishments in Latin America can be expected to carry on their good work. They know from experience that good health is good business. They know also that the example value of their accomplishments is tremendous. It has already been heeded by most or all Latin-American governments. It can well be heeded by our own government.

Inter-American defense against disease can be continued and expedited by increased trade. It can be benefited by many other means which await further study and experimental proof.

One possibility, for example, would be a severance tax on Latin-American resources, with the resulting impoundment of money committed and assured to public health departments of the country from which the resources are removed. Another might be a sort of inter-

American plague insurance: a central revolving fund to which American nations would contribute in proportion to their national incomes, a fund from which the authorized health authorities of any nation involved could draw funds and expert counsel for combating epidemics within its boundaries.

It seems easily possible and highly advisable to increase the appropriations and service personnel of the Pan American Sanitary Bureau, which is already established and supported by voluntary contributions by American nations. It would be possible and, I believe, highly advisable to increase greatly the strength and the budgets of the Gorgas Memorial Institute, Hospital, and Laboratories, admirable institutions which have already proved their value.

It would probably be beneficial to establish a quasi-official Pan American Medical Congress with representative membership to serve as a long-term planning and policy group. It would be possible to establish an inter-American pool of specialists with necessary facilities for selecting and dispatching particularly well-qualified medical men to perform needed services in time of need regardless of national boundaries. That such personnel is available in many parts of the hemisphere is suggested by the fact that about 240 Latin Americans are now fellows of the American College of Surgeons.

Better reciprocity in medical licensing rules is needed, and it is unquestionably attainable. Manifold increase in the exchange of government and private scholarships for medical students would be desirable and is also attainable. While receiving more Latin-American medical students in our own medical colleges it would be beneficial to dispatch more of our own students to universities and research institutions in Latin America.

The primary solution of Latin America's mighty health problem is common willingness to face the issue and to seek its solution at a time when the defense of health is not only an obligation of neighborliness but a necessity if the Americas are to survive.

We can never be, even if it were desirable to hope for such an eventuality, entirely free of the rest of the world. The outcome of a sound, well-planned, amply funded, and energetically prosecuted plan for Western Hemisphere health, however, would have the effect of consolidating in one great healthy body of great nations the strength and resources which they can command, of giving to the Americas a voice in world affairs which shall be able to make itself heard in time of future crisis and prove itself capable of leading all nations away from such a catastrophe as that in which we are now embroiled.

Let us have more ambassadors in white and more American dollars, minds, and hands to move in behind them.

NOTES

Chapter One. SICK MAN'S SOCIETY

1. William C. Gorgas, *Sanitation in Panama*. D. Appleton, New York, 1918.
2. *Bulletin of the Pan American Union*, Vol. LXXV, No. 9, September, 1941, p. 540. Estimate of average life span in Mexico is based on 1941 statistics issues by the Mexican government.
3. Aristides A. Moll, "Half a Century of Medical and Public Health Progress," *Bulletin of the Pan American Union*, Vol. LXXIV, No. 4, April, 1940, p. 344.
4. These estimates are based on statistical compilations of the United States Public Health Service.
5. *Bulletin of the Pan American Sanitary Bureau*, Washington, D. C., Vol. 20, No. 9, September, 1940.
6. *Ibid.*, p. 695.
7. *Bulletin of the Pan American Union*, Vol. LXXIV, No. 4, April, 1940, p. 345.
8. George Cheever Shattuck and Collaborators, *The Peninsula of Yucatan*, Publication No. 431, pp. 61-62, Carnegie Institution of Washington, Washington, D. C., 1933.
9. Aristides A. Moll, "Disease and Population in Latin America," *Bulletin of the Pan American Union*, Vol. LXXV, No. 9, September, 1941, pp. 539-540.
10. *Annual Medical Reports* (unpublished). United Fruit Company, New York, 1935-1939.
11. Letter to author, dated Buenos Aires, November 8, 1941.

Chapter Two. PAST AND PRESENT

1. For much of the foregoing information I am indebted to *Medical Research in Latin America*, by Aristides A. Moll, Education Series No. 16, The Pan American Union, Washington, D. C.
2. Aristides A. Moll, "Hospital Development in Latin America," *Hospitals*, Vol. 13, No. 11, November, 1939, pp. 25-35.
3. *American and Canadian Hospitals*, Directory. Physicians Record Company, Chicago, 1937.
4. *Hospitals*, Vol. 13, No. 11, November, 1939, pp. 25-35.
5. *Ibid.*

Chapter Three. *DITCHES, BIG AND LITTLE*

1. William Crawford Gorgas, *Sanitation in Panama*, p. 73 ff. D. Appleton, New York, 1918.
2. *Ibid.*, p. 158.
3. *Ibid.*, p. 204.
4. *Ibid.*, p. 223.
5. *Ibid.*, p. 275.
6. *Ibid.*, p. 292.
7. *American Journal of Public Health*, Vol. XXIII, November, 1933, p. 1132.

Chapter Four. *CARLOS FINLAY OF CUBA*

1. Carlos E. Finlay, *Carlos Finlay and Yellow Fever*, pp. 46-57. Institute of Tropical Medicine of the University of Havana, and Oxford University Press, New York, 1940.
2. *Ibid.*, p. 17.
3. *Ibid.*, p. 17.
4. *Ibid.*, p. 21. Also Carlos Finlay, *Trabajos Selectos*, p. 575. Havana.
5. *Ibid.*, p. 211.
6. La Roche, *Yellow Fever*, p. 62. Philadelphia, 1885.
7. Herrera, *Decadas de las Indias*, Dec. 1, Lib. 11, Cap. X, XVIII.
8. *Ibid.*, Dec. 1, Lib. V, Cap. 11.
9. Quoted from *Carlos Finlay and Yellow Fever*, pp. 183-184.
10. Herrera, *Decadas de las Indias*, Dec. IV, Lib. IX, Cap. VIII.
11. *Carlos Finlay and Yellow Fever*, p. 189.
12. Quoted from *Carlos Finlay and Yellow Fever*, pp. 206-208.
13. Pezuela, *Dicta. de la Isla de Cuba*, p. 182.
14. *Carlos Finlay and Yellow Fever*; also Carlos J. Finlay, *Trabajos Selectos*, p. 39.
15. Carlos J. Finlay, *Trabajos Selectos*, p. 39. Havana.
16. Protocol No. 7, Session of February 18, 1881, Washington, D. C.
17. "El Mosquito hipoteticamente considerado como Agente de Transmision de la Fiebre Amarilla," *Anales de la Real Academia de Ciencias Medicas, Fisicasm y Naturales de La Habana*, 48:4, 1881.
18. Conference of State and Provincial Boards of Health of North America, New Haven, Conn., Oct. 28, 1902.
19. *British Medical Journal*, Sept. 8, 1900, pp. 656-657; *Thomas Yates Laboratory Reports*, Vol. IV, Part 11, 1902.
20. *Carlos Finlay and Yellow Fever*, p. 96.
21. *Carlos Finlay and Yellow Fever*. Letter is produced in photostat on pages 98-99.
22. *Ibid.*, p. 97.

23. *Ibid.*, p. 108.
24. *Ibid.*, pp. 37-38.
25. *Journal of Experimental Medicine*, Vol. 63, No. 6, June 1, 1937, pp. 787-800.

Chapter Five. REED OF VIRGINIA

1. Howard Atwood Kelley, *Walter Reed and Yellow Fever*, pp. 125-126. McClure, Philips & Company, New York, 1906. See also "The Propagation of Yellow Fever: Observations Based on Recent Researches," *Medical Record*, Aug. 10, 1901.
2. *Walter Reed and Yellow Fever*, pp. 10-11.
3. *Ibid.*, pp. 12-15.
4. *Ibid.*, pp. 15-16.
5. *Ibid.*, pp. 19-20.
6. *Ibid.*, pp. 32-33.
7. *Ibid.*, pp. 42-49.
8. *Ibid.*, p. 51.
9. *Ibid.*, p. 108.
10. *American Journal of Public Health*, Vol. XXIII, No. 11, November, 1933, pp. 1127-1135; also *Walter Reed and Yellow Fever*, p. 135.
11. *Walter Reed and Yellow Fever*, p. 139.
12. *Ibid.*, pp. 141-142.
13. *Ibid.*, pp. 142-143.
14. Walter Reed, "Etiology of Yellow Fever: An Additional Note," *Journal of the American Medical Association*, Feb. 16, 1901.
15. *Walter Reed and Yellow Fever*, p. 152.
16. *Ibid.*, p. 153.
17. *Ibid.*, p. 163.
18. Walter Reed Memorial Association, Washington, D. C., 1902.

Chapter Six. GORGAS OF ALABAMA

1. Marie D. Gorgas and Burton J. Hendrick, *William Crawford Gorgas*, p. 22. Doubleday, 1924.
2. *A Journal of Josiah Gorgas* (unpublished). Library of Congress, 1871.
3. *Ibid.*, p. 23.
4. *William Crawford Gorgas*, p. 31. Doubleday, 1924.
5. *Ibid.*, pp. 40-41.
6. *Ibid.*, p. 52.
7. *Ibid.*, p. 17.
8. *Ibid.*, p. 88.
9. *Ibid.*, p. 92.
10. James Anthony Froude, *Growth of Empire*, p. 93. McClure, Chicago, 1885.
11. *William Crawford Gorgas*, p. 164.

12. *Ibid.*, p. 186.
13. *Ibid.*, p. 187.
14. Charles A. L. Reed, *Panama Notes*, Cleveland (privately published), 1906.
15. William Crawford Gorgas to Mrs. Josiah Gorgas, Tuscaloosa, Ala., August 1, 1911, *Gorgas Journal*, Library of Congress, Washington.
16. *William Crawford Gorgas*, p. 281. Doubleday, 1924.
17. *Ibid.*, p. 287.
18. *Ibid.*, p. 290.
19. *Ibid.*, p. 313.

Chapter Seven. DEEKS OF CANADA

1. I am indebted to Mrs. William E. Deeks, of New York, for most of the information regarding Dr. Deeks's earlier and private life.
2. W. E. Deeks and W. M. James, *A Report on Hemoglobinuric Fever in the Canal Zone*. Mount Hope, Canal Zone, 1911.
3. *Ibid.*, pp. 19-20.
4. *Ibid.*, p. 64.
5. *Ibid.*, p. 72.
6. "Sonderdruck aus Abhandlungen aus dem Gabiete der Auslandskunde," *Hamburgische Universität*, Bd. 26, Recke D., Medizin Bd. 2, p. 68.
7. Quoted from an interview with Mrs. William E. Deeks, New York, July 25, 1941.
8. W. E. Deeks, *A Review of the Digestive Functions and Food Requirements for the Maintenance of Health with Particular Reference to the Tropics*. United Fruit Company, New York, 1925.
9. W. E. Deeks, "Hookworm Disease," *Medical Insurance* (November, 1924), and *The Cause of Hookworm Disease and Its Prevention* (New York, 1925).
10. W. E. Deeks, "Influence of Nutrition on Deformities and Decay of the Teeth, *Dental Cosmos*, Vol. LXVI, April, 1924.
11. W. E. Deeks, "The Significance of Chronic Pharyngitis," *Clinical Medicine and Surgery*, July, 1928; *Journal of the American Medical Association*, Vol. LIX, Oct. 26, 1912.
12. *American Journal of Tropical Medicine*, Vol. IV, No. 2, March, 1925.
13. *Southern Medical Journal*, Vol. IX, No. 2, pp. 123-124.

Chapter Eight. NOGUCHI OF JAPAN

1. Gustav Eckstein, *Noguchi*, p. 344. Harper & Bros., New York, 1931.
2. *Ibid.*, pp. 362-363.
3. *Report of the First Expedition to South America of the Harvard School of Tropical Medicine*, Harvard University Press, Cambridge, 1915.
4. *Ibid.*, p. 364.

For information regarding the life and works of Hideyo Noguchi I am particularly indebted to Dr. Gustav Eckstein; the late Mr. H. E. Morrow and the late Dr. F. B. Rice; also to Dr. Edward Irving Salisbury, renowned surgeon of Costa Rica and former executive of the American College of Surgeons; to Mr. Thomas Bradshaw of Kingston, Jamaica; to Dr. L. A. Knight, now of the British Royal Army Medical Corps; and to the various published works of Dr. Noguchi, including *Monograph No. 26*, Rockefeller Foundation, New York; *Journal of Experimental Medicine*, 29:585 (June), 1919; 30:1, 9, 13, 87, 95 (August), 1919; 30:401 (October) 1919; 31:35, 159 (February), 1921; A. E. Cohn, and H. Noguchi, *Ibid.*, 33:683 (June), 1921; H. Noguchi and W. Pareja, *Journal of the American Medical Association*, 76:96 (January), 1921; H. Noguchi and I. J. Kligler, *Journal of Experimental Medicine*, 33:239, 253 (February), 1921, and *Journal of Experimental Medicine*, 33: 239, 235, February, 1921; H. Noguchi, *The Lancet*, 202:1185 (June), 1922; H. Noguchi, *American Journal of Tropical Medicine*, 4:131, March, 1924; *Journal of Experimental Medicine*, 25:755 (May), 1917, and 30:95 (August), 1919; and *Journal of the American Medical Association*, 77:181 (July), 1921.

Chapter Nine. MICROBE TOURISTS

1. H. H. Bancroft, *History of Central America*, Vol. VII, pp. 345-347, 352, 619-620. See also *Journal of the American Medical Association*, May 4, 1935, p. 1663.

2. *History of Central America*, Vol. VIII, p. 123.

3. Henry R. Carter, *Yellow Fever*, p. 101. Johns Hopkins, Baltimore, 1931.

4. Fuentes y Guzmán, *Historia de Guatemala y Recordacion Florida*, Vol. II, pp. 111-112. Madrid, 1882.

5. Don Domingo Juarros, *The Kingdom of Guatemala in Spanish America*, translation by Lieut. J. Bailey, p. 157. London, 1923.

6. Hans Zinsser, *Rats, Lice and History*, p. 157. Little, Brown, Boston, 1935.

7. *Ibid.*, p. 264.

8. Bernal Diaz, *True History of the Conquest of Mexico*, translated by Maurice Keating, p. 299. Salem and London.

9. *The Kingdom of Guatemala in Spanish America*, p. 148.

10. *Ibid.*, p. 149.

11. *Historia de Guatemala y Recordacion Florida*, Vol. II, p. 112.

12. *Ibid.*, p. 157.

13. Thomas Gann, *In an Unknown Land*, p. 40. New York, 1924.

14. *Physiological and Medical Observations Among the Indians of the Southwestern United States and Mexico*, American Ethnology Bulletin No. 34, p. 108. Smithsonian Institution, Washington, D. C., 1908.

15. *U. S. Navy Medical Bulletin*, No. 26, pp. 801-833. Washington, D. C., 1928.

16. George Cheever Shattuck and Collaborators, *Medical Survey of the Republic*

of Guatemala, p. 46. Carnegie Institution of Washington, Washington, D. C.,
1938.

17. *Ibid.,* p. 47.

18. August Hirsch, *Handbook of Geographical and Historical Pathology,* Vol. I,
pp. 6-7. New Sydenham Society, London, 1883.

19. Henry R. Carter, *Yellow Fever,* p. 54. Johns Hopkins, Baltimore, 1931.

20. *Ibid.,* p. 200.

21. *United States Public Health Reports, 1919,* p. 484. Washington, D. C.

22. *Royal Society of Medicine,* 1929-1930. Vol. XXIII, Part 11, pp. 165-177,
Section on Tropical Diseases. London, 1929.

23. Henry R. Carter, *Yellow Fever,* p. 64.

24. *Annual Epidemiological Reports: 1934.* League of Nations, Geneva, 1936.

25. George Cheever Shattuck and Collaborators, *The Peninsula of Yucatan,* Publication No. 431, pp. 61-62, Carnegie Institution of Washington, Washington, D. C., 1933.

26. *Ibid.*

27. *Ibid.,* pp. 65-66.

28. *Ibid.,* p. 448.

Chapter Ten. *"FIERCE, DEEP, BLACK MYSTERIES"*

1. E. R. Stitt, *Diagnostics and Treatment of Tropical Diseases* (5th edition),
p. 388 (Blakiston, Philadelphia, 1929); also Richard P. Strong, *Stitt's Diagnosis, Prevention and Treatment of Tropical Diseases* (6th edition), Chap.
XXIX, pp. 997-1012. Blakiston, Philadelphia, 1942.

2. *Diagnostics and Treatment of Tropical Diseases,* p. 388.

3. *Ibid.,* pp. 388-394.

4. *Ibid.,* pp. 391-393; see also *Stitt's Diagnosis, Prevention and Treatment of
Tropical Diseases,* pp. 1007-1012.

5. *Diagnostics and Treatment of Tropical Diseases,* p. 391; also *Stitt's Diagnosis,
Prevention and Treatment of Tropical Diseases,* p. 1012.

6. Eduardo Urueta, "Pinta or Carate," *International Conference on Health
Problems in the American Tropics,* pp. 524-532. United Fruit Company,
Boston, 1924.

7. *Ibid.,* p. 527.

8. *Ibid.,* pp. 526-527.

9. Sir Aldo Castellani, "Medical Mycology," *Journal of Tropical Medicine and
Hygiene,* Vol. XXVII, March 1, 1924, p. 49. See also *Stitt's Diagnosis, Prevention and Treatment of Tropical Diseases,* pp. 1140-1141.

10. *Diagnostics and Treatment of Tropical Diseases* (5th edition), p. 362.

11. *Ibid.,* p. 364. See also *Stitt's Diagnosis, Prevention and Treatment of Tropical
Diseases* (6th edition), Vol. II, pp. 927-961.

12. *Diagnostics and Treatment of Tropical Diseases,* p. 364.

13. *Stitt's Diagnosis, Prevention and Treatment of Tropical Diseases*, pp. 948-952.

14. *Diagnostics and Treatment of Tropical Diseases*, p. 97.

15. *Ibid.*, p. 99. See also *Stitt's Diagnosis, Prevention and Treatment of Tropical Diseases*, Vol. I, pp. 207-227.

16. *Diagnostics and Treatment of Tropical Diseases*, pp. 138-142. See also *Stitt's Diagnosis, Prevention and Treatment of Tropical Diseases*, pp. 357-377.

17. *Diagnostics and Treatment of Tropical Diseases*, pp. 143-146.

18. *Ibid.*, pp. 552-564.

19. *Ibid.*, p. 554.

20. *Stitt's Diagnosis, Prevention and Treatment of Tropical Diseases* (6th edition), Vol. II, pp. 1294-1341.

21. *Diagnostics and Treatment of Tropical Diseases*, pp. 595-613.

22. *Ibid*, p. 174.

23. *Ibid.*, pp. 186-187.

24. *Ibid.*, p. 190. See also *Stitt's Diagnosis, Prevention and Treatment of Tropical Diseases*, Vol. I, pp. 474-523.

25. *Diagnosis and Treatment of Tropical Diseases*, p. 197.

26. *Ibid.*, pp. 200-201.

27. *Ibid.*, p. 220.

28. *Ibid.*, p. 225. See also *Stitt's Diagnosis, Prevention and Treatment of Tropical Diseases* (6th edition), Vol. I, pp. 541-589.

29. Sir Aldo Castellani, "Medical Mycology," *Journal of Tropical Medicine and Hygiene*, Vol. XXVII, March 1, 1924, p. 49.

30. Dr. Richard P. Strong, *American Journal of Tropical Medicine*, Vol. IV, 1924, p. 345.

31. Albert R. Patterson, Chief Sanitation Officer, Colony and Protectorate of Kenya; *International Conference on Health Problems in Tropical America*, p. 581. United Fruit Company, Boston, 1924.

32. *Ibid.*, pp. 586-588.

33. *Ibid.*, p. 587.

34. *Ibid.*, pp. 588-589.

35. Dr. Friedrich Füllerborn refers to hookworm casualties reported from plantations of the Netherlands Indies.

36. Siler, Garrison and MacNeal, "Studies in Pellagra," *Archives of Internal Medicine*, Vol. XIV, p. 293.

37. Goldberger, *Cause and Prevention of Pellagra*, United States Public Health Service Reports Nos. 218 and 311, Washington, D. C.

38. W. E. Deeks, "Carbohydrates as Etiological Factors in Stomach Disorders," *New York Medical Journal*, June 25 and July 2, 1904.

39. William McCollum, *The Newer Knowledge of Nutrition*, Macmillan, New York, 1922.

40. R. McGarrison, "Faulty Food in Relation to Gastro-Intestinal Disorder," *Journal of the American Medical Association*, Vol. 78, No. 1, p. 1.

41. Records of Dr. Herbert C. Clark, Superintendent Gorgas Memorial Hospital, Panama City, Panama.

42. Sir Leonard Rogers, "The Treatment of Leprosy," *Lancet* (London), June 29, 1924.

43. Sir Arthur Newholme, "A Note on the Cause of Historical Reduction of Leprosy," *International Conference on Health Problems of the American Tropics*, pp. 791-796. United Fruit Company, Boston, 1924.

44. *Ibid.*, p. 791.

45. F. L. Hoffman, "Leprosy as a National and International Problem," *Journal of Sociological Medicine*, Vol. VII, No. 2, April, 1931.

46. Interview by the author.

Chapter Eleven. DAMN THOSE MOSQUITOES

1. *New York Times Magazine*, New York, July 20, 1941, p. 9.

2. *International Conference on Health Problems in Tropical America*, pp. 154-164. United Fruit Company, Boston, 1925.

3. Dr. Henry R. Carter, "Anopheles and Malaria Control," *International Conference on Health Problems in Tropical America*, pp. 165-168. United Fruit Company, Boston, 1925.

4. *Ibid.*, p. 167.

5. *Ibid.*, pp. 163-164.

6. *Ibid.*, pp. 103-104.

7. M. E. M. Walker, *Pioneers in Public Health*, pp. 235-236. Oliver and Boyd, London, 1930.

8. *American Anopheles and Malaria*, unpublished and unrevised lecture by Dr. Francis Metcalf Root, Associate in Medical Entomology, Johns Hopkins University, Baltimore.

9. *Report of International Conference on Health Problems in the American Tropics*, pp. 229-230. United Fruit Company, Boston, 1925.

10. Lecture by Dr. Henry R. Carter, United States Public Health Service, Johns Hopkins University School of Hygiene and Public Health, Baltimore.

11. *Report of International Conference on Health Problems in the American Tropics*, p. 237. United Fruit Company, Boston, 1925.

Chapter Twelve. BANANA MEDICINE

1. Medical Department, *Eighteenth Annual Report*, p. 335. United Fruit Company, Boston, 1929.

2. *Ibid.*, Recklinghausen's Disease, pp. 181-182.

Chapter Thirteen. WANTED: ANOTHER WALTER REED

1. J. Ragnal, *Anales de Medicine y de Pharmacia Coloniales* (Guatemala), Vol. 30, No. 59, pp. 63-66.
2. Dr. George Cheever Shattuck, *A Medical Survey of the Republic of Guatemala*, p. 78. Carnegie Institution of Washington, Washington, D. C., 1938.
3. *Annual Report*, 1940, Rockefeller Foundation, Division of International Health, New York. Also Associated Press, March 8, 1941.
4. Letter from Dr. Neil P. Macphail, Qiurigua, Guatemala, July 2, 1941.
5. *Foreign Agriculture*, Vol. 5, No. 3, p. 87, March, 1941. Office of Foreign Agricultural Relations, U. S. Department of Agriculture, Washington, D. C.
6. Dr. M. G. Mira, *Anti-malarial Campaign in Guatemala*, Guatemala City, 1936.
7. *Ibid.*, pp. 95-96.
8. E. R. Stitt, *Diagnostics and Treatment of Tropical Diseases* (5th edition), Chap. I, Sec. I, pp. 1-64. Blakiston, Philadelphia, 1929.

Chapter Fourteen. LOOKING FORWARD

1. Quoted from *New York Times*, Vol. XCI, No. 30,721, March 5, 1942.
2. *Foreign Agriculture*, May, 1941. Office of Foreign Agricultural Relations, U. S. Department of Agriculture, Washington, D. C.
3. This estimate is by Harvey Firestone, Jr., of Akron, Ohio.
4. News Release, National Geographic Society, Washington, D. C., Feb. 24, 1942.
5. See discussions of Tropical Climates and Medicine; E. R. Stitt, *Diagnostics and Treatment of Tropical Diseases* (5th edition, Blakiston, Philadelphia, 1929); also Richard P. Strong, *Stitt's Diagnosis, Prevention and Treatment of Tropical Diseases* (6th edition), Blakiston, Philadelphia, 1942.

Appendix A

ACKNOWLEDGMENTS

For assistance and counsel in the preparation of this book I wish to acknowledge my deep gratitude to the following: Dr. R. C. Connor, General Superintendent of the Medical Department of the United Fruit Company, formerly Chief of Clinic for the Ancon Hospital; Dr. Edward Irving Salisbury, of the United Fruit Company Medical Staff, fellow and pioneer executive of the American College of Surgeons; Dr. Herbert C. Clark, Superintendent of the Gorgas Memorial Hospital of Panama; Dr. Neil P. Macphail, Superintendent of the Quirigua Hospital of Guatemala, veteran of British and American tropical medicine; Dr. Aristides A. Moll, Secretary of the Pan American Sanitary Bureau of Washington; Dr. Joseph White, renowned sanitary expert and friend of Gorgas; the late Dr. M. E. Connor, "last of the great yellow fever fighters"; Dr. Carlos E. Finlay, of Havana; Dr. O. L. Drennan, of Santa Marta, Colombia; Dr. Gustav Eckstein, author, scientist, and biographer of Noguchi; Dr. Jaime de la Guardia, of Panama and Cuba; Dr. Teodore de la Torre, a great sanitary expert of Cuba; and Dr. M. A. Barber, of the United States Public Health Service. I am also deeply grateful for assistance received from: Dr. George C. Shattuck and Dr. Richard P. Strong, of Harvard University; Rear Admiral E. R. Stitt, of the United States Navy; the Rockefeller Foundation; and the Carnegie Institution of Washington.

Appendix B

GENERAL BIBLIOGRAPHY

1. Stitt, E. R., *Diagnostics and Treatment of Tropical Diseases* (5th edition). Philadelphia: Blakiston, 1929.
2. Gorgas, Marie D., and Burton J. Hendrick, *William Crawford Gorgas*. New York: Doubleday, Page, 1924.
3. *A Journal of Josiah Gorgas* (unpublished). Washington: Library of Congress, 1871.
4. Froude, James Anthony, *Growth of Empire*. Chicago: McClure, 1885.
5. Reed, Charles A. L., *Panama Notes*. Cleveland, 1906.
6. Stitt, E. R., *Diagnosis, Treatment and Prevention of Tropical Diseases* (6th edition), edited by Richard P. Strong. Philadelphia: Blakiston, 1942.
7. Regnal, J., *Anales de Medicina et de Pharmacia*, Vol. XXX, No. 59, p. 83. Guatemala City, 1934.
8. Shattuck, Dr. George Cheever, *A Medical Survey of the Republic of Guatemala*. Washington: Carnegie Institution of Washington, 1938.
9. *Foreign Agriculture*, Vol. 5, No. 3, March, 1941. Office Foreign Agricultural Relations, U. S. Department of Agriculture, Washington, D. C.
10. *Journal of the American Medical Association*, Vol. LIX, Oct. 26, 1912.
11. Mira, Dr. M. G., *Anti-Malarial Campaigns in Guatemala*. Guatemala City, 1936.
12. *Southern Medical Journal*, Vol. IX, No. 2.
13. "Use of Condensed, Evaporated and Powdered Milk for Feeding Infants in the Tropics," *American Journal of Tropical Medicine*, Vol. IV, No. 2, March, 1925.
14. Deeks, W. E., and W. M. James, *Report on Hemoglobinuric Fever in the Canal Zone: A Study of Its Etiology and Treatment*. Mount Hope, Canal Zone, 1911.
15. Deeks, W. E., and Associates, *Malaria, Its Cause, Prevention and Cure*. Boston: United Fruit Company, 1930.
16. Deeks, W. E., *A Review of the Digestive Functions and Food Requirements for the Maintenance of Health with Particular Reference to the Tropics*. New York: United Fruit Company, 1923.
17. *The Cause of Hookworm Disease and Its Prevention*, edited by W. E. Deeks. New York: United Fruit Company, 1925.

18. DEEKS, W. E., "The Significance of Chronic Pharyngitis," *Clinical Medicine and Surgery*, July, 1928.

19. CARTER, HENRY ROSE, *Yellow Fever*. Baltimore: Johns Hopkins, 1931.

20. FUENTES Y GUZMÁN, *Historia de Guatemala y Recordacion Florida*. Madrid, 1882.

21. JUARROS, DON DOMINGO, *The Kingdom of Guatemala in Spanish America*, trans. J. Bailey. London, 1923.

22. ZINSSER, HANS, *Rats, Lice and History*. Boston: Little, Brown, 1935.

23. DIAZ, BERNAL, *True History of the Conquest of Mexico*, trans. Maurice Keating. London, 1568.

24. GANN, THOMAS, *In an Unknown Land*. New York, 1924.

25. *Physiological and Medical Observations Among the Indians of Southwestern United States and Mexico*, Smithsonian Institution, American Ethnology Bulletin 34, Washington, D. C., 1908.

26. *United States Navy Medical Bulletin No. 26*, Navy Dept., Washington, D. C., 1928.

27. HIRSCH, AUGUST, *Handbook of Geographical and Historical Pathology*. London: New Sydenham Society, 1883.

28. *United States Public Health Reports*, Government Printing Office, Washington, D. C., 1919.

29. *Annual Epidemiological Reports for the Year 1934*, League of Nations, Geneva, 1936.

30. *Proctor Royal Society of Medicine*, Section on Tropical Diseases, London, 1929.

31. SHATTUCK, GEORGE CHEEVER, and COLLABORATORS, *The Peninsula of Yucatan*, Carnegie Institution of Washington, No. 431, Washington, D. C., 1928.

32. GORGAS, WILLIAM CRAWFORD, *Sanitation in Panama*. New York: D. Appleton and Company, 1918.

33. *American Journal of Public Health*, Vol. XXIII, No. 11, 1933.

34. CHAMBERLAIN, WESTON P., *Twenty-five Years of American Medical Activity in the Isthmus of Panama*, U. S. Public Health Service, No. 923, Washington, D. C.

35. ECKSTEIN, GUSTAV, *Noguchi*. New York: Harper, 1931.

36. KELLEY, HOWARD, *Walter Reed and Yellow Fever*. Chicago: McClure, 1909.

37. FINLAY, CARLOS E., *Carlos Finlay and Yellow Fever*. Havana and New York: Oxford University Press, 1940.

38. LAWRENCE, JAMES COOPER, *The World's Struggle with Rubber*. London-New York: Harper, 1931.

39. *International Conference on Health Problems in Tropical America*. Boston: United Fruit Company, 1924.

40. *Annual Reports* (26 volumes), Medical Department, United Fruit Company, Boston, 1903-1929.

41. "Studies in Pellagra," *Archives of Internal Medicine*, Vol. XIV, 1914.

42. CASTELLANI, SIR ALDO, "Medical Mycology," *Journal of Tropical Medicine and Hygiene*, Vol. XXII, March 1, 1924.

43. GOLDBERGER, *The Cause and Prevention of Pellagra*, U. S. Public Health Service Reports, Nos. 218 and 311. Washington, D. C.

44. McCOLLUM, WILLIAM, *The Newer Knowledge of Nutrition*. New York: Macmillan, 1922.

45. DEEKS, WILLIAM E., "The Carbohydrates as Etiological Factors in Stomach Disorders," *New York Medical Journal*, June 25 and July 2, 1904.

46. "Faulty Food in Relation to Gastro-Intestinal Disorders," *Journal of the American Medical Association*, Vol. 78, No. 1.

47. ROGERS, SIR LEONARD, "The Treatment of Leprosy," *Lancet*, June 29, 1924.

48. FINLAY, CARLOS, *Garceta medica de la Habana*, Vols. I and II. Havana, 1879.

49. *Anales de la Real Academia de Ciencias*, Vol. IX, Havana, 1872.

50. *Annual Report, 1902*, Secretary of War, Government Printing Office, Washington, D. C.

51. MacCAW, W. D., *Walter Reed, a Memorial*. Washington: Walter Reed Memorial Association, 1904.

52. BOYCE, RUPERT, "Witness at New Orleans," *Southern Magazine*, October, 1905.

53. *Thompson Yates Laboratory Reports:* Report of the Yellow Fever Expedition to Para, Brazil, Vol. IV, Part 2. London, 1902.

54. *Boletin del Departmento de la Secretaria de Estado y Justicia*, Vol. 4. Havana, 1907.

55. BERENGER-FÉRAUD, *Traité de la Fièvre Jaune*. Paris, 1890.

56. GUITERAS, *Cronica Medico*. Havana: Quirugica de la Habana, 1894.

57. *Selected Papers of Carlos Finlay*. Havana, 1917.

58. FINLAY, CARLOS, "El Mosquito Hipoteticamente Considerado como Agente de Transmision de la Fiebre Amarilla," *Anales de la Real Academia de Ciencias Medicas Fisicas y Naturales de la Habana*, 1881.

59. *Conference of State and Provincial Boards of Health of North America*, New Haven, Conn., October, 1902.

60. DOMINGUEZ, FRANCISCO, *Carlos J. Finlay—Son Centenaire—Sa Découverte.* Paris, 1933.

61. *American Journal of Hygiene*, Vol. 16, No. 1, July, 1932.

62. *New Orleans Medical and Surgical Journal*, November, 1916.

63. *New Orleans Medical and Surgical Journal*, May, 1898.

64. *British Medical Journal*, Sept. 8, 1900.

65. *Philadelphia Medical Journal*, Oct. 27, 1900.

66. *Journal of the American Medical Association*, Nov. 23, 1901; June 30, 1903.

67. GUITERAS, *Boletín de Sanidad y Beneficencia*. Havana, January, 1909.

68. *Revista de Medicinia Tropical*, Havana, October, 1902.

69. *Anales de l'Institut Pasteur,* Tome 17, November, 1903.

70. *Bulletin No. 13,* Bureau of Public Health and Marine Hospital Service, Yellow Fever Institute, March, 1903.

71. *Annals of Tropical Medicine and Parasitology,* Vol. 24, 1930.

72. *American Journal of Tropical Medicine,* Vol. 17, No. 1, January, 1937.

73. *Journal of Experimental Medicine,* Vol. LIV, 1931.

74. *Southern Medical Journal,* March, 1932.

75. *Annual Report,* Rockefeller Foundation. New York, 1916.

76. *Files of the Rockefeller Foundation,* Unpublished Memorandum No. 748, 1914.

77. *Journal of Tropical Medicine and Hygiene,* Vol. 28, 1925.

78. *American Journal of Tropical Medicine,* Vol. XVII, No. 1, 1937.

79. *Gaz. de Notitian da Rio Janeiro,* Rio de Janeiro, 1883.

80. *Gaz. de Hospitaux,* Rio de Janeiro, 1883.

81. STERNBERG, LT. COL. GEORGE M., *Report on the Etiology and Prevention of Yellow Fever.* Washington, D. C., 1890.

82. *Journal of Pathology and Bacteriology,* Vol. XV, 1910.

83. *Journal of Tropical Medicine and Hygiene,* Vol. XXVIII, 1927.

84. *Memoirs of Oswaldo Cruz.* Rio de Janeiro: Cruz Institute, 1928, 1931.

85. *Memoirs of Butatan Institute,* Vol. 30. Rio de Janeiro, 1929.

86. *Royal Society of Tropical Medicine and Hygiene,* Vol. 29, 1936.

87. *Bull. de L'Office International d'Hygiène Publique,* Vol. 28, No. 12, December, 1936.

88. *Bulletin,* Academy of Medicine, Vol. 105. Paris, 1931.

89. SOPER, J. L., *Jungle Yellow Fever, a New Public Health Problem in Colombia.* Bogotá, 1935.

90. SOPER, J. L., "The New Epidemiology of Yellow Fever," *American Journal of Public Health,* Vol. XXVI, No. 1, January, 1937.

91. LAS CASAS, *Historia de las Indias,* Vol. II. Madrid (date unknown).

92. HERRERA, *Decadas de las Indias,* Dec. 1, Libs. II, V. Madrid, 1688.

93. *The Inscription at Copan,* Washington, D. C.: Carnegie Institution of Washington, 1920.

94. LANDA, *Relaciones de las Cosas de Yucatán.* Madrid, 1556.

95. COGULLODO, *Historia de Yucatán,* Lib. XII. Madrid, 1688.

96. *Proceedings of the Entomological Society of Washington,* Vol. 38, No. 4. Washington, D. C., 1936.

97. CARROLL, JAMES, "Without Mosquitoes There Can Be No Yellow Fever," *American Medicine,* March 17, 1906.

98. REED, WALTER, "Remarks on Cholera Spirillum," *Northwest Lancet,* Vol. 13, No. 9, May 1, 1893.

99. REED, WALTER, "The Parasite of Malaria," *Journal of Practical Medicine,* Vol. 6, No. 9, April, 1896.

100. *Character, Prevalence and Probable Causation of the Malarial Fevers at Washington Barracks and Fort Myer*, Report of the Surgeon General. Washington, D. C.: U. S. Printing Office, 1896.

101. *An Investigation into the So-Called Lymphoid Nodules of the Liver in Typhoid Fever*, Johns Hopkins Hospital Report No. 5. Baltimore, 1895.

102. REED, WALTER, "The Contagiousness of Erysipelas," *Boston Medical and Surgical Journal*, Vol. 126, 1892.

103. REED, WALTER, "On the Appearance of Certain Amoeboid Bodies in the Blood of Vaccinated Monkeys (Rhoesus) and Children, and in the Blood of Variola," *Journal of Experimental Medicine*, Vol. II, No. 5, September, 1897.

104. REED, WALTER, *Serum Diagnosis in Typhoid Fever*, Report of Surgeon General, United States Army, Washington, D. C., 1897.

105. REED, WALTER, *Report on the Practical Use of Electrozone as a Disinfectant in the City of Havana*, Report of Surgeon General, United States Army, Washington, D. C., 1900.

106. UNITED STATES ARMY COMMISSION, "Recent Researches Concerning the Etiology, Propagation and Prevention of Yellow Fever," *Journal of Hygiene*, Vol. 2, April, 1902 (Cambridge, England).

107. REED, WALTER, and GEORGE M. STERNBERG, *Report of Immunity Against Vaccination Conferred upon the Monkey by the Use of the Serum of the Vaccinated Calf and Monkey* (Vol. 10). Association of American Physicians, Philadelphia, 1895.

108. "Malaria in Southeast Russia," *Lancet*, Vol. 55, No. 1225, 1923.

109. HUNTINGTON, ELLSWORTH, *Civilization and Climate*. New Haven: Yale University Press, 1915.

110. ROSENAU, M. J., *Preventive Medicine and Hygiene*. New York: D. Appleton & Company, 1924.

111. LOVELACE, C., "The Etiology and Treatment of Haemoglobinuric Fever," *Archives Internal Medicine*, Vol. XI, No. 6, 1922.

112. GUERERO, PASTOR, *La Juventud Medica*. Guatemala City, 1922.

113. O'CONNOR, *Research in the Western Pacific*. Research Memoirs, London School of Tropical Medicine, Vol. 4. London, 1923.

114. Low and MANSON-BAHR, "Filariasis," *Transactions of the Royal Society of Tropical Medicine and Hygiene*, Vol. 16, No. 7, January 18, 1923.

115. BYRAM and ARCHIBALD, *Practice of Medicine in the Tropics* (Vol. 3). London, 1924.

116. DOBELL, C., *The Amoebia Living in Man*. London: John Bale Sons and Danielssons, 1919.

117. KAUFMANN-WOLF, M., "Fungus Diseases of the Hands and Feet," *Dermatologische Zeitschrift*, 1914 (Berlin).

118. STITT, E. R., *Practical Bacteriology, Blood Work and Parasitology*. Philadelphia: Blakiston, 1923.

119. SIMPSON, W. J., *A Treatise on Plague.* Cambridge, England: Cambridge University Press.

120. SIMPSON, W. J., *Report on Sanitary Matters on the East Africa Protectorate,* British Colonial Office, African Report No. 1025, London, 1915.

121. McCARRISON, R., "Faulty Food in Relation to Gastro-Intestinal Disorder," *Journal American Medical Association,* Vol. 78, No. 1, 1922.

122. CUMMINS, S. L., "Primitive Tribes and Tuberculosis," *Transactions of the Society of Tropical Medicine and Hygiene,* Vol. V, No. 7, 1912 (London).

123. PHALEN and KILBORNE, *Reports of U. S. Army Board for Study of Tropical Diseases.* Washington, D. C.: Government Printing Office, 1909.

124. DAVIS and PILOT, *Collected Studies from the Department of Pathology and Bacteriology.* Chicago, 1923.

125. *Anales de la Faculty de Medicine,* Vol. VIII. Montevideo, 1923.

126. STRONG, R. P., *The Clinical and Pathological Significance of B. Coli.* Bulletin No. 26, Bureau of Government Laboratories, Manila, P. I., 1904.

127. *Publications of Biological Laboratory,* Bureau of Science, Manila, P. I., 1904.

128. *Report of the Origin and Spread of Typhoid Fever in United States Army Camp during the Spanish American War* (2 vols.). Washington, D. C.: Office of the Surgeon General, U. S. Army, War Department, 1904.

129. DEVEZE, JEAN, *An Inquiry into and Observations upon the Causes and Effects of the Epidemic which Raged in Philadelphia from the Month of August till toward the Middle of December, 1793.* Philadelphia, 1794.

130. NUTTALL, G. H. F., *On the Role of Insects . . . as Carriers in the Spread of Bacterial and Parasitic Diseases,* Johns Hopkins Hospital Reports, Vol. III. Baltimore, 1899.

131. REED and CARROLL, "The Prevention of Yellow Fever," *Medical Record,* Vol. 60, No. 17, Oct. 26, 1901.

132. PATTERSON, ROBERT V., "Work of Walter Reed," *American Journal of Public Health,* Vol. XXII, No. 11, November, 1933.

133. WHITMORE, E. R., *Observations on Bird Malaria and the Pathogenesis of Relapse in Human Malaria,* Johns Hopkins Hospital Bulletins Nos. 39, 62. Baltimore, 1918.

134. FREIMAN, M., "Plasmoquin, etc., in Malaria," *Journal of Tropical Medicine and Hygiene,* Vol. 32, No. 165, 1929 (London).

135. JAMES, S. P., and P. G. SHUTE, *Report on the First Results of Laboratory Work on Malaria in England,* Malaria Commission, League of Nations Health Organization. Geneva, 1926.

136. YORKE and WARRINGTON, "Further Observations on Malaria Made During Treatment of General Paralysis," *Transactions of the Royal Society of Tropical Medicine and Hygiene,* Vol. XIX, No. 3, June 18, 1925 (London).

137. CLARK, H. C., *Some Notes on Animal Diseases in Panama with Special Reference to Blood and Muscle Parasites.* Mount Hope, Canal Zone: Panama Canal Press, 1920.

138. GOLDMAN, EDWARD A., *Mammals of Panama*, Smithsonian Miscellaneous Collections, Vol. 69, No. 5. Washington, D. C.: Smithsonian Institution, 1920.

139. WENYON, C. M., *Protozoology*. New York: William Wood and Company, 1926.

140. *The Works of Thomas Sydenham, M.D.*, edited and published by Benjamin Rush. Philadelphia, 1815.

141. VORSCHUTZ, J., and B. TENCKHOFF, "Treatment with Autohemotherapy," *Deutsche Ztschr. f. Chir.*, Vol. CLXXXIII, 1923-1934 (Leipzig).

142. CLARK, H. C., *The Pneumococci by Types, in Cultures from Seventy-one*, Sixteenth Annual Report, Medical Department, United Fruit Company. Boston, 1927.

143. LEGGE, R. T., and L. BONAR, "Ringworm of the Feet," *Journal of the American Medical Association*, Vol. 92, No. 18, May 4, 1929.

144. CASTELLANI and CHAMBERS, *Manual of Tropical Medicine* (3rd edition). London, 1919.

145. MANSON-BAHR, PHILIP H., *Manson's Tropical Diseases* (8th edition). London, 1925.

146. GAGE, ALFRED, *The Machete Versus the Microbe in Central America*, Fifteenth Annual Report, Medical Department, United Fruit Company. Boston, 1926.

147. PIERSOL, GEORGE A., *Human Anatomy*. Philadelphia: J. B. Lippincott, 1908.

148. CHAGAS, C., "Sobre um trypanosoma do tatu, Tatisia novemcincta, transmittido pela Triatoma geniculata Latr," *Brazilian Medicine*, Vol. XXVI, 1912.

149. ROGERS, LEONARD, *Recent Advances in Tropical Medicine*. London: J. & A. Churchill, 1929.

Appendix C

A CHRONOLOGICAL LIST OF LATIN AMERICAN EPIDEMICS

Date	Disease	Probable Source	Countries Victimized	Comments
1450 (?)	pneumonia	Europe (?)	Mexico	Caused extensive migration of Toltecs and Maya Indians.
1490 (?)	yaws	indigenous (?)	Mexico	....
1494	scurvy	Spain	Santo Domingo	....
1496	yellow fever (?)	Europe (?)	Santo Domingo	Alleged to have killed one-third of native population (Herrera).
1510–1520	yaws and malaria	Africa (?)	Panama to Peru	Caused death of 40,000 Spaniards en route to Peru (Herrera).
1515	yellow fever (?)	Europe (?)	Central America and West Indies	....
1521–1572	typhus, malaria and smallpox	Europe (?)	Mexico	At least nine severe epidemics during this period.
1530–1533	diphtheria, measles, and scarlet fever	Europe	Peru, Cuba, and Venezuela	Responsible for countless fatalities.
1541	smallpox	Spain	Mexico	.... (*Historia Ecclesiastica Indianas*.)
1545–1595	typhus	Europe	Mexico	Ravaged Bogotá Settlement.
1558	smallpox	Europe	Colombia	
1560–1595	mumps	Europe	Mexico	Killed one-third of the population (Pimentel).
1577	smallpox and measles	Europe	Venezuela	
1587–1589	smallpox	Europe	Colombia	Estimated to have destroyed 90 per cent of the Indians.
1590–1610	smallpox, measles and other of the "ten plagues of Spain"	Europe	Bolivia, Chile, and Argentina	Killed at least 2,000,000 natives (Moll).
1591 (?)	smallpox and measles	Europe	Paraguay and Uruguay	....
1609	anthrax	Europe	Argentina	Responsible for death of many Indians.
1620	yellow fever and malaria	Europe or Africa (?)	Cuba	Caused heavy losses to both life and shipping.
1620–1630	influenza	Europe	North, Central, and South Americas	....

354

Date	Disease	Origin	Location	Notes
1621-1645	typhus (?)	Europe	Guadeloupe	Reported to have killed three out of every four arrivals.
1630	typhus	Europe	Colombia	Believed to have killed about 80 per cent of Sabana Indians.
1635-1640	yellow fever	Europe or Africa	Haiti and West Indies	Caused large numbers of deaths (Dutertre).
1648-1649	yellow fever	controversial	Yucatan, Guatemala, and Campeche	" " " " "
1648-1649	yellow fever	Europe or Africa	Martinique and Guadeloupe	" " " " "
1649	yellow fever	American continent	Cuba	Killed one-third of population between May and October.
1665-1667	"cocoliztle"— probably yellow fever	Europe or Africa	Mexico	Caused large numbers of deaths.
1719	smallpox	Europe	Rio de la Plata area	Reported to have killed 17,000 Indians.
1720	Carrión's disease	indigenous (?)	Peru	Reduced Incan populations by 1,000,000 (Unanue).
1720	malaria	controversial	Venezuela, Ecuador, etc.	....
1750-1790	measles and smallpox	Europe	Peru	Greatly reduced Indian population in the Andes.
1798-1803	yellow fever	Europe or Africa	Haiti	Killed seven-eighths of French army of 25,000; ruined France's attempt to subdue the slave rebellion.
1820-1830	typhus and yellow fever	Europe	Ecuador, Colombia and Venezuela	Large numbers of deaths reported by Spanish armies and defending forces of Bolívar.
1836-1840	scarlet fever	Europe	Mexico	Caused innumerable fatalities.
1840	smallpox	Europe	Mexico	
1845-1846	yellow fever and typhoid	Europe (?)	Mexico	Of U. S. soldiers lost in the Mexican War 1,549 were killed in battle and 10,951 died of disease.
1846-1847	typhus	Europe	Mexico	Caused large numbers of deaths.
1847	yellow fever, typhus, etc.	Europe (?)	Mexico	Out of 20,000 Spanish soldiers at Veracruz garrison 17,000 died of disease.
1858	smallpox	Europe	Mexico	Caused large numbers of deaths.
1860	typhus	Europe	Mexico	" " " " "
1870	measles	Europe	Mexico	" " " " "
1874	typhus	Europe	Mexico	Caused large numbers of deaths.
1874	smallpox	Europe	Mexico	" " " " "
1880	scarlet fever	Europe	Chile	" " " " "
1883	amoebic dysentery	controversial	Venezuela	Toribio González, Venezuelan scientist, reported amoebic dysentery for first time in Western Hemisphere.
1886-1896	yellow fever and malaria	controversial	Isthmus of Panama	Out of 86,000 employees of French Panama Canal Company roughly 52,000 suffered yellow fever.

355

Date	Disease	Probable Source	Countries Victimized	Comments
1890-1898	smallpox	Europe	Chile	Killed 27,000; motivated founding of Chile's Institute of Hygiene.
1890-1899	bubonic plague	Europe	Brazil (São Paulo)	Led to founding of Butantan Institute by State of São Paulo to manufacture vaccine and serums.
1890-1901	yellow fever	controversial	Cuba and Panama	Helped crush Spain's hold on Cuba; prompted work of U. S. Army Yellow Fever Commission.
1891	malaria	controversial	Venezuela	Led to discovery of Risquez method for rapid diagnosis of malaria.
1895	paratyphoid	Europe (?)	Venezuela	Enabled Mosquera and Risquez of Venezuela to identify paratyphoid for first time in the Western Hemisphere.
1899	bubonic plague	Europe	Brazil	Let to founding of Federal Institute of Serum-Therapy (later Oswaldo Cruz Institute) to manufacture vaccine and serum.
1904-1914	yellow fever and malaria	controversial	Isthmus of Panama	Motivated the sanitation of Panama which made possible the completion of the Panama Canal.
1910	yellow fever	controversial	Venezuela and Ecuador	Helped to interest Rockefeller Foundation in sanitation efforts.
1922-1925	hookworm	controversial	Jamaica, Ecuador, Venezuela, etc.	Led to collaboration between the Rockefeller Foundation and the respective governments in a model antihookworm campaign.
1923-1924	yellow fever	controversial	Guatemala, Nicaragua, Honduras, etc.	Motivated a commendable public health campaign.
1933	typhus	Europe	Chile and Bolivia	Led to extension of public health training and sera manufacture.
1933	leprosy	Europe	Colombia, Brazil, and Panama	Led to founding of Federico Lleras Institute of Medical Research at Bogotá in 1934.

Courtesy of Pan American Sanitary Bureau, Washington, D. C.

Appendix D

LATIN-AMERICAN POPULATIONS*

| Country | CENSUS TOTAL OR APPROXIMATION | | | | | | |

Argentina
1800	1869	1900	1914	1920	1930	1942
1,000,000	1,830,000	5,000,000	7,900,000	8,500,000	12,000,000	13,000,000

Bolivia
1900		1938	
1,640,000	(estimated)	3,426,296	(estimated)

Brazil
1585	1600	1700	1800	1872	1900	1942
55,000	70,000	750,000	2,500,000	10,000,000	18,000,000	50,000,000

Chile
1800	1850	1870	1900	1920	1930	1941
800,000	1,400,000	2,000,000	3,000,000	3,730,000	4,300,000	4,700,000

Colombia
1800	1835	1905	1920	1930	1940
1,500,000	1,700,000	4,150,000	5,900,000	7,900,000	8,700,000

Costa Rica
1850	1900	1927	1942
80,000	250,000	475,000	640,000

Cuba
1793	1827	1889	1907	1919	1931	1940
272,000	704,478	1,572,792	2,004,900	2,889,004	3,962,244	4,227,579

Dominican Republic
1845	1940
270,000	1,581,248

Ecuador
1800	1942
700,000	3,000,000

El Salvador
1910	1939
682,000	1,704,497

Guatemala
1778	1825	1872	1903	1921	1941
369,164	512,120	1,190,750	1,842,134	2,004,900	3,284,269

Haiti
1800	1941
700,000	3,000,000(?)

Honduras
1800	1940	
465,000	1,140,000	(estimated)

Mexico
1793	1800	1900	1930	1941
4,483,569	6,000,000	13,607,259	16,550,000	20,000,000

* Authority: Population Association of America, Ninth Annual Meeting, Princeton, N. J., May 16, 1941; Dr. A. A. Moll, Secretary, Pan American Sanitary Bureau, Washington, D. C., *Bulletin of the Pan American Union*, Vol. LXXV, No. 9, September, 1941, pp. 537-541.

Country		CENSUS TOTAL OR APPROXIMATION		
	1890	*1938*		
Nicaraugua ..	942,000	1,172,324		
	1910		*1920*	*1930*
Panama	196,000	(estimated)	361,000	467,459
	1791	*1876*	*1900*	*1940*
Peru	1,100,000	2,700,000	4,000,000	6,760,000
	1793	*1829*	*1852*	*1900*	*1940*
Uruguay	30,685	75,000	131,969	915,647	2,125,000
	1800	*1845*	*1941*	
Venezuela ...	800,000	1,250,000	3,500,000	

ESTIMATED PERCENTAGES OF INCREASE OF POPULATION

1800-1900

Country	*Increase*
Uruguay	2990
Brazil and Cuba	700
Costa Rica and Guatemala	500
Peru	400
Chile	375
Mexico	320
Colombia	270

ESTIMATED PERCENTAGES OF INCREASE OF POPULATION

1800-1941

Country	*Increase*
Uruguay	6900
Brazil	2000
Cuba	1600
Argentina	1300
Guatemala	900
Costa Rica	800
Peru	700
Chile and Colombia	600
Haiti and Venezuela	400
Ecuador	350
Mexico	300

Since 1890 the population of the United States has increased from 62,000,000 to about 132,000,000; that of Latin America, from about 53,000,000 to about 120,000,000.

INDEX
